Disc--- debate disaders
vs —
Sanchez

Negotiating Disability

Miranda — disclosure
uxiz. bad if
insttalzd

→ Disability Adv.
→ Fem adv. (Ⓔ of externalization
via rez)

→ Queerness (via disclosure)

Corporealities: Discourses of Disability

Series editors: David T. Mitchell and Sharon L. Snyder

Recent Titles

Negotiating Disability: Disclosure and Higher Education
by Stephanie L. Kerschbaum, Laura T. Eisenman, and James M. Jones

Portraits of Violence: War and the Aesthetics of Disfigurement
by Suzannah Biernoff

Bodies of Modernism: Physical Disability in Transatlantic Modernist Literature
by Maren Tova Linett

War on Autism: On the Cultural Logic of Normative Violence
by Anne McGuire

The Biopolitics of Disability: Neoliberalism, Ablenationalism, and Peripheral Embodiment
by David T. Mitchell with Sharon L. Snyder

Foucault and the Government of Disability, Enlarged and Revised Edition
by Shelley Tremain, editor

The Measure of Manliness: Disability and Masculinity in the Mid-Victorian Novel
by Karen Bourrier

American Lobotomy: A Rhetorical History
by Jenell Johnson

Shakin' All Over: Popular Music and Disability
by George McKay

The Metanarrative of Blindness: A Re-reading of Twentieth-Century Anglophone Writing
by David Bolt

Disabled Veterans in History
by David A. Gerber, editor

Mad at School: Rhetorics of Mental Disability and Academic Life
by Margaret Price

Disability Aesthetics
by Tobin Siebers

Stumbling Blocks Before the Blind: Medieval Constructions of a Disability
by Edward Wheatley

Signifying Bodies: Disability in Contemporary Life Writing
by G. Thomas Couser

Concerto for the Left Hand: Disability and the Defamiliar Body
by Michael Davidson

The Songs of Blind Folk: African American Musicians and the Cultures of Blindness
by Terry Rowden

Disability Theory
by Tobin Siebers

Fictions of Affliction: Physical Disability in Victorian Culture
by Martha Stoddard Holmes

A complete list of titles in the series can be found at www.press.umich.edu

Negotiating Disability

Disclosure and Higher Education

Stephanie L. Kerschbaum
Laura T. Eisenman
James M. Jones, Editors

University of Michigan Press
Ann Arbor

Copyright © 2017 by Stephanie L. Kerschbaum, Laura T. Eisenman,
and James M. Jones
All rights reserved

This book may not be reproduced, in whole or in part, including illustrations, in any
form (beyond that copying permitted by Sections 107 and 108 of the U.S. Copyright
Law and except by reviewers for the public press), without written permission from the
publisher.

Published in the United States of America by the
University of Michigan Press
Manufactured in the United States of America
⊛ Printed on acid-free paper

2020   2019   2018   2017   4   3   2   1

A CIP catalog record for this book is available from the British Library.

Library of Congress Cataloging-in-Publication data has been applied for.

ISBN: 978-0-472-07370-2 (Hardcover : alk paper)
ISBN: 978-0-472-05370-4 (Paperback : alk paper)
ISBN: 978-0-472-12339-1 (ebook)

Cover description for accessibility: A multi-colored abstract design with strong brush
strokes in many directions covers the front of the book. The energy and movement of
colors, forms and lines invoke passion and complexity. A dark gray horizontal band
cuts across the cover and includes the book title and editors' names.

To J, R, and RUS—SLK

To Erik, whose unending support makes many things possible—LTE

To all who share their disability stories, and teach us
about their and our human capacity—JMJ

Contents

IV. Institutional Change and Policy

Acknowledgments

We would like to formally thank two anonymous reviewers who gave considerably of their time and feedback to strengthen the contributions made by the scholars and activists who populate this collection. Our acquisitions editor at the University of Michigan Press, LeAnn Fields, along with Jenny Geyer, Christopher Dreyer and the many press staff who have helped bring this collection to life have been an absolute dream to work with, and we are grateful for their advice, guidance, and wisdom. Throughout this entire process, Bess Davis and Lisa Schulz have provided invaluable editorial assistance. Alison Kafer was a sounding board and gave feedback at several critical junctures, and John Ernest provided steadfast encouragement at every stage. Thanks to Bess Davis, Margaret Price and Karl Booksh for their work on the 2013 Disability Disclosure in/and Higher Education Conference, where this collection had its origins. And thanks to those who attended the conference and shared their scholarship, wisdom, and personal stories, all of which inspired us to undertake this volume.

The editors would like to acknowledge financial support and assistance for this collection, including for the conference that helped initiate this project, from the following offices and groups: the University of Delaware Center for the Study of Diversity, the University of Delaware President's Diversity Initiative, the University of Delaware Interdisciplinary Humanities Research Center, the University of Delaware Office of the Provost, the University of Delaware College of Arts and Sciences, the University of Delaware Department of English, the University of Delaware Office for Disability Support Services, the Delaware Developmental Disabilities Council, the Delaware State Council for Persons with Disabilities, the Delaware Governor's Advisory Council for Exceptional Citizens, the National Institute on Disability and Rehabilitation Research, the Association on Higher Education And

Disability, the American Psychological Association, and the University of Delaware Center for Disabilities Studies.

Permission to reprint Lynn Manning's poem "The Magic Wand" was granted from Taylor and Francis.

Cover image from ArtFest 2012. Courtesy of Art Therapy Express and University of Delaware's Center for Disabilities Studies.

Negotiating Disability

Disability, Disclosure, and Diversity

STEPHANIE L. KERSCHBAUM

LAURA T. EISENMAN

JAMES M. JONES

In/visible disability. Passing. Masquerade. Coming out. Covering. As the range of these terms suggests, disability disclosure is not a singular event, not a once-and-for-all action but, rather, an ongoing process of continuously, in a variety of settings and contexts, performing and negotiating disability awareness and perceptibility. This collection takes as a central focus what it means to disclose a disability, and it situates that inquiry within the experiences and spaces of higher education. Its motivating questions include: What does it mean to (not) disclose a disability? What is involved in that process? What is and is not disclosed and with what costs, benefits, or risks? What are the consequences and the implications of disability disclosure? How do disclosures—as well as the potential for disclosures—shape individual and collective experiences? Theorizing these questions is needed in order to understand the ways that disability might entail changes in the cultures and environments in which higher education is designed, delivered, and negotiated.

Arguments about disability disclosure are often tied to claims about the transformative potential of such disclosures, suggesting that conceiving disabled identities as integral to higher education is necessary to creating more inclusive and welcoming environments. Indeed, we have witnessed many times over how acts of identifying shared experiences can engender moments of solidarity that enable continued persistence in ableist and discriminatory institutions. However, it is necessary to also acknowledge that disability disclosures are complicated by the fact that disabled identities always intersect with other identities and that the risk-taking that accompanies disclosure is not experienced equally or in the same ways by all people, as many of the contributors to this volume emphasize (see Samuels, this volume). With disability disclosure as a central point of departure, this collection builds on scholarship that highlights the deeply rhetorical nature of disclosure and embodied movement, emphasizing disability disclosure as a complex calculus in which degrees of perceptibility are dependent on contexts, types of interactions that are unfolding, interlocutors' long- and short-term goals, disabilities and disability experiences, and many other contingencies (see Kerschbaum 2014).

While the policy climate and environment for disability in higher education is somewhat developed for students (e.g., resources available through the Association on Higher Education And Disability as well as the prevalence of campus disability support offices), it is almost non-existent for other populations, such as faculty and staff. Indeed, for this latter group, little national guidance is available aside from a well-intentioned but problematic report issued by the American Association of University Professors in 2012 (for more detailed critiques, see Kerschbaum et al. 2013; Oswal 2016). Much of what currently exists regarding disability and higher education does not engage multiple higher education constituencies. Instead, pockets of disability knowledge are tucked away in different places on different campuses and, sometimes, in different places on the same campus for different groups. For example, sometimes disability services offices help facilitate classroom and educational accommodations while human resources offices might handle employee and workplace accommodations. And within such institutional structures, some constituencies, such as graduate students, are caught in a liminal space as both students and employees (Carter, Catania, Schmitt and Swenson, this volume). In exploring questions surrounding disability disclosure, this collection highlights how issues related to disability in higher education are not only relevant to those who have disabilities but have far-reaching consequences across higher education and beyond. Considering disability holistically, across the spectrum of experiences in higher education, will have broader impact than focusing on a specific demographic population.

Some of the essays in this collection were first developed for the Disability Disclosure in/and Higher Education Conference held at the University of Delaware in October 2013, but the collection here is not a conference proceedings. Instead, while this collection is inspired by the conversations, talks, and forms of engagement sponsored by the conference, it extends well beyond the conference space itself. The collection thus seeks to critique the many issues raised at the conference from new temporal and spatial vantage points. In assembling the essays featured here, we have explicitly invited attention to gaps, omissions, and absences that were part of the physical and conceptual spaces created by the Disability Disclosure in/and Higher Education Conference. Those gaps included representation of and by disability scholars of color; multiply minoritized disabled people; the experiences of faculty, students, and staff across diverse experiences and dynamics; and deeper social-scientific exploration of sites, conceptions, and experiences of disability disclosure within higher education. Despite these efforts to address gaps, there remain constituencies and perspectives not represented in this collection. For instance, none of the essays in this collection address the experiences of disabled employees other than faculty: custodial, food service, secretarial and skilled tradespeople, to name just a few, are not taken up, a key question at a time when more colleges and universities are tracking the number of disabled people they employ. And only one essay (Seelman) directly addresses questions about the intersections between disability and poverty. We cannot address every relevant issue in this one volume, so we hope that readers of this collection will identify further gaps and continue to open spaces for new theorizing and connections around disability and disclosure within higher education.

That these new connections are needed is evident in our attention to disability as an important aspect of diversity. While diversity often specifically refers to race and ethnic diversity, we take the view that diversity—including disability—is broad, complex, multileveled, intersectional, and dynamic. This perspective is grounded in five core principles articulated by the University of Delaware Center for the Study of Diversity (UDCSD), which one of us (Jones) directs. We understand these five core principles as necessary for diversity to make a meaningful difference in the life of institutions of higher education. First, *diversity has to be valued.* By value, we mean that diversity has to be central to the core mission of an institution. However, having it as a value is not enough, which leads to the second core principle: *diversity must also be a priority.* What we mean by priority is that diversity must have sufficient value and importance that institutional resources are directed to it. This is especially important in times of austerity or difficulty, when it may be quite challenging or difficult to find or generate the kind of support that allows diversity programs and projects to go forward.

The third principle is that *diversity is complex.* The complexity of diversity is without doubt the biggest challenge facing those working on behalf of social justice and institutional change in higher education. When people say "diversity," they can mean many different things. And the way in which different people approach diversity is so multivariate and multifaceted that diversity discourses can run the risk of simultaneously saying so much and saying nothing. We don't want diversity to say nothing. It is a principle, a concept that has application to a variety of relationships among people and a variety of challenges that institutions and people face. In order to deal with such a complex concept and circumstance, we need to be smart, to be analytical, and to have understanding and information.

Our fourth principle is that *diversity must lead to institutional change*. Institutional change is a core principle because if we are to address diversity issues, we have to be prepared for big changes. We cannot talk about diversity and keep doing things the way we have always done them. We have to change—but how? The answers are not always obvious, but we nevertheless have to be prepared and to strategically work with information, people, and leadership to make effective and appropriate change. This collection is a big part of making necessary information available to sponsor productive new directions for disability and higher education. And finally, the fifth principle that we abide by is that *to do diversity work, you must engage your campus as well as other local, regional, and national communities*.

We see both the Disability Disclosure in/and Higher Education Conference and this collection as the embodiment of these principles. They represent diversity as broad and multifaceted, with disability considered as an integral part of diversity. Unfortunately, this is currently not well-understood across higher education institutions. Through the work of the conference and this collection, we signal that disability is a priority, as demonstrated by the amount of time, energy, and financial and human resources that have gone into bringing them both to life. The sensitivity and resources that a disability-related conference requires are extraordinary, and we all learned so much from figuring out how to make them happen and what kinds of things need to be taken into account and prioritized (see, e.g., Kerschbaum and Price 2014; Fink 2014). All of these issues are highly complex, and any attempt to make positive change requires the kind of knowledge, data, analysis, and testimonies that emerged from the conference and that appear in this collection. We see the issues that arise in disability analyses also giving rise to other areas of diversity. The notion of accommodation is one important example. While accommodation is often associated with disability, it is also useful when thinking more generally about diversity on campus. With accommodation, we can ask questions such as, "what accommodations do we need to make in order to help people learn better and to be more successful?" and we can connect disability-related accommodations to the need for classrooms to be culturally sensitive and inclusive in order to engage broad communities and enact inclusion (see Jones, Dovidio, & Vietze 2014).

Collection Overview

The collection has four key thematic sections; in what follows, we briefly describe these sections and give an overview of how each chapter contributes to the section's theme. As a whole, the chapters represent a robust set of interdisciplinary perspectives, and they engage different intersections among disability and other forms of identity. In working through this collection, then, readers will find some aspects of disability emphasized more at different times and less at others. Throughout, however, all of the chapters work to situate disability within conversations about the many contextual complexities that shape how disability is read, engaged, and negotiated.

Identity

While disability studies has worked to affirm disability as a positive and important element of identity, it nevertheless remains important to carefully explore disability's positive *and* negative valences, including pride and shame—both of which were recurring themes at the Disability Disclosure in/ and Higher Education Conference. Disability brings with it a complex web of interconnected and deeply held, internalized, and institutionalized orientations to disability, and resisting ableism within identity remains significant to disability studies today.

This section opens with "Passing, Coming Out, and Other Magical Acts," which was first shared as Samuels' powerful closing keynote at the Disability Disclosure in/and Higher Education conference. Her remarks served to close the 2013 conference while offering significant staging for subsequent conversation and dialogue, an effort that this collection forwards. Samuels calls for us all to address social justice issues and "find ways to disclose and unclose disability . . . and that we do so in dynamic interchange and critical awareness of other axes of identity and privilege: class, gender, sexuality, and race."

In "A Hybridized Academic Identity," Alshammari narrates the interrelationships between disability, culture, race and ethnicity, class, and gender in her experiences of ableism as she fights first to pursue higher education and then to secure employment as an academic. Not only does she find herself negotiating a hybridized identity as a Bedouin Kuwaiti woman but again when she is diagnosed as a young woman with multiple sclerosis, itself a hybrid disease. Throughout the chapter, disclosure is an ever-present reality, always involving disability as well as the other privileged and marginalized identities that shape her experiences.

Perceptions of disability and orientations toward disclosure are deeply affected by orientations to disability within society. Barragan and Nusbaum weave the results of a survey of sixty-four disabled students regarding disability on a college campus along with Barragan's personal reflections on themes emerging in the survey analysis to theorize the significance of self-love (drawing on social philosopher Erich Fromm's work) when addressing oppression and stigma.

Picking up on the fear and anxiety that often accompany disclosures, Knight turns to her own performances of disclosure and sharing of her own disability experiences with her classes. Theorizing these experiences through the lens of vulnerability, following feminist theorist bell hooks's work, Knight suggests four ways that teachers might find value in creating spaces for vulnerability with their students, while recognizing that such vulnerability must also be situated within complex intersectional matrices of identity and self-representation.

Wood reports on an interview study involving thirty-five disabled students at a large U.S. university to identify key strategies students use as they negotiate teachers' perceptions of their disability. Insisting on a complex orientation to stigma that recognizes moments of resistance and of rhetorical agency, Wood forwards two strategies students used to manage the risks around disclosure: strategic genericism, in which participants disclosed as disabled but did not offer information about their specific disability, and selective disclosure, in which students shared one diagnosis or a partial diagnosis while avoiding a more full discussion.

Intersectionality

Essays in this section focus on ways that disability identities intersect with, emerge within, and are influenced by myriad aspects of embodied presence and experience. How, and in what ways, does disability infuse the experiences of abled and disabled bodies alike? In what ways does disability converge with gender, race, ethnicity, and sexuality, as well as other aspects of identity performance, to shape the way disabilities are disclosed in a variety of ways and within numerous contexts in higher education?

"Bodyminds Like Ours: An Autoethnographic Analysis of Graduate School, Disability, and the Politics of Disclosure" opens this section with an invitation to join the four authors, Carter, Catania, Schmitt, and Swenson, in personal explorations and disclosures of their experience as graduate students, marginalized by disability dynamics and compounded by intersections with queer, race, and gendered identities. They dare, in—"risking the personal"—to share the wisdom borne of struggle and visions of change that they hope will increase access and visibility, and more importantly, "promote holistic transformation."

The intersectionality theme continues with "Complicating 'Coming Out': Disclosing Disability, Gender and Sexuality in Higher Education." Authors Miller, Wynn and Webb conducted a qualitative study of undergraduate (seventeen) and graduate (fourteen) students using a "situational analysis"—a postmodern extension of grounded theory. Their study revealed disability and sexual identities were disclosed *contextually* (contingent on who, when, where, and why); *strategically* (as a means of accomplishing personal goals), *avoidant* (intentional *non*disclosure) and *comparatively* (selective disclosure of one's disability *or* gender identity, depending on the context). This carefully developed study demonstrates convincingly that disability closure is affected by intersectional identities and follows fluid and evolving processes.

In "Students with Disabilities in Higher Education: Welfare, Stigma Management and Disclosure," Seelman offers a different view of intersectionality, one that includes the dual stigmas of disability and public welfare. Noting the limited research on this topic, she suggests that students who must disclose their disability to receive welfare benefits (e.g., supplemental security income) might face an additional stigmatized burden of perceived poverty, further undermining their chances for success. By exploring multiple conceptualizations of stigma, Seelman draws out important considerations for higher education administrators who must oversee the policies that govern these dually stigmatized processes. This exploratory chapter highlights for us the urgency of additional research and data-gathering at these intersections in order to develop deeper answers to the questions it raises.

Harbour, Boone, Heath, and Ledbetter present a colloquy on the meaning of "overcoming" in their essay "'Overcoming' in Disability Studies and African American Culture, and Implications for Higher Education." The intersection of disability studies, in which overcoming has a negative connotation based in a deficit framework, and African American Civil rights movement, famously characterized by the rallying song "we shall overcome," provides a context for meaningful dialogue. Sharing perspectives and arriving at a series of policy and program recommendations that honor "both/and" points of view is a significant and exemplary achievement.

In the final essay of this section, "Risking Experience: Disability and Disclosure," Kaul provides an engaging journey through the perils of disclosing a disability against disclosing an impairment. Should or shouldn't I disclose a visible or not-visible disability and/or impairment? Kaul shares her experiences as a contract professor whose ties to the academy are already precarious, and disclosing her impairment along with her disability is risky business, as well as institutionally incoherent. Demanding that disability be disclosed to receive accommodations (such as, in Kaul's case, an accessible classroom) can be harrowing.

Representation

How are disabilities represented within institutions of higher education? How do representations of higher education—in popular media, literature, film, television, and advertising, among others—imagine disability? How do representations of disability intersect with race, gender, class, and other forms of identity? Given that these representations matter to the ways that disabilities are read and understood by those within higher education, and to the ways that various participants perform and enact disability, how do these different representations matter to experience(s) of and around disability in higher education?

In "Postmodern Madness on Campus: Narrating and Navigating Mental Difference and Disability," Lewis examines the broad cultural terrain of mental disability and representation on college campuses in the early twenty-first century, showing how neoliberalism seeps into every aspect of higher education to exacerbate mental stress and distress while simultaneously marketing solutions to that distress. Ultimately, Lewis calls for mad studies programs that can involve students, faculty, and staff in creating new possibilities for disability representation and avenues for positive change vis-à-vis mental difference and disability.

In "Doing Disability with Others," Sanchez upends the very concept of disclosure, querying whether, as a word, disclosure can effectively point to what it purports to describe. Through attention to three artifacts: a DeafBlind and Badass button, colored lights on a wheelchair, and a piss on pity T-shirt, Sanchez problematizes the singular moment of disclosure and considers instead language for ongoing processes of "doing disability."

Representation is often a means for recognition, as Lukin shows in his analysis of Philip K. Dick and Vandana Singh's presentations of disability in wide-ranging science-fiction texts. A significant part of such work means validating—*recognizing*—shame and pain as part of the disability experience. Indeed, Lukin notes, "Read or taught in a disability studies context, science-fictional tales of shame and anguish over changing abilities offer nuanced perspectives that question whether we can always redefine disability as a Good Thing or understand it via epiphanies gained through the social model."

Attention to disability representation must also uncover silences and erasures, as Pickens shows in her analysis of Mat Johnson's *Pym*, which opens with the story of a tenure denial involving the novel's central character, Chris Jaynes, an African American English professor. Pickens argues that attention to such representations highlights how current tenure processes, in necessitating "intellectual production of a certain kind" alongside "reproduction . . . of the norms of the institution" ultimately "create a fundamentally unsafe space for faculty who identify as mad and those against whom madness is mobilized as insult or disciplining practice."

Vidali turns to the complexities of potential disclosure in students' research writing and explores one such assignment in her own class. Vidali's attention to her own teaching reveals how representations of disability and disease find their way into students' writing as they research symptoms and diagnose (even hypothetical) conditions using internet resources. As she writes, "we must more thoughtfully evaluate the disclosures that research requires from teachers and students; examine the ways that research discloses certain ideas of disability, disease, and disorder to students; and develop approaches for more productively realizing the progressive goals of disability studies when teaching students to research disability topics and perspectives."

Institutional Change and Policy

This section explores how attention to disability invites reconsideration of institutional environments and policies. What does—or would—it mean for higher education to truly, as Jay Dolmage (2008) has put it, "invite disability in the front door"? The essays in this section look at past and current practices as well as imagine future directions for disability in institutional policy. What policies are needed? How have past and how do present policies address disability? What kinds of minds and bodies are imagined and addressed within such policies? What does disability disclosure ask us to consider in light of such policies?

In "Access to Higher Education Mediated by Self-Disclosure: 'It's a *Hassle*,'" Carroll-Miranda introduces six students attending an institution of higher education in Puerto Rico who participated in a study of the process of inclusion and the role of assistive technologies. Students revealed the complexities of self-disclosure, including how their identities as disabled students often clashed with the ways in which institutional policies and bureaucratic processes constructed their disability.

Freedman, Eisenman, Grigal, and Hart examine implications of access to higher education for a new student population. In "Intellectual Disability: Expanding the Conversation about Diversity and Disclosure," they provide an overview of college initiatives for youth with intellectual disability. Following a discussion of unique disclosure issues arising from interactions of students' goals, program structures, and campus systems, they suggest practical responses based on principles of inclusion, self-determination, and person-centeredness.

"Disclosure and Accommodations for Faculty Members with Mental Health Disabilities" are the subjects of the chapter by Kerschbaum, O'Shea, Price, and Salzer. To date, most data on faculty members and accommodation has been anecdotal. This chapter draws on a national survey of faculty members with a broad range of mental health issues to offer knowledge about these faculty members' reported familiarity with and use of various accommodations, as well as those accommodations' perceived helpfulness. The authors conclude by discussing avenues for further research as well as suggestions regarding faculty members and accommodation.

Rocco and Collins describe "An Initial Model for Accommodation Communication between Students with Disabilities and Faculty." This chapter provides an adult education perspective on the roles, processes, and structures within these communications and discusses why they may break down and what makes them more likely to succeed. The authors suggest that faculty and students should avoid assuming that their institutions' policies and practices around disclosure are "correct." They conclude with suggestions for ways that faculty and students can proactively enhance their communications.

Finally, Breneman, Schoolcraft, Ghiaciuc, and Vandeberg use a conversational frame in their essay, "I am Different/So Are You: Creating Safe Spaces for Disability Disclosure (A Conversation)" to expose the highly personal, complicated nature of disability disclosures that are experienced within the legal and procedural approaches taken by many institutions of higher education. This chapter brings together the director of a disability services office, two faculty members who address disability in the classroom, and a social work student and disability advocate. This collaborative, multi-voiced chapter in its presentation performs the uncertainty often experienced around disability and disclosure as the writers (at least initially) leave open the question of their own disability identifications. As they examine their own relationships to disclosure, they also emphasize the value of creating accessible, inclusive, safe spaces through various means, including campus partnerships and interdisciplinary disability curricula. The authors conclude by inviting readers to explore their own relationships with disclosure, while encouraging them to envision ways of building institutional community.

This collection reflects our belief that the work we need to do around disability and higher education is work all of us need to do together, engaging scholars, activists, and constituencies from diverse areas, fields of inquiry, and modes of analysis. We see such coalitions as necessary for broadening knowledge about disability and helping that knowledge take root within the cultures, institutions, and practices of higher education. *Negotiating Disability* does this by facilitating some of these connections, in hopes of motivating further and deeper partnerships and new avenues for exploration and knowledge dissemination.

References

Dolmage, Jay. 2008. "Mapping Composition: Inviting Disability in the Front Door. *Disability and the Teaching of Writing.* Edited by Cynthia Lewiecki-Wilson and Brenda Brueggemann with Jay Dolmage, 14–27. Boston: Bedford/St. Martin's.

Fink, Margaret. 2014. "Comment from the Field: Disability Disclosure in/and Higher Education, University of Delaware, Newark." *Journal of Literary and Cultural Disability Studies* 8 (2): 219–24.

Jones, James M., Dovidio, John F. and Vietze, Deborah L. 2014. *The Psychology of Diversity: Beyond Prejudice and Racism.* New York: Wiley/Blackwell.

Kerschbaum, Stephanie. 2014. "On Rhetorical Agency and Disclosing Disability in Academic Writing." *Rhetoric Review* 33 (1): 55–71.

Kerschbaum, Stephanie and Margaret Price. 2014. "Perils and Prospects of Disclosing Disability Identity in Higher Education." *Diversity US: A Blog of the Center for the Study of Diversity.* 03 March 2014. http://sites.udel.edu/csd/2014/03/03/perils-and-prospects-of-disclosing-disability-identity-in-higher-education/

Kerschbaum, Stephanie L., Rosemarie Garland-Thomson, Sushil K. Oswal, Amy Vidali, Susan Ghiaciuc, Margaret Price, Jay Dolmage, Craig A. Meyer, Brenda Brueggemann, and Ellen Samuels. 2013. "Faculty Members, Accommodation,

and Access in Higher Education." *Profession*. http://profession.commons.mla.
org/2013/12/09/faculty-members-accommodation-and-access-in-higher-ed-
ucation/

Oswal, Sushil. 2016. "Disabling Policies and Exclusionary Infrastructures: A Critique of the AAUP Report." *Disability, Avoidance, and the Academy: Challenging
Resistance*. Edited by David Bolt and Claire Penketh. London: Routledge. 21–32.

I

———

Identity

Passing, Coming Out, and Other Magical Acts

ELLEN SAMUELS

———

I'm going to start with a story. With a story and a poem, really.

The story is about a conference, the Modern Language Association Convention, which I attended in January 2013 in Boston. Like all MLA conventions, this one was exhausting—physically, intellectually, and even spiritually—and my physical exhaustion was exacerbated by the fact that technical failures kept me from bringing my mobility scooter as planned, and I had to walk around the sprawling, multi-building convention site for four days. By the time I left for the airport, I was truly and literally on my last legs.

Fortunately, the cab driver dropped me off right at the curbside check-in station—but then the skycap told me I was at the wrong terminal. He started to give me a long string of directions: go in these doors, go downstairs, catch a shuttle, and I had to interrupt him to say, "I can't do that. I need a wheelchair, please." He nodded silently and turned away to get my baggage tag, leaving me standing there on the sidewalk, swaying a bit as I tried to keep my balance. So I reached inside my purse for my folding cane and pulled it out so it automatically snapped together.

Immediately, the skycap stopped what he was doing and grabbed a walkie-talkie, speaking in urgent tones: "I need a wheelchair at door seven." "You go inside and sit down," he added to me, looking in my eyes for the first time. Gratefully, and slowly, I walked inside leaning on my cane, my cane which had functioned, in this case, like a virtual magic wand.

When I think back on this experience, I always connect it to Manning's remarkable poem, "The Magic Wand" (in Fries 2014, 165):

Quick-change artist extraordinaire,
I whip out my folded cane
and change from black man to blind man
with a flick of my wrist.
It is a profound metamorphosis—
From God-gifted wizard of roundball
dominating backboards across America,
To God-gifted idiot savant composer
pounding out chart-busters on a cockeyed whim;
From sociopathic gangbanger with death for eyes
to all-seeing soul with saintly spirit;
From rape deranged misogynist
to poor motherless child;
From welfare-rich pimp
to disability-rich gimp;
And from "white man's burden"
to every man's burden.

It is always a profound metamorphosis.
Whether from cursed by man to cursed by God;
or from scriptures condemned to God ordained,
My final form is never of my choosing;
I only wield the wand;
You are the magicians.

Why do I begin with this story and this poem? To remind us all that disability disclosure never happens in only one direction, or on only one level
of communication, interpretation, and meaning. When I transformed from
a nondisabled-seeming young white woman into an invalid lady leaning on
a cane, or when Manning's narrator is transformed from an embodiment of
white America's stereotypes of black men into its stereotypes of blindness,
that transformation takes place at the intersection of multiple identities, locations, and assumptions. Not only disability but also gender, sexuality, race,
and class play into these moments of transformation, and when we talk about
disclosure, we need to talk about all of those sites of embodied social power
relationships. In particular, Manning's poem highlights the role of racializa-
tion in the perception of his identity as both confirming and confounding
stereotypes regarding not just black men or blind men, but black blind men,
a representational space haunted by those "God-given idiot savants," Stevie

Wonder and Ray Charles, who supposedly "overcame" the "handicaps" of racial and ability difference through their musical talent.

How, Manning's poem challenges us, do we apprehend multiple and intersecting identities of marginalization in resistance to stereotypes? I am reminded of a phrase O'Toole (2015), a white, disabled lesbian mother, once used when talking about how people would see her wheeling along with her disabled, Asian-American daughter and "flip through their rolodex of stereotypes," trying to find one to fit. For that is often how the process of disclosure works: while in our ideal scenarios the disabled person should be able to simply disclose their disability status and be recognized and perhaps accommodated, such disclosures do not take place in a vacuum. Rather, they are issued into a complex representational realm in which each person at the other end of disclosure tends to do their best to fit the revealed identity into a preexisting matrix of meanings and assumptions. Thus, disclosure functions interactionally, with the fear of negative reception or misrecognition often stifling the impulse to disclose or, as it is often called, to "come out." And I also suggest that while passing, in terms of disability identity, is more possible for some of us than for others, passing too has to be understood as taking place inside such a complex matrix where disability status is never the only identity under pressure and where nondisabled status is never the only identity at risk.

At the end of the Disability Disclosure in/and Higher Education Conference, I found myself returning continually to certain main themes: intersectionality and diversity, risk-taking, privilege, representation, pride—and the other face of pride, shame. I start here with intersectionality because I think it was both present and not present at the conference and in the wider disability community: so many of us live at the margins of multiple normative structures, not only in terms of mental and physical ability but also in terms of gender, sexuality, class, and race. Seelman, in her opening keynote (this volume), highlighted how this intersectionality of class and race functions in the lives of higher education students who receive public benefits and who are often hesitant to disclose that fact due to the tremendous stigma attached to it. Her presentation pointed to the convergence of complex racial, economic, and disability factors when she noted that disabled undergraduate students receiving Social Security Insurance (SSI) benefits are nearly three times more likely to be African American than those disabled students who do not receive such benefits. Since SSI, unlike SSDI (Social Security Disability Insurance), is a means-tested benefit, this statistic indicates that students who are both African American and disabled are far more likely to come from families living in poverty or near-poverty than other disabled students.

This should not be surprising to those of us who are aware of the racialized income gap in this country or how sharply it has widened since the beginning of the financial downturn in 2008. The postmodern, neoliberal conditions under which we live (Lewis, this volume) mean that we live in an increasingly fragmented and unequal world, one in which each of us is imagined to be responsible for our privilege or lack of privilege. Yet the presentations at this conference have vividly demonstrated how privilege functions as a regulatory force that supports institutional power structures even as it impacts each of us in our daily lives (see Chen 2014; Haraway 1988).

Who has the privilege to disclose disability? I do, apparently, since I do so in this essay and in many of my published works (Samuels 2003; 2011). So did quite a few of us at the conference—although, as Kafer (2016) pointed out in her keynote, many of us expressed considerable fear about doing so, even in the protected space of the conference. We arrived into a space of privilege, bringing our privilege with us: the privilege of holding status in higher education, as faculty, administrators, and graduate students, part of a chosen few. We brought the privilege of class, spending money—our own or our institution's—on travel, and our time on attending a conference rather than working at wage labor. And many of us brought the privilege of whiteness, as Chen (2014) so importantly and necessarily reminded us: the conference, like most disability studies conferences, was predominantly white and that is a problem the entire field needs to address, and needs to address better, if we are not to remain a truly segregated—and I use that term advisedly—field of endeavor (see Bell 2005).

We even brought the privilege of ability: while many at the conference had impairments and identified with disability, those who traveled to that conference, by definition, were not the disabled people who are too disabled to leave their homes or for whom leaving their homes is disabling, whether due to chemical toxins, emotional trauma, or sensory overload. We were not the disabled people in state-run institutions, or in the overcrowded prisons that so often function as carceral institutions for disabled people in the United States today (see Ben-Moshe, Chapman, and Carey 2014). We did not represent the full range of disabilities or impairments in the nation or in the world, and so we must always remember who is not here and to challenge ourselves not to remain immersed in the bubble of privilege but always to reach outside it, to reach across it.

One of the themes that emerged and re-emerged in the conference was the greater difficulty and stigma of coming out about mental and cognitive disability in the higher education setting. While Seelman (this volume) pointed out the growing numbers of undergraduate students whose disabilities can be classified as "mental, emotional, or cognitive," tremendous stigma still attaches to those categories across educational and social settings (see also American College Health Association). And for graduate students and faculty alike, it clearly remains a highly risky endeavor to reveal any form of mental or cognitive difference or vulnerability: our minds, our justifications for being here, must run like steely machinery, always reliable, always stable.

I thank those who talked about the impossibility of maintaining that state of normative mindfulness and the toll taken when we try to conceal our mental vulnerabilities. I thank Ibby Grace for talking about the costs of trying to pass as neurotypical and the importance of claiming her autistic self with pride. I thank Chen (2014) for talking about brain fog and states of "not-knowing" and the crushing denial of those common conditions within the rarefied space of the academy. I thank Kafer (2016) for speaking about trauma and the restrictions of "safe space" even within—especially within— the worlds of disability studies and disability culture. I especially thank Price (2011) for taking a groundbreaking risk in her research and writing to give us crucial tools for thinking through these issues from a disability studies perspective.

This is an absolutely essential conversation to have now because mental distress is becoming the norm, not the exception, in higher education today. When Lewis (this volume) told us that a 2010 survey of students by American College Health Association showed that 45.6 percent reported feeling things were hopeless, and 30.7 percent were so depressed it was difficult to function, I—and likely many of you reading this—felt these statistics simply confirmed what I have seen in my own campuses and classrooms (see also American College Health Association).[1] When the very endeavor to which we have dedicated our lives appears to be transforming into a laboratory of despair, how can we think about disclosure as merely a transaction between one individual and another, or between an individual and an institution? Surely each of these individual students deserves support and accommodations and biomedical treatment if they so desire. But sometime soon, we are going to run out of Band-Aids, and we need to start thinking about structural solutions and about the meaning of access on a whole different plane.

What would mental and emotional access look like? It would by necessity include financial access: sufficient financial aid and graduate student support so that students are not working two jobs while taking too many credits to save on tuition dollars. Such access must also include social access, a diversity of residential and extracurricular structures so that students can find support and acceptance on campuses rather than a set of additional strictures and demands. And finally, such access needs to include representational access, to provide students with critical skills to interpret the onslaught of cultural representations that makes up our postmodern digital world, to combat stigma and to imaginatively project themselves into new forms of representation.

I work in the field of cultural studies, and my training is in literary studies and visual culture. I believe in the power of cultural representation to make change in the world, and I also believe in the importance of critically interpreting and resisting cultural representations. I think it is just as essential for a disabled child to see diverse and positive representations of herself in the world as for her to have an IEP or an occupational therapist. Such images are loaded with power and history, and especially in the case of disability, where representation has so often been driven by stereotype and stigma, it is crucially important that we give critical context to the representations that we use in our work.[2] In fact, I will go so far as to suggest that everyone who works in disability studies, or disability policy, or special education, or rehabilitation, should take at least one class on disability and representation. Literature, film, visual art: these are the ways all of us, disabled and nondisabled, apprehend our worlds and imagine new ones, and it is vitally important to uncover their meanings.

Turning now to my last point, which is about diversity, I was thrilled that the conference was sponsored by the University of Delaware Center for the Study of Diversity. Like many of us, I struggle to get my own institution to recognize disability as part of diversity. In fact, I have kind of a funny story about how these issues play out at my university. In my first week there, at a new faculty workshop, I heard a presentation on something called the Inclusivity Initiative. After about ten minutes, I still couldn't figure out what it was, so—being me—I raised my hand and asked. The presenters explained that it was an initiative to address climate issues on campus for LGBTQ people. Then it was explained to me: "At the UW, inclusivity means LGBT. Equality means women. Diversity means race, and access means disability."

No wonder I was confused.

If we are to address social justice issues with any kind of meaning or efficacy, I suggest, we need models that move beyond such segregated thinking. James Jones, director of the Center for the Study of Diversity, in his opening remarks for the conference, listed five principles that guide the meaningful work of diversity (see editors' introduction, this volume). They are: (1) value, (2) priority, (3) complexity, (4) institutional change, and (5) engagement with communities: campus, local, regional, national, global. At the end of the conference, in my closing keynote, I asked the audience to imagine how revolutionary it would be if we all returned to our home campuses with the goal of applying these principles to disability: to work toward our campuses giving disability value, making it a priority, addressing its complexity, committing to institutional change, and making disability a central point of community engagement. Such an endeavor would demand that we move beyond the limited model of individual accommodation and think in terms of disability justice and universal accessibility.

This endeavor would also, I suggest, demand that we find ways to disclose and unclose disability: our own disability status, our relationships to disability, our investments in disability; and that we do so in dynamic interchange and critical awareness of other axes of identity and privilege: class, gender, sexuality, and race. I don't think we can achieve justice only by disclosing, by telling stories, but I do believe stories are powerful and they are necessary.

So I'm going to close, just as I started, with a story and a poem. This time, the poem is my own, which I had promised to the conference organizers as part of my official bio: my disability, disclosed in haiku form:

Connective tissue
disorder: Ehlers-Danlos.
I break easily.

There it is. All the information you would get in my multi-page medical documentation distilled into seventeen syllables. You probably still have questions, but you would after reading that documentation too, I assure you. For one thing, medicine just doesn't have all the answers.

But more importantly, that's not how people really communicate with each other, with the language of bureaucracy. We communicate with stories. So here's my last story.

When I read this poem during my keynote, I accompanied it with a picture of a toy called a "push puppet." This particular push puppet is a jointed human figure atop a round platform, its body held together with string. When you push the bottom of the platform, the string is loosened and the figure collapses at its joints. I used the image of the push puppet to get a badly-needed accommodation from my university in my third year of working there. Now this was an accommodation my university had agreed to in writing during my hire and one that was perfectly ADA-compatible and reasonable. But a new dean had come in and she wanted to take it away. Many meetings ensued, during which I and my advocates explained over and over in legalistic, bureaucratic, and medical terms why I needed this accommodation and why it had to work this way. Still, the dean resisted.

Finally, in the umpteenth of these meetings, frustrated and exhausted, I turned to her and said, "You know those toys where all the joints are connected by string and you push the bottom and it just collapses? That's what my joints do. That's why I need this."

Her face changed and her mouth opened. Somehow that story had persuaded her, when all of my doctor's notes about collagen defects and functional limitations, and the equity office's explanations about reasonable accommodations and undue burdens, had failed. She signed off on the accommodation immediately.

Now in a way, this story is absurd. It certainly felt so at that time. But with the passing of years, I have come to see it in a different light. I see that sometimes disclosure is not enough. There has to be shared communication and understanding—and, often, there has to be metaphor. This toy, this push puppet, is my metaphor. It is a representation, a story that does work in the world.

So to close, I invite all of you reading this to ask yourselves two things: What is your story, your metaphor, and how will it help you to do your work? And what is the story of this collection and what work has it given us to do?

References

American College Health Association. 2014. *American College Health Association-National College Health Assessment II: Undergraduate Students Reference Group Executive Summary Spring 2014.* Hanover, MD: American College Health Association.

Bell, Christopher. 2005. "Is Disability Studies Actually White Disability Studies?" *The Disability Studies Reader*, 3rd ed., edited by Lennard J. Davis. New York: Routledge, 374–82.

Ben-Moshe, Liat, Chris Chapman, and Allison C. Carey, eds. 2014. *Disability Incarcerated: Imprisonment and Disability in the United States and Canada.* New York: Palgrave Macmillan.

Chen, Mel Y. "Brain Fog: The Race for Cripistemology," *Journal of Literary and Cultural Disability Studies* 8, no. 2 (2014): 171–84.

Garland-Thomson, Rosemarie. 1997. *Extraordinary Bodies: Figuring Physical Disability in American Culture and Literature.* New York: Columbia University Press.

Grace, Elizabeth J. n.d. "TinyGraceNotes." Accessed 18 May 2016. http://tinygracenotes.blogspot.com/

Haraway, Donna. 1988. "Situated Knowledges: The Science Question in Feminism and the Privilege of Partial Perspective," *Feminist Studies* 14 (3): 575–99.

Kafer, Alison. 2016. "Un/Safe Disclosures: Scenes of Disability and Trauma." *Journal of Literary and Cultural Disability Studies* 10 (1): 1–20.

Kerschbaum, Stephanie L., Laura T. Eisenman, and James M. Jones. This volume.

Lewis, Bradley. This volume.

Longmore, Paul. 2003. "Screening Stereotypes: Images of Disabled People in Television and Motion Pictures." *Why I Burned My Book and Other Essays on Disability*. Philadelphia: Temple University Press, 131–46.

Manning, Lynn. 1997. "The Magic Wand" in *Staring Back: Disability Experience from the Inside Out*, ed. Kenny Fries. New York: Plume, 165.

Mitchell, David T. and Sharon L. Snyder. 2000. *Narrative Prosthesis: Disability and the Dependencies of Discourse*. Ann Arbor: University of Michigan Press.

Osteen, Mark, ed. 2010. *Autism and Representation*. New York: Routledge.

O'Toole, Corbett Joan. 2015. *Fading Scars: My Queer Disability History*. Autonomous Press.

Price, Margaret. 2011. *Mad at School: Rhetorics of Mental Disability and Academic Life*. Ann Arbor: University of Michigan Press.

Samuels, Ellen. 2003. "My Body, My Closet: Invisible Disability and the Limits of Coming Out Discourse." *GLQ* 9 (1–2): 233–55.

Samuels, Ellen. 2011. "Examining Millie and Christine McKoy: Where Enslavement and Enfreakment Meet." *Signs* 37 (1): 53–81.

Seelman, Katherine. This volume.

A Hybridized Academic Identity

*Negotiating a Disability
within Academia's Discourse of Ableism*

SHAHD ALSHAMMARI

I have always been very aware of my body. As a Kuwaiti Bedouin woman, I grew up in a culture that viewed my body as taboo, as something to be hidden, concealed, and, mostly, regulated. At a very early age, I was informed by my father that I was to protect my body, that the entire tribe's honor laid within me. If I was a "good girl," I would be able to understand how sacred my body was. I was always conflicted while growing up because I was caught between three very different, disparate cultures. My father was Bedouin, my mother was Palestinian, and I was educated in American, co-ed schools. In this environment, race and identity were two issues I was forced to negotiate. Language itself was terrifying—I was bullied for speaking a hybridized language, bits of Kuwaiti Bedouin, bits of Palestinian, and, of course, English.

By the age of sixteen, I had developed a sense of immunity toward society's expectations of me. I merely existed in my world, choosing to be alone, and focusing only on my education. Unlike most women in my tribe, I was fortunate to be educated: my mother had consistently fought for me to be given the opportunity to study. To be educated was the first step in overcoming tribal and patriarchal oppression. Education would secure my future and grant me financial and social status. However, my position as a hybrid left me constantly shifting between two worlds: because I was a woman, I was expected to remain "good" and "modest" while at the same time trying to reclaim rights that I had been denied because I was born a woman. Born into a Bedouin family, I knew that although I was older, my younger brother had freedoms and rights that I could only fight for. I was constantly trying to prove that although I was a girl, I could be just as competent as my brother, and that I could make a difference in the world. I was always fighting for a sense of individuality, a sense of being, set apart from the family and the tribe.

But then, when I was eighteen and about to head to college, the biggest blow of my life hit: I was diagnosed with multiple sclerosis (MS), an auto-immune illness. The diagnosis further complicated an already complex situation and left me feeling even more marginalized and inferior than before. I was now a woman, a hybrid, and diagnosed with an illness that people in my society knew very little about. How would I ever find my place in a society that upholds normativity and rejects an ambiguous state of being?

MS is itself a hybrid disease, in the sense that it is completely random, indeterminate, and presents itself between the juncture of abled/disabled, healthy/sick. MS patients may go days or months or even years feeling relatively stable and healthy, and then one day, out of the blue, they may wake up blind, deaf, or unable to walk. Just like that, without any warning, people with MS may move between the boundaries of abled/disabled. Because MS is sometimes an invisible illness, it can be concealed. Not all symptoms are apparent, and certainly not all symptoms are permanent. You may be walking one day just fine, and the next, you may need a cane, or even a wheelchair. This invisibility can make it hard for people with MS to claim a disabled identity. Thus, for me, MS has always occupied an ambivalent, ambiguous space. It is a hybridized disease. Allow me to quote Mairs (1996) on the mechanisms of MS:

> The hypothesis is that the disease process, in which the protective covering of the nerves in the brain and spinal cord is eaten away and replaced by scar tissue . . . is caused by an autoimmune reaction to a slow-acting virus. . . . In effect, living with this mysterious mechanism feels like having your present self, and the past selves it embodies, haunted by a capricious and mean-spirited ghost, unseen except for its footprints, which trips you even when you're watching where you're going . . . and weights your whole body with a weariness no amount of rest can relieve. An alien invader must be at work. But of course it's not. It's your own body. That is, it's you. (83–84)

With such attacks, every sense of a stable self is called into question. Who am I and how has my body attacked me? If the mind is superior to the body in the Western mind/body dualism, then how is it that MS, a disease that originates in the central nervous system, is able to control the body and one's sense of self? No amount of positive thinking can change the reality of a failing body. My body was protesting, and it was reminding me and everyone around me of its existence, its visibility. At the same time, there were many years when my MS was not visible at all. I was passing as "normal" and "healthy," although I was in pain most of the time and required medication to keep some of the symptoms in check.

For the longest time, I believed it was important for me to pass as "normal" if I wanted to prove myself worthy. According to McRuer (2006), able-bodiedness is deemed as important and compulsory as compulsory heterosexuality (10). This pull towards compulsory able-bodiedness led me to struggle with both aspects of my identity. Various systems of societal discipline seek to control and regulate identities and bodies, constantly emphasizing the fictive necessity of achieving normalcy in all aspects of life. Disability holds negative connotations and is associated with lack, failure, and loss. Socially, it is often interpreted as unfeminine and chaotic, even subhuman. This set of terms is complex and needs unpacking—although they are shared by different cultures and communities—they are not strictly universal.

The Western tradition of viewing the body as morally inferior and the mind as superior has infiltrated our conscious and unconscious perceptions of a cohesive identity. The supposed split between the mind and body is too simplistic and reductive. Similar to Western ideologies that suggest the mind is a powerhouse and treat the body as controlled by the mind, Eastern conceptions of the body remain stigmatizing. The mind is supposedly capable of willing the body into place, of setting it straight; positive thinking can change your reality, and the shameful corporeality of the body is deliberately ignored. Yet despite the public eye's neglect of the body, "physical pain is highly unpredictable and raw as reality. It pits the mind against the body in ways that make the opposition between thought and ideology in most current body theory seem trivial" (Siebers 2008, 64). If MS is a disease of the central nervous system and affects motor control and limbs, then is it the mind or the body that is falling short?

Generally speaking, MS is uncommon in the Arab world. We are told by scientists that it mostly affects "Caucasians" and occurs mainly in areas of the globe where there is hardly any sun exposure. I come from the desert, literally, a country that has high temperatures year round. My diagnosis made very little sense. I was seen by British neurologists who were utterly baffled. I was a healthy teenager, I had never tasted alcohol in my life, and I had never tried any form of drugs. I had never been ill before, and I was suddenly unable to walk and needed help doing most of the everyday chores I had taken for granted. My body had called attention to itself; it was in crisis. I was now undeniably immersed in my body, and it was choosing to fail me.

My father had always insisted that by the time I started menstruating, I would have to cover my hair. My mother kept fighting for the opposite, claiming that it was my choice whether I would ever want to be veiled or not. He agreed reluctantly and said that we would wait until I was a freshman at college. After all, that was the real world. The world really begins at college, he said, and that was when my identity as a Bedouin woman would really flourish. I would have to represent the family and the tribe. I was now part of the larger public sphere, and college was the first initiation into it. But because my MS diagnosis decided to join me as I entered the "real world," this further complicated matters. My curly hair could not be tamed; I could not brush it myself, let alone cover it. Not only that, but I would also have to face the world with my wild hair, an unbalanced gait, slurred speech, and a twitching eye. Not very feminine, not exactly an ideal body, let alone an "ideal woman." My father let the issue of regulating my body go—now there was something worse to deal with.

I had been accepted to study Literature at the American University of Paris, but because of my new diagnosis, I was unable to travel or live on my own. I stayed home, attending Kuwait University, where I majored in English Literature. I did not inform the school of my disability for many reasons: partly because it was an invisible disability, partly because I was ashamed, partly because my family refused to let me claim a disabled identity, and mainly, because I was afraid of what this new-found identity might do to my career. I had a goal. I wanted to become an academic, and I believed wholeheartedly that disclosing would destroy my career. Each year, our English department chose the best candidates and sent them on a scholarship to earn a PhD from England or the United States. I feared that if the news ever spilled that I had MS, I would no longer be eligible. Indeed, one of the rules of the scholarship explicitly stated that the applicant should be "healthy." And so I spent the next four years hiding my disability, passing, and refraining from sharing any details of my illness with anyone, even when such sharing might have really made my life easier. For instance, I would claim I had injured my leg playing soccer, when in reality, I was suffering from an MS relapse and my legs were numb and not functioning normally. I would claim that my handwriting was naturally awful, but my hands were actually suffering from a persistent tremor, and I required more time to take my examinations. I had to deal with comments like "that's why girls shouldn't play soccer" and "you need to fix your handwriting, bad handwriting is a sign of bad character" and "you can't be that clumsy." In all of this, I preferred dealing with criticism of my character rather than risk being discriminated against because of my disability.

As an undergraduate student, for a time, I had to use a cane. All heads turned. I was suddenly a spectacle, both admired and pitied, found both fascinating and repulsive, and I was sometimes asked many questions by my peers and professors, while at other times, I was simply ignored. I began noticing that the public's attitude toward the sick female body differed from the way men with disabilities were viewed. There were many male students with disabilities, but I observed that they were not stared at. Tension would arise when I would enter a classroom, cane in hand, feet shuffling. A professor once looked up from his desk and asked me why I insisted on coming to class. In front of the entire classroom, I had to mumble a few incoherent words—I said I needed to take notes for the upcoming exam. I felt the need to *excuse* my behavior and my presence. My presence made others uncomfortable, and I was apologetic for failing to meet the image of both ideal womanhood and a "good student." I was constantly trying to prove my social worthiness and academic abilities. When MS remained invisible, socially awkward situations like the former example were avoided. However, there were times when no matter how much I wanted to hide, to be sheltered from exposure, my body demanded to be seen, to be made visible.

During these years, I tried to set myself apart from the "disabled" and did not seek their company. I was aware that MS support groups existed, but I could not bring myself to associate with them. They were mostly older people, and ageism was an issue of which I was not aware. I was the youngest patient, and I was not severely disabled. I felt a strange feeling overcome me, one that I later recognized as guilt. I felt as an imposter would, as if I was an able-bodied individual seeking to be included in a community that was supportive and understanding. I did not yet understand that there were varieties of disabilities and that I was still subscribing to the binary division of able-bodied/disabled. I truly wanted to be perceived as "normal" so that I could, in the same vein, be considered academically proficient.

After graduating with a high GPA, I convinced my parents that I deserved a chance to pursue my higher education. There was one condition: I needed someone to live with me, in case my MS decided to attack. Fortunately, at the time, a friend was interested in pursuing the same education, and so we traveled together. Eventually, I earned my MA degree from the University of Exeter in England. While a postgraduate student there, I received support from my professors, and one suggested that I work on Disability Studies research. I brushed off the suggestion, unable to claim a disabled identity and not yet ready to face the world. I was still trying to be the "best" image of myself. If I failed to live up to normative ideas of womanhood, then I would at least be a successful academic. I applied for numerous jobs but never landed a full-time offer. The "heartbreak in academia" as I like to call it, took place one day when I informed the interview panel at a local university that I had MS and that I would sometimes be unable to perform at my level best. The head of the committee responded warmly, but after a teaching observation, they decided against hiring me. They shared a list of reasons why I was not fit for the job, but the one that left me dumfounded and angered was that I was criticized for teaching while sitting down, rather than walking around the classroom. This, to the committee, meant that I was not "engaged" or "engaging."

I filed a complaint, of course, and attempted to take the issue to the dean, to the newspapers, but I never pulled through. My complaints had little effect, and I was not ready to fight. I was not ready to have my career killed: I was only twenty-five, and I was still planning on staying within academia. This was the first in a series of disappointments with the "real world" and the academic world. I began to understand that my job was to protect my career, just like I had attempted to protect myself as an undergraduate. I told myself I would embrace passing, and I would do my utmost to keep MS at bay, to keep it as invisible as possible. My identity over the years had become founded on education; it was all that I had carried within me along the years. Education set me apart from my tribe, and it was the only reason I had come as far as I had. I needed to survive in academia; my identity as a woman rested entirely on my ability to land (and keep) a job, to be financially independent, and to break free from patriarchal oppression.

Over the last few years, I have managed to work as an adjunct faculty member in various universities, while at the same time completing my PhD. Completing a PhD, of course, has been a challenge, as my cognitive abilities have begun to fail me and my body struggles to maintain a teaching job and do research at the same time. Yet somehow, I still only find solace in academia, and I find that my career as an academic is inextricably linked to my identity. I have, however, also begun to come to terms with the possibility that being an independent scholar might one day be the most valid option for me.

Passing as a concept can have different meanings depending on racial, social, and gender ideologies. Disability passing, crossing the boundaries between able-bodied/disabled, normal/abnormal, and visible/invisible disabilities is a complex act that challenges rigid dichotomies that attempt to fix an otherwise fluid identity. Because disability passing is multifaceted, and certainly not universal, one needs to remain vigilant to its nuances and complexities. However, as Brune and Wilson note, "nearly all disabled people confront, often routinely, the choice of hiding their disability or drawing attention to it and the question of what to do when others overlook it. Going to the root of a disability identity, their decisions weigh issues of stigma, pride, prejudice, discrimination, and privilege but rarely put the matter to rest" (2013, 1). In academia, passing is even more daunting. Though many academics might protest and deny this, academia relies heavily on presenting an intellectual, coherent, and productive identity that emerges as distinctive and distinguished. The psychological effects of such passing, however, can be traumatic, especially when finally acknowledging what Wilson has termed the "impossibility of passing as normal" (2013, 31). To recognize this impossibility is to come to terms with a newfound identity that is not based on simplistic and reductive definitions that continue to isolate and exclude people whose bodies are marked as deviant or different. Reaching this stage is not a straightforward process and requires constant revision and renegotiation.

Working as an academic with a disability has been problematic at times. I have become experienced with the art of hiding pain, of hiding a huge part of me, that is, of my body. Not only do I know that my body may well be the end of my career, but I also recognize the discomfort that people feel when the "disabled" body is brought to their attention. Frank (1997) reminds us of the double-burden that the person with the illness or disability must carry:

> When adult bodies lose control, they are expected to attempt to regain it if possible, and if not then at least to conceal the loss. . . . Thus the work of the stigmatized person is not only to avoid embarrassing himself by being out of control in situations where control is expected. The person must also avoid embarrassing others, who should be protected from the specter of lost body control." (31)

My students, for instance, never see me limp or double over from the chest pain that sometimes attacks me (known, ironically, as the MS hug). At times, my eye twitches uncontrollably, my hand shakes from a tremor, and I must put the red pen down, hide my hand under the desk, and wait for it to pass. Sometimes it does. Other times, I have to dismiss the class. The ultimate question remains to pass or not to pass. Keeping a huge part of one's identity hidden is a form of closeting. Siebers (2008) notes that "[c]loseting involves things not merely concealed but difficult to disclose—the inability to disclose is, in fact, one of the constitutive markers of oppression" (97). There is too much at stake upon disclosure. And so closeting becomes yet another duty to carry out. Passing as non-disabled requires effort, dedication, and the ability to manipulate others' perception of you. Passing also becomes manageable because other people assist in this performance. But there might be no desire to pass if society provided equal opportunities for the disabled. As Carey puts it:

> Perhaps at a macro level, a positive culmination of social justice movements would be a society that resists sharp demarcations of identity and related resources and instead meets the individual needs of its people without imposing bounded identities on them, thereby removing the structural constraints that shape individuals' choices regarding, and understandings, of passing. (2013, 160)

Access to elevators, offices that are not too far from the department's classrooms, and flexible work hours all count as means for inclusion within the workforce. However, there are other, not-so-visible issues that arise. Chronic fatigue, for example, is yet another symptom of MS, and because the fatigue is invisible, it places you at the juncture of normal/abnormal. Disabled people fall into many categories, but when the impairment/disability is invisible, it adds to the indeterminacy. Chronic fatigue is a vague state of being that is often misunderstood, even in the medical community. More often than not, it is associated with depression and a general lack of interest in the world. This misrepresentation of a very real, and often disabling, condition marks the person complaining of chronic fatigue as lazy, unproductive, and even "dramatic." Other disabled women have shared with me their experience of being considered liars or "drama queens" because their fatigue is invisible. In a society that remains very patriarchal and oppressive, these women are fighting to establish an autonomous identity. As an academic, my experience is that a debilitating symptom such as fatigue is difficult to explain to the general public, even as it can alter one's productivity, energy, and concentration levels.

Because MS is a hybrid disease, claiming disability with MS can be problematic. If, as Siebers writes, disability "does not yet have the advantage of a political interpretation because the ideology of ability remains largely unquestioned" (2008, 81), how are we to call for an understanding of an invisible disability? He continues,

> There is no term for the prejudicial reduction of a body to its disability. Disability activists have proposed the term ableism to name this prejudice, but it has not been accepted into general usage. Its use elicits scowls and smirks, even in progressive society. There is little sense either in the general population or among scholars that words like blind, crippled, stupid . . . or dumb carry social meanings having an interpretation, history, and politics well beyond the particularities of one human body. (2008, 81)

If scholars are still unaware of the importance of disability studies, then how can we expect more from the general population?

When I express my interest in Disability Studies to colleagues, some still smirk at both the existence of such a field as well as my insistent academic and personal interest in it. Accused thus of narcissism, the disabled individual is left trying to explain and rationalize their behavior. Siebers (2008) contends that "the accusation of narcissism is one of the strongest weapons used against people with disabilities (and other minorities who pray that consciousness-raising will bring an end to their oppression)" (37). As I have taken an interest in the creation of disability politics and problematics of identity, I find myself having to defend that choice to other able-bodied academics who are not yet convinced of the category of Disability Studies. Much like Women's Studies and Queer Studies, Disability Studies does not have a viable market in the Middle East. Disability Studies calls for intersectionality and inclusivity, but still faces contempt from both academics and the general public. While such attitudes may be changing in the West, it remains difficult to work in this field from an Arab woman's perspective. I find it difficult to locate academic resources that address disability in the Middle East. Upon walking into one of the best Arabic bookstores in Kuwait, I asked the salesman if I could find anything relevant, and he laughed. There was something in my question that unsettled him and made him giggle. I frowned, confused with his reaction. He managed to compose himself, but his initial reaction remained with me for months after.

To consider disability, we cannot ignore gender or race. A disabled individual is not genderless, and personal circumstances are not separated from gender and race. A disabled man living in Kuwait will likely be able to maintain a

social network and lead a fulfilling life. Although he will also be stigmatized and deemed less desirable than an able-bodied man, he will still retain
some of his pride and dignity. For example, marriage is not completely ruled
out. For disabled women, the situation is different. Many disabled women in
the Middle East do not get married, and gender ideology works to oppress
them, leaving them excluded from their communities (Abu-Habib 1997, 20).
Indeed, as Abu-Habib (1997) notes, "disability should be understood as actually reinforcing inequalities between men and women" (21). Disabled women
fail to maintain Middle Eastern society's ideal image of womanhood, and
as such, their quality of life is affected. They are denied basic human needs,
including emotional satisfaction. A dear friend of mine who also has MS,
a thirty-year-old male, has not been through the same prejudice I have encountered. His issues were different, centering on his ability to have satisfying
sexual relations. Marriage for a disabled man is accessible, while for a disabled
woman, it is almost unheard of. Women are expected to reproduce, take care
of children, and carry multiple burdens. If a woman is disabled, her ability
to be a caretaker is questioned. This social stigma further destroys one's self-
image and ability to function in society.

Western culture has more often than not, attached symbolic meanings
to illness and disability. As Wendell (1996) writes, cancer and AIDS have
often been viewed as "cosmic punishment for immorality (AIDS) or for living unhealthy lives (Cancer and AIDS)" (62). These Western assumptions
in some ways parallel Islamic interpretations of disability. For instance, in
Islam, disability is understood as a form of punishment and purification. As
a punishment for committing sins, disabilities are also viewed as having a
"cathartic function by purging the sinner of his sins and bringing him relief
from greater torment in the Hereafter" (Ghaly 2010, 44). Disability, then,
does not afflict good people; it is reserved for immoral ones and strives to
correct, to purify. Such ideology can fuel individual self-hatred and guilt as it
brands the disabled individual as immoral, dirty, and deserving of pain and
punishment. Following this line of thought, then, I have brought this onto
myself. Wendell (1996) explains:

> Most people are deeply reluctant to believe that bad things happen to
> people who do not deserve them, or seek them, or risk them, or fail to
> take care of themselves. To believe this as a general proposition is to
> acknowledge the fragility of one's own life; to realize it in relation to
> someone one knows is to become acutely aware of one's own vulner-
> ability. (107)

Instead of accepting the randomness of illness/disability, societies across different continents and cultures try to rationalize and make sense of a sometimes nonsensical affliction. Should one be grateful for the disability since it supposedly purifies the soul and saves you from "greater torment in the Hereafter," as Ghaly (2010, 44) puts it? Islamic thought says that a good Muslim ought to thank God for everything, be it a blessing or a curse: one is not to question Allah's choices. Such restricting ideologies further silence minorities, women, and individuals with disabilities. I found no consolation anywhere. Society and religion marked me as the "Other," almost invisible, and these societal oppressions led me to immerse myself in education and the pursuit of an academic career.

In Bedouin culture, the body is closely associated to shame and honor. The body is to be hidden, purified, it is both sacred and a burden. A very crucial and significant concept in Bedouin culture is *Hasham*. It connotes several meanings, but mainly it suggests maintaining honor, modesty, shyness, and being "good" overall. It can also simultaneously be tied to shame:

> *Hasham* as the experience of shame arises in interpersonal interactions between social unequals or strangers; it is conceptualized in the idiom of exposure and manifests itself through a language of formality, self-effacement, and the cloaking of the natural weaknesses or sources of dependency, which includes anything having to do with bodily needs, sexuality, and so forth. (Abu-Lughod 1999, 234)

Following Abu-Lughod's argument, I argue that *hasham* is tied to disability and illness. To be ill and/or disabled is to lack *hasham*, to be lacking in ideal womanhood. Because "honor is attained through embodying the cultural ideals" (Abu-Lughod 1999, 130), then illness and disability conjure images of lack and shame, and they corrupt the ideal image that the tribe attempts to maintain, thus threatening its honor.

Ahmed aptly notes that "Family love may be conditional upon how one lives one's life in relation to social ideals. . . . Shame secures the form of the family by assigning to those who have failed its form the origin of bad feeling ('You have brought shame on the family')" (2004, 107). Shame, in Ahmed's formulation, functions like *hasham*: both control and regulate the individual's body and social position. Coming out with a disability affects both the individual and the family. Another important concept in Bedouin culture and ideology is *asil*. *Asil* is an important concept that determines one's lineage and purity of origin, and it determines one's social class and tribal affiliation. While my Bedouin origins were considered noble, my other Palestinian half marked me as the product of a deviant or taboo marriage. Both of my parents had chosen to marry someone outside of their familial and social circle. My father, specifically, had committed a huge transgression: marrying a non-Bedouin, a Palestinian city-dweller, or *hadar*. It is no surprise then, that their children were not embraced socially. When MS came into the picture, the presence of illness within the family further ostracized my immediate family. I was urged to keep my disability hidden and not admit to it when asked by family members or friends what was "wrong" with me while continuing to pass.

I still alternate between periods of disabled visibility and invisibility, between inclusion and exclusion, and I have come to terms with this always hybridized state of being. My body and my identity have both claimed me as a hybrid, always both inside and outside the margins, always speaking multiple languages of existence. My focus on Disability Studies as a scholar is one way I am claiming my identity as a disabled academic who is affected by MS but who, nevertheless, is not fully disabled. I find myself occupying different spaces and attempting to "come out" with my identity by speaking and verbalizing my experience within my body and within academia. I am writing to negotiate what my hybridized body as an academic could possibly mean. It is a constant struggle, a continuous attempt to develop new understandings and meanings of how I present myself to the world and how I am perceived in the academic (as well as the public) sphere.

References

Abu-Habib, Lina. 1997. *Gender and Disability: Women's Experiences in the Middle East*. UK: Oxfam.

Abu-Lughod, Lila. 1999. *Veiled Sentiments: Honor and Poetry in a Bedouin Society*. Berkeley: University of California Press.

Ahmed, Sara. 2004. *The Cultural Politics of Emotion*. New York: Routledge.

Brune, Jeffrey A. and Daniel J. Wilson. "Introduction." *Disability and Passing: Blurring the Lines of Identity*, edited by Jeffrey A. Brune and Daniel J. Wilson. Philadelphia: Temple University Press, 1–12.

Carey, Alison C. 2013. "Sociopolitical Contexts of Passing and Intellectual Disability." *Disability and Passing: Blurring the Lines of Identity*, edited by Jeffrey Brune and Daniel J. Wilson. Philadelphia: Temple University Press: 142–66.

Frank, Arthur W. 1997. *The Wounded Storyteller: Body, Illness, and Ethics*. Chicago: University of Chicago Press.

Ghaly, Mohammed. 2010. *Islam and Disability: Perspectives in Theory and Jurisprudence*. New York: Routledge.

Mairs, Nancy. 1996. *Carnal Acts: Essays*. Boston: Beacon.

McRuer, Robert. 2006. C*rip Theory: Cultural Signs of Queerness and Disability*. New York: New York University Press.

Siebers, Tobin. 2008. *Disability Theory*. Ann Arbor: University of Michigan Press.

Wilson, Daniel J. 2013. "Passing in the Shadow of FDR." *Disability and Passing: Blurring the Lines of Identity*, edited by Jeffrey Brune and Daniel J. Wilson. Philadelphia: Temple University Press, 13–35.

Wendell, Susan. 1996. *The Rejected Body: Feminist Philosophical Reflections on Disability*. New York: Routledge.

Perceptions of Disability
on a Post-Secondary Campus

Implications for Oppression and Human Love

EDUARDO BARRAGAN

EMILY A. NUSBAUM

The research described here explored how disability was understood and perceived on a public university campus in California. A survey of questions related to disability in the public space of the university was distributed online. A subset of responses to the question "what is your perception of disability at this university?" from those who self-identified as being disabled were analyzed using methods consistent with grounded theory (Charmaz 2006; Strauss and Corbin 1990). Findings indicated an array of conceptual categories, all of which were linked to both internal and external forms of oppression, thus showing that disability perception and forms of oppression were intimately connected. Following the inductive analysis, data were further interpreted utilizing Fromm's (1956) writings on the art of loving and his description of the human need to love and be loved. According to Fromm, disowning, oppressing, detaching or any other means of separating from oneself represents an inability to totally and genuinely love oneself and others. Rejecting a part of one's lived experiences, a central part of one's identity, is to reject the existence and make-up of oneself.

This essay highlights the potential impact of disability perception and forms of oppression on respondents' sense of self and, more specifically, their ability to self-love and love others. To deepen these insights, and consistent with constructivist grounded theory methodology (Charmaz 2003, 2006), one of the researchers presents personal reflections on the research process and how these analytic categories were reflected in his lived experience to demonstrate how his experiences on campus reinforced and legitimized the internalized oppression accumulated through his life.

Fromm and "The Art of Loving"

As Fromm (1956), psychoanalyst and social philosopher, explains in his book *The Art of Loving*, humans have the unique gift of reason. People have the ability to reason beyond oneself and become fully aware of their time and surroundings, of their own entity as a human being, separated from others and nature. Fromm describes this as the ability to become aware "of the fact that without his will he is born and against his will he will die, that he will die before those whom he loves, or they before him, the awareness of his aloneness and separateness, of his helplessness before the forces of nature and of society" (1956, 8). This unique gift of reason can also represent a source of great distress. According to Fromm, to experience this profound human disunity and separation with life, humans, and nature is to live a life of imprisonment: "Being separate means being cut off, without any capacity to use my human powers . . . to be helpless, unable to grasp the world—things and people—actively, it means that the world can invade me without my ability to react" (1956, 8). Furthermore, this sense of imprisonment can culminate in feelings of guilt and shame. This is the kind of prison-life that everyone attempts to escape on a daily basis by connecting and bonding with the outside world. As a consequence, Fromm suggests that humans will pay whatever price necessary to escape this imprisonment. We can identify examples of this sense of terror and prison-life, for example, when a family disowns a child. To the child, not being united with the outside world (her/his family is the world) means s/he is left helpless and separated cut off from everything and everyone. The ultimate solution to this state of anxiety and imprisonment lies in the ability to love.

Cultivating such an art of loving, according to Fromm (1956), like any other art, requires discipline, concentration, and patience. The different forms of love Fromm identifies all require care, responsibility, respect, and knowledge. On practicing the art of love he wrote, "love, being dependent on the relative absence of narcissism, it requires the development of humility, objectivity, and reason" (1956, 111). This means that we need to be objective with other people and acknowledge the other person's reality without any distortions of that person's reality and behaviors. This requires putting aside one's interests, needs, and fears. Mastering the art of love requires rational faith—to have a firm faith in oneself and in others, as well as in the potentialities of what one can hope to be and achieve for self and for others. Thus, Fromm's work would lead us to the need to learn the art of love that is rooted in the genuine blending of human souls.

In contrast to the art of love that Fromm describes, in our modern world, one could argue that the culture of love mirrors that of the culture of buying items in the market. Fromm noted that "love develops usually only with regard to such human commodities as are within reach of one's own possibilities for exchange . . . human love relations follow the same pattern of exchange which govern the commodity and the labor market" (1956, 3–4). An object has as much value as the value that the majority of the people place on it. As things in the market world go down or up in price depending on the demand at hand, similarly, the value of individual qualities that are deemed "valuable" go up or down. The market world of love thus has a self-determined understanding of what success must look like, of what worth must look like, of what beauty must look like, and of what love must look like. If a person is determined by the market world to have little or no value, then they are out of the market world, disposed and forgotten as if they were merely an object with no innate worth or purpose. The market world of love has no space for the human soul. Too often, people are not pursuing the art of love; rather, they are after the buying of love—obsessively preoccupied with being loved—at the expense of ever finding the kind of unity with oneself and the outside world that would liberate them from imprisonment.

The portrayal of love that Fromm offers describes the ultimate concern and drive of humankind—the hunger for human love and unity in a broken world. Faced with a desperate need for love (versus genuine love), reason gets distorted and so does love. People become lost and trapped, and they do not cultivate the innate capacity to love that is in every human being. In turn, they unconsciously foster hate, neglect, and indifference. This leads to an unending cycle of oppression—both by oppressors (those who determine "value" in the market world of love) and within those who are oppressed because they do not possess valued qualities. People with disabilities have historically been marginalized because of the devalued status of their embodied experience in the world. Further, in order to love and be loved completely, one needs to accept oneself and others in entirety; one cannot actively love the self or others if certain qualities about the person are denied, rejected, and devalued by others.

Students with disabilities on a college campus are not exempt from this reality. The research reported here shows that student respondents who self-identify as disabled on one college campus experience that their lives are surrounded by a transparent, yet fierce, bubble of external and internal oppression that can be difficult to detect but almost impossible to eradicate. More so, according to this analysis, perceptions of disability shared by participants indicate both external and internal oppression in the form of detachment and disowning of one's own and others' disabilities. Rejecting parts of one's embodied self and lived experience, both central to an individual's identity, make the attainment of love (from the self and others) almost impossible, according to Fromm. And without love from the self and others, a person experiences a life of anxiety, aloneness, and disconnectedness—what Fromm refers to as a *state of existential crisis.*

Surveying Perceptions of Disability on Campus

The original purpose of this research was to capture the atmosphere around disability-related issues at one university using an open-ended online survey. At the time this research was conducted, the second author (Nusbaum), a non-disabled white woman, was a new assistant professor on the campus where the first author (Barragan), a disabled Latino man, was a graduate student in rehabilitation counseling. Our motivation was the revival of a defunct, disabled students' campus group, and thus, we wanted to gain a sense of the presence of disability on campus and its impact on student life. We believed that our analysis would bring disability visibility to campus, provide voice around disability-related discrimination and disability perception, and provide opportunities for further research.

Participants received an electronic email stating the purpose of the survey, confidentiality protections, estimated time completion, and the survey link. Flyers about how to complete the survey were also distributed on campus and posted on several buildings. Four of the seven colleges on campus sent out emails through their listservs. Participants completed the survey instrument via Survey Gizmo. The survey questions focused on disability perception, disability-related discrimination, on-campus participation, possible interest in joining a disabled students' campus group, and peer mentoring.[1]

For this essay, we focused on responses to the question "what is your perception of disability at this university?" from participants who self-identified as disabled. Of 418 total respondents, 64 self-identified as disabled. These 64 respondents also identified as Caucasian (42 percent), Hispanic (23 percent), other/multiracial (11 percent), and Native American/Alaska Native (2 percent). The majority (67 percent) were female and the rest (33 percent) were male. In terms of education level, 55 percent were undergraduates, 44 percent were graduates, and 2 percent were prospective students. Data analysis consistent with a grounded theory approach was used. Analytic categories and concept development gradually evolved from the data through an iterative process of coding and movement between codes and data with attention to premises of credibility, dependability, and trustworthiness, all indicators of rigor and transparency in qualitative research (Strauss and Corbin 1990; Glesne 2006; Charmaz 2006).

The analytic categories that first emerged illuminated how respondents who identified as disabled perceived disability on campus: external attitudes, internalized attitudes, deviance, impairment, obstacle, special, natural characteristic, and description. Concepts and relationships developed through a second level of axial coding (Strauss and Corbin 1990) pointed to oppression, physical and social inaccessibility, deviance and loss, detachment, turmoil with the divine, and natural. These concepts were then related to Fromm's writing about self-love and love of others in the stage of selective coding (Strauss and Corbin 1990). We considered the barriers to these authentic forms of love within our analytic categories, as well as evidence of what could facilitate the attainment of authentic self/brotherly love.

The First Author's Role as Researcher and Reluctant Participant

EDUARDO: *Identifying as a person with a disability, as a student with a disability, was the primary lens that guided my research work. I went through most of my school years at (the university where data were collected) feeling invisible and excluded in the classroom, in the cafeteria, and in the events held on campus. My school activity consisted mostly of going to class and heading back home. I did not fit anywhere or so I felt. It hurt deeply to see my limited life reflected by my other peers with disabilities. I ached seeing some of them alone disconnected from both disabled and non-disabled students. It was distinctively sad to see that there was not any acknowledgment, any bond among disabled students. We all had a common experience, yet it felt as if that common experience only pushed us more apart from each other instead of uniting us. I found it more shocking once I dived into the survey, getting pulled in deep into the experiences of these students with disabilities. In analyzing the data gathered from the survey, I felt conflicted and uneasy.*

I found myself detaching from the respondents. It felt, in looking at the data, as if I were wearing an "objective" lens, an outside lens that made me appear, or perhaps wanting, to have no personal connection with the content of the responses. I had even thought that the data I was analyzing was from those respondents who self-identified as not having a disability. Feelings of shock and confusion settled in as I realized that the responses were in fact from the respondents with disabilities. I could not help but to feel empathy and sadness toward myself and the respondents—and, at the same time, anger at the way disabled people have been victims of an indifferent society. Reflecting on my lived experiences, I wonder if I may have detached from the data because the voices and perceptions of some of the respondents required that I relive some of my own, deep internal struggles, thoughts, and feelings surrounding my disability and being in the world.

Considering how intimate I became with this research and the voices of these respondents, I decided to incorporate my own experiences in relation to the contextual analysis. At a personal level, this was a moment to take back my dignity as a person and with a disability, which was taken from me at a very young age. This process helped re-shape my understanding of myself, my peers, and the very concept of disability. Via my work as a researcher, I ventured into a journey of self-determining and self-redefining.

Analysis

The remainder of this manuscript presents concepts that emerged through our multistage analysis. Each subsection includes a summary of the findings, illustrative quotes from the participants in the research, and then personal reflections in italics from the first author that deepen the analytic concept by discussing how it resonates with him.

Inaccessible Physical Spaces

External separation from physical environments on campus mediated respondents' perception of disability. These environments included campus buildings and classrooms, as well as course materials and pedagogical methods used in classes. This is evident in statements such as: "My perception of disability is not being able to focus on school work or lectures because the way that the materials are presented to me is not the way that I can access them most effectively." Other respondents used words such as "should" to describe the use of the physical space on the campus and a belief that disabled students "should have the same opportunities" to access campus spaces as non-disabled students. Another respondent moved issues of inaccessibility from physical spaces to the disabled individual by stating that "certain citizens, due to a physical or mental limitation, require intervention on their behalf . . . to be in environments." Each of these responses points to real issues the disabled students on this campus have accessing physical space—and, as importantly, where the "problem" of access issues can be identified (within the space or within the individual).

EDUARDO: *As a disabled Hispanic male, I grew up in physical spaces—my home, community, and society—that were inaccessible and deplorable. I was born and raised in a Catholic family with eight siblings in a small town in Mexico. There were no health, education, or economic resources. During my first 12 years, I did not receive the appropriate medical care that my health condition needed. Dragging myself around the house was my means of mobility because I did not have a wheelchair. My family hardly ever took me outside the house—only every so often to go to church or grandparents' house. I was not permitted to attend school. My home became my world. I was isolated and outcast. It gave me first-hand experience of the deepest forms of external separation and oppression.*

Everything in my home was practically out of my reach or strength, which forced me to depend on others for most of my daily activities (e.g., showering, dressing, eating, etc.). Within my community, buildings appeared even more inaccessible (e.g., schools, churches, neighbor's houses). I immigrated to the U.S. at age 12—this was when I obtained a wheelchair and began school. The environment, though more reachable, was relatively inaccessible. The physical spaces of the classroom served as another barrier in the separation between me and the other students. It was incredibly painful to have to sit within the classroom at a corner in my own distinctive desk away from the rest of the students. Everything from classrooms to restrooms, cafeteria, water fountains, basketball/volleyball courts, and concrete were not designed for my use. It felt as if I did not belong there. I eventually feared venturing outside of my home because I did not want to experience the humiliation of people watching me unsuccessfully navigate my surroundings. Even more damaging to my being was the surrounding social spaces that governed my life.

Inaccessible Social Spaces

We defined social spaces as the attitudes that individuals bring into social interactions—and we see these attitudes as a key element in the accessibility of human relations. These attitudes, shaped by families, histories, cultures, institutions, and opportunities determine the degree of accessibility in social interactions. Social spaces as an additional layer of separation in addition to inaccessible physical spaces were evident in responses that articulated attitudinal barriers: "Everyone should be treated equal . . . disability isn't a barrier but attitudes are," "how different people react to seeing disability is frustrating," and "people who are insensitive and ignorant are the problem." Another respondent noted the intersections of disability with gender and race by indicating the "need for adjustments to live fully within a narrowly defined society designed for and by white able-bodied males." Attitudinal barriers were also attributed to professors, as evidenced by one student's experience with self-disclosure: "Learning disability, it takes me longer to comprehend things the way they're presented, but I don't like letting people and professors know because they look at me like I'm stupid." The barriers disabled students described in social spaces point to the impossibility of genuine social relations free of imposition and stigma within an environment that fails to embrace all individuals as equally deserving and equally human.

EDUARDO: *I grew up in a family, culture, and society that were extremely ignorant of disability or of anything that appeared unfamiliar. I felt pity, rejection, neglect, anger, disgust, disappointment, and ambivalence from my family. Such attitudes and feelings were mirrored within my community—a community that rejected and pitied me, a community that felt repulsed and humiliated by my mere presence. The experience of these social spaces left me voiceless, mindless, and heartless.*

In the Mexican culture, people attach religious, mystical explanations to the "unnatural," to the unknown; I still remember witch doctors approaching my parents believing whole heartedly that they could "cure" me, as if something evil or divine had taken over me. I also had to deal with the notion that the physical body symbolizes personhood/manhood and ability to carry a family—something that I clearly did not possess. In addition, there is a paternalistic view of disability in which people perceived as "sick" are meant to be children forever and to be taken care of until death. Then, to see the societal values of beauty and physical appearance, independence and self-sufficiency, and work and productivity represent a person's sense of worth, pushed me further six feet underground. My disability within these social spaces symbolized pathology, unholiness, and sinfulness. It trapped me in a perpetuated ideology that imprisoned my life needs, wants, and desires.

In the U.S., I had some teachers who treated me with pity and curiosity, assured I was not going to get far in life. But here I was mainstreamed into regular school. The schools I attended in the U.S. lacked resources and adequate education in meeting the needs of people with disabilities (PWD). The only Disabled Students' Program assistance I requested throughout my college years was an accessible desk. I am sure I could have benefited from other assistance, one way or another, but I was used to doing things on my own without any outside help. I also wanted to show myself and everyone else that I was quite capable of achieving things in life just like anybody else. And, I did not want to be stigmatized further by becoming associated with the disability services program (DSP) office. When I first visited the DSP office in college, I felt uncomfortable. The atmosphere was one of both apologetic and superior, as if they were "gods" providing special services to "the poor students who cannot do it on their own." Apologetic in the sense that I felt as if they were doing a pitiful favor to us, students with disabilities, for having such unfortunate and pessimistic lives. Superiority in the sense that I felt as if they were "normal" and functioning people helping those students with disabilities who are unable to take care of themselves, and thus, I felt their feelings of superiority were apparent in their work with me and other students with disabilities who registered with the DSP office for accommodations.

Internalized Oppression

External barriers—those in physical and social spaces—impact internalized oppression in disabled students, which can, in turn, impact the ability to self-love: "I associate pain, embarrassment, and guilt with my disability . . . I am embarrassed by and hide my (disability). This caused me anxiety. And I also feel guilty because many people have much greater disabilities and I feel as though I shouldn't feel disabled." Other respondents similarly described internalized oppression with statements such as "disability is frustrating for the individual with the disability" and disability being about "learning to deal with your limitations."

EDUARDO: *It was existentially painful to see and feel the world revolving while I remained motionless and detached from everyone else. I felt unprotected, unloved, and abandoned by a family, community, culture, and society who regarded me as not part of the human race. I was stripped away of my freedom, responsibility, independence, autonomy, and empowerment to decide what was to become of my life. So I came to learn to be obedient, passive, child-like, and complacent. I had no voice—I could not voice the pain, anger, disappointment, confusion, and loneliness that slowly consumed me. I felt the ultimate rejection—I didn't feel like a human being but just another creature out in the wilderness, deserving nothing more than food and shelter just to keep breathing. A waste of mankind. My innocence, my self-love, my hopes, and my dreams all had been shattered, leaving me wounded, empty, and senseless. I soon become my own oppressor—I passionately hated myself as much as I hated the universe, as much as I hated God. My experience and understanding of disability and myself occurred through the lens of other people.*

Navigating through my surroundings felt like a maze, clueless about where to start and where to end. At a very young age, I developed intense frustration and alienation toward my disability. I blamed all of my misery to the way I was born—deformed and crippled. I had come to believe that my physical condition was the wall that kept me from human life. I was frustrated because I did not know why I had been cursed, what I could possibly have done to deserve this punishment. Later on in my life, my frustration shifted more toward society. After coming to terms that my disability was not the problem but society's intolerance and non-acceptance, I detested the world for its lack of love, respect, and compassion to fellow men. Then I found myself shifting frustration toward myself and my lack of self-love. I could not make sense of why I could not accept, why I could not love myself no matter how hard I tried even when, in my mind, I knew I was just as human as anyone can be. It is frustrating to feel on the verge of self-transcendence only to get sucked back into the black hole. It is a vicious cycle of experiencing disability between my own lens and those of the external world.

Deviance and Loss

Deviance from a norm and a sense of loss were evident in many responses. Throughout many survey responses were statements that described disability as "someone who struggles physically or mentally compared to another person," "disability is something that keeps someone from being able to do certain things the same way the average person does," and "unable to do things other students can." These responses are particularly interesting because they not only articulate deviance from a known norm, but in each case, the respondent moved to using a third-person pronoun, detaching themselves from disability (this will be further taken up in the following section). Also present in responses that articulated deviance were descriptors such as "an ailment that hinders," a condition that "limits one's ability to participate," "hinders a person's ability to function or associate with others," and "creates a disadvantage." Detachment of the self from disability continues to be evident, as respondents discussed "persons" versus themselves.

EDUARDO: *I felt my disability keeping me away from "normal" daily activities that most everyone around me enjoyed. Anger, resentment, and sadness overshadowed my days. My body was the definitive categorical marker that separated me from the rest of the "normal" human bodies. In school (U.S.), I would come across other students with similar physical bodies as mine, which only added to my shame and stigmatization and my pitifully lonely world. This was so because I had intensely internalized and personified the accepted norm of being. Anything differing from what was perceived as desirable (e.g., medical devices, physical appearance) I rejected. Being in a wheelchair, I rolled while everyone else walked. I watched sports while others actually played. I remained seated while others danced and jumped. I starved for companionship while others self-indulged. I day-dreamed while everyone around me achieved. I looked down while everyone looked up. I ached while others laughed. All these experiences defined me. My way of life belonged on the other side of the wall with the rest of my kind.*

I could not make sense of my life; it all seemed so fragmented and disturbing. Back in Mexico, I could not even peek through the front doors. The minute I peeked, people in the block would respond subtly to me as if something monstrous had been unleashed from its cage. Even in college, there was a time when a student coming my way made a detour to avoid crossing my pathway. I came to believe I was not meant to self-actualize. My body was alive but nonfunctional, and it felt dead as if I had been born into an old-aged body. That perceived physical loss came with many other losses, which left me in a state of chronic depression for a long time. In the eyes of those around me, I was not capable of leading the loving, self-sufficient, productive, and fulfilling live that comes with

getting an education, working, dating, marrying, forming a family, and the enjoyment of the many other gifts of life. Society's impressions of disability have been the ultimate human marker that categorized and boxed me in as something distinctively separate from mankind.

Detachment from the Disabled-Self and Disabled Others

The detachment of the self that is evident in respondents' connection between disability and deviance/loss reflects Freire's (1970/2000) and Memmi's (1991) discussions about oppressed groups becoming oppressors of themselves and others. When an individual leads a life disconnected from the self, this same disconnectedness is projected on others of the same group, leading to greater tension within the self and projected onto others. This detachment is reflected in repeated statements about "overcoming" and "conquering" disability within responses. One respondent succinctly reflects self/other detachment: "I think a true disability needs to be accommodated, but there is also something to be said for those of us who are able to overcome these problems without any special requests."

EDUARDO: *For a long time, I had no solid intrapersonal/interpersonal relationships, particularly with disabled individuals. I lived a life absent of congruence, transparence, and genuineness. All of my friends were abled-bodied individuals and rarely, if ever, I related with my disabled group members. In them I saw myself reflected, and I did not want to be reminded of my disability. I felt they would only bring more pity, shame, and disgrace to my existence. I did not want to be seen as one of them because unlike them, or so I thought, I did have feelings and dreams. I oppressively related to other disabled people, devaluing and dehumanizing their way of being. My projection onto others was a reflection of my own being, of my lack of self-love and brotherly love.*

So many times tears streamed down my face wishing my disability would be gone, wishing that somehow I could overcome it and be limitless. But I knew that would only be possible if I was reborn, which was totally out of the question (though in my mind that became a fantasy). Perhaps if I did not relate to other disabled people, I would be treated as not one of them. And when I related to my disabled peers, I thought I was better than them. Throughout most of my education, I refused to rely on accommodations because I wanted to prove to myself and everyone that I was like the rest of the "normal," non-disabled students. It was my thought or hope that this would be a sign of overcoming my disability and limitations. But I still felt and was treated as a disabled student despite my academic achievements. This was devastating. There came a point in my life when I finally realized that I was never going to overcome my disability. I was meant to live with this intoxicating reality. I was stuck with my disabled peers.

Turmoil with the Divine

Rejection of one's self (and disability) is evidence of one kind of oppression. Marking disability as a form of mystical, divine intervention reinforces other, stereotypical notions of disabled individuals possessing supernatural qualities. This was noted in a few responses, such as: "I believe that the word disability should not exist. I have not met one person with a disability who does not demonstrate some above average ability . . . persons with disabilities have perceptions and talents above and beyond others." This response might reflect disability as providing a unique perspective that is foundational to the human experience and that adds to the enrichment of human difference. It may also, however, reflect the making of disability as something to be more understood as the supernatural.

EDUARDO: *Growing up, I came to believe wholeheartedly that disability was a punishment, a curse from God for the wrongdoing my ancestors had caused in a past "life." Though I have grown out of this mentality, sometimes, when my physical and mental pain gets too unbearable, I go back to this divine/demonic feeling. Even my accomplishments I tend to discredit. In spite of my many achievements, I do not hold myself in high regard for how far I have traveled in such short time. My achievements and academic standing defy many of the statistics for Latino, male, disabled immigrants. I cut myself short just like I do with my disabled peers. I used to relate to my group in such a way that I felt they had no potential to achieve things in life. My belief was that they could not engage fully in school, work, socialization, and recreational activities. What for, I thought? They are not able to and probably are not interested. But unlike them, I did desire to learn, get a career, establish relationships, and enjoy leisure time. It hurts deeply, but the reality was that I have been extremely oppressive not only to myself but to my disability community.*

Disability: From the Unnatural to the Natural

It is in human connectedness, as Fromm (1956) claimed, where one finds
wholeness, union, peace, congruence, and purpose. It is the answer to a person's internal aloneness and vulnerability. The ingredient to achieving this
connectedness is love, as described by Fromm, which symbolizes and requires care, responsibility, respect, and knowledge. This kind of love cannot
be achieved without embracing one another in totality and in-depth—to recognize and appreciate another's essence. Disability is deeply connected and
foundational to a person's inner essence. Thus, human connectedness, inner
essence, and disability are intertwined and cannot exist without the others.
In this relationship, disability is a natural and integral part of human life,
foundational to an individual's experience and society. This was reflected in
some respondents, who embraced disability and positioned it as a natural and
needed variation: "it is a way of life, a culture" and "it is a culture that brings
people of all walks of life together." It should be noted that there were few
responses such as these, which demonstrated what is needed for the self and
brotherly-love as described by Fromm.

EDUARDO: *My disability was not at all a piece of my life puzzle. My life
experiences left scars and wounds too painful and deep to mend. Life
with a disability could never be a natural aspect of human life. Something as bad and threatening as disability could not be part of nature.
As I entered the journey of healing, of accepting my disability as part
of an entity, I came in touch with my inner essence. This allowed me
the experiencing of myself and the world in a more transparent and
congruent lens. I am no longer defined solely by my disability, though it
plays a central role in my persona. As I embrace myself in my totality, I
am finding that inner/outer peace and connectedness that fills my heart
with joy and humanity. I have come to find love, comfort, and identity
within the disability community. I am blending in with the world in
such ways that every new experience, every instance of being transforms
me into something bigger than myself. I am in a place of growth and
transformation where the life puzzle without disability does not make
sense. Disability is a more natural and integral part of human life than
I had ever imagined it to be.*

*It has been through my disability that I have discovered the unique-
ness and complexity that lies within the human being. It is a priceless
feeling to witness the outcome of the blending of my own uniqueness*

with the uniqueness of mankind. It is in this blending where the ultimate creation and appreciation of diversity lies. Disability is to humanity as trees are to forest. Much like disability, a tree is not identical to another tree. Every tree is different in form, shade, scent, color, and strength. But it is still a tree. It is still part of the forest. Its essence and purpose is still intact. PWD are still part of the human race. Disability does not make a person less or more of a human. I am still part of the human creation.

Final Thoughts from the First Author

EDUARDO: *Medical and health challenges are much a natural aspect and course of human life just like any other challenges a person faces. It is frightening to be faced with a medical condition or life situation that is unpredictable, uncontrollable, life altering, and life threatening. But that does not make it unnatural. What is natural is to feel the good and the bad that is in life. What is not natural is to suppress realities that we all in one form or another will face. We are not immortal; we are not exempt from life-changing experiences. But we live as if we are immortal, as if nothing eminent can break us, as if we are immune to pain and suffering. What is not natural is for us to distance so much away from those facing life alterations that we lose perspective of the situation and the persons at hand. In reality, we are so terrified of life-altering experiences and the unknown that we choose to run away from acknowledging these experiences even if it means unconsciously oppressing others.*

The way my body is formed is just as natural as any other body, but people try to make it unnatural. I cannot accept the concept of disability because that is not something that is natural in me. Disability is a person-made concept made to justify and rationalize people's inability or struggle to love and unite with those who are made a little different, with those whose life has taken on a different turn. What I have come to fear most is not so much my own medical condition and mortality but people's fears and the ugliness that can come out of it and what that can do to my existence. I fear the years passing, my health deteriorating all while my heart and soul yearns for lost dreams, for companionship, for love. I fear withering away in a bed, in a room alone and forgotten, knowing that I could have offered so much more to life, that I could have made so many more memories.

Discussion and Implications for University Campuses

We acknowledge highly individual experience of lived disability and also that an individual's perceptions about any given phenomena are an accumulation of historical and current experiences. They influence thinking, feeling, behaving, and interacting. In our data, the perceptions of disability, as expressed by students who identify as disabled, were deeply reflective of external and internal forms of oppression—and communicated a sense of anger, rejection, shame, anxiety, and heroism. Understanding this leads to considerations of how the respondents' perceptions are amplified by the ways that disability-related issues are addressed/not addressed on campus. Implications for disabled student support services, disability and classroom climates, and the presence of disability in public spaces on campus should be considered.

The visibility and presence of disability on university campuses is too often relegated to those spaces designed to "respond" to disability (such as DSP offices). These spaces require medicalized "proof" of disability from students and, in turn, require "compliance" with provision of accommodations and supports from faculty. This cycle of proof/compliance limits the ways that students and faculty communicate (communication is initiated based on the letter that a student presents to an instructor—a letter that contains "proof" of their disability and which outlines the provision of supports that an instructor must comply with). This deters more authentic communication (and thus relationship and care) between students and faculty. The relegation of disability on many post-secondary campuses to those academic and curricular areas that are designed to "fix" or remediate disability (departments such as rehabilitation or special education, for example), coupled with the absence of disability from broader diversity efforts on most campuses, limits ways of understanding disability as deficit or pathology that exists within the individual student and prevents critical and intersectional engagement with disability.

There is a very real tension between the lens of compliance described above and the need to enact acceptance, genuine care, and support, as our analysis and the writing of Fromm point to. As such, we believe that this research points to the need for institutions of higher education to more specifically confront and effectively address the manner in which disability is responded to in academic and social contexts, as well as represented in curriculum and in other campus spaces.

References

Charmaz, Kathy. 2003. "Grounded Theory: Objectivist and Constructivist Methods." In *Strategies of Qualitative Inquiry*. Eds. Norman K. Denzin & Yvonna S. Lincoln, 2nd ed. London: Sage Publications Limited, 249–91.

Charmaz, Kathy. 2006. *Constructing Grounded Theory: A Practical Guide through Qualitative Analysis*. Thousand Oaks, California: Sage.

Freire, Paulo. 1970/2000. *Pedagogy of the Oppressed*. New York: Bloomsbury.

Fromm, Erich. 1956. *The Art of Loving*. New York: Harper and Row.

Glesne, Corrine. 2006. *Becoming Qualitative Researchers: An Introduction (3rd edition)*. New York: Pearson.

Memmi, Albert. 1991. *The Colonizers and the Colonized*. Boston: Beacon Press.

Strauss, Anselm L. and Juliet M. Corbin. 1990. *Basics of Qualitative Research: Grounded Theory Procedures and Technique*. London: Sage.

Feminism, Disability, and the Democratic Classroom

AMBER KNIGHT

Regardless of the subject matter, the first day of class follows a familiar script. I welcome students to the course, introduce myself, and pass out the syllabus. In those relatively uneventful minutes, however, an extraordinary dynamic always develops. Many students stare at my left hand, or lack thereof. Some students uncomfortably avert their gaze and fixate on the syllabus. Others try so hard not to stare at my "stump" that they smile politely, nod enthusiastically, and appear entirely too interested in information about office hours. Although students' initial responses vary considerably, one thing always seems clear: nobody quite knows what to do about the "deviant" body on display at the front of the room.

Initially, these types of encounters made me self-conscious, and my self-consciousness inhibited my ability to concentrate on the material and develop a rapport with students. In fact, it is still common for me to stutter on the first day of class or occasionally lose my train of thought; it is downright overwhelming to realize that my body is a public spectacle. Over the years, however, I have become more used to this reaction, and I have developed various tactics to navigate the discomfort. In the classroom, as with many other public spaces, my visible disability demands some sort of recognition and explanation. In order to shape my body's narrative and create open interpersonal relationships with my students, I find it necessary to immediately "come out" to them within the first few minutes of class.[1] I answer the question underpinning their stares—"What happened to your hand?"—and say something along the following lines:

I also want to briefly note that I was born without a left hand. I bring this up for a few reasons. First, it relates to my research interests. As a political theorist who is interested in disability studies, my work explores the political nature of disability and the often disabling nature of politics. Second, my impairment impacts your life insofar as I will give you feedback on your written assignments via voice file, instead of writing notes in the margins. I have carpal syndrome from overusing my right hand, so verbal feedback allows me to be more thorough. If you ever have any additional questions about my disability, or my research, please feel free to ask.

The students' reactions are usually anticlimactic. Once I "put it out there," so to speak, we just move on to the next topic. Occasionally a bold and curious student will raise his or her hand to pose a question ("How do you . . . with one hand?"), or offer a comment ("That one-handed pitcher, Jim Abbott, was my favorite baseball player"). But generally, students are satisfied with my brief explanation, and, in turn, I am satisfied with their satisfaction. After coming out, I can confidently turn to the task at hand: empowering students to learn and think for themselves.

I recount this teaching experience in writing because this is ultimately an essay about the instructive power of sharing personal stories. Let's imagine that I candidly discuss my feelings about such first-day-of-class disclosures with students in a disability studies course in order to illustrate how ableism manifests in the daily lives of those with impairments. Given that my students have seen me in my role as a professor and were themselves present on the first day of class, the example may be particularly instructive because it may give them a new vantage point into an experience that we shared. Perhaps some students noticed my nervous behavior on the first day of class, while others could not detect my self-consciousness. Perhaps some students were surprised to see a visibly disabled professor at the front of the classroom, while others found the experience unremarkable. In light of my confession that being in front of a new group of students can make me uncomfortable and slightly impact my behavior, as a group we might consider some of the following questions:

- Whose bodies are disproportionately stigmatized and scrutinized in public space, and why?
- How does social stigmatization impact a person's capacity for self-realization?

- Do you think that the act of disability disclosure was personally empowering? Was it politically subversive? Or, did it reinforce the problematic expectation that bodies marked as "deviant" need to be explained in a way that puts able-bodied people at ease?
- How can we revise social scripts so that interactions between disabled and able-bodied strangers are not strained?
- Is the "coming out" process different for people with invisible disabilities? What is at stake in revealing an invisible disability?

In such a way, then, an accessible discussion about my experience might serve as the entry point into a broader inquiry about how power relations influence even the most commonplace social interactions. What is often required for this kind of discussion to take place, however, is for me to be willing to disclose my experiences and perspectives to my students, many of whom have able-bodied privilege and are largely unfamiliar with disability injustice.

For decades, feminist theorists have extolled the virtues of personal narrative, and one of the central tenets of feminist pedagogy is the idea that teachers and students should disclose lived experiences in the classroom in order to illuminate how "the personal is political." hooks persuasively advances this idea in *Teaching to Transgress: Education as the Practice of Freedom* (1994). In this work, hooks argues in favor of engaged pedagogy, which encourages teaching practices that promote self-actualization and holistic well-being (13). According to hooks, engaged pedagogy intends to "educate for critical consciousness," which requires that professors approach education in a way that empowers students to draw connections between the course material and their everyday lives, think for themselves, find their "voices," and make progressive social change. Ultimately, as hooks (1994) envisions it, teaching is a political practice: it is a practice that can either reinforce the status quo, or it can promote multiculturalism, validate experiential knowledge, and emancipate students from an oppressive educational system that rewards obedience and conformity (36).

Critical to hooks's (1994) views on engaged pedagogy is her emphasis on the concept of vulnerability. I will argue that her treatment of vulnerability, among other things, distinguishes her work within the literature on feminist pedagogy, where much attention has been given to how professors should go about establishing authority in accordance with feminist principles.[2] Vulnerability is a multidimensional concept, with multiple meanings. For compelling reasons, feminists have predominantly depicted vulnerability as a forced, and undesirable, state of being. Under patriarchy, women, as a group, have disproportionately been *made vulnerable* to unjust practices and conditions—such as sexual violence, domestic abuse, and poverty. Thus, it is hardly surprising that those seeking to empower members of historically marginalized groups, in the classroom and elsewhere, have rarely discussed vulnerability as a virtue.

While hooks would undoubtedly find the above examples of structural *forced* vulnerability objectionable, she nevertheless encourages feminist educators to *choose* to make themselves vulnerable in the classroom. In her discussion of why students and professors should disclose lived experiences in relation to the course material, she writes,

> Any classroom that employs a holistic model of learning will also be a place where teachers grow, and are empowered by the process. That empowerment cannot happen if we refuse to be *vulnerable* while encouraging students to take risks. Professors who expect students to share confessional narratives but who are themselves unwilling to share are exercising power in a manner that could be coercive. In my classrooms, I do not expect students to take any risks that I would not take, to share in any way that I would not. . . . It is often productive if professors take the first risk, linking confessional narratives to academic discussions so as to show how experience can illuminate and enhance our understanding of academic material. But most professors must practice being *vulnerable* in the classroom, being wholly present in mind, body, and spirit. (1994, 21, emphases added)

For hooks, being vulnerable in the classroom primarily requires professors to acknowledge that they are whole, embodied, subjective persons, with particular histories and identities. Such an acknowledgment challenges bourgeois educational structures committed to the public/private distinction, a rigid mind/body split, and the attendant assumption that good professors are basically free-floating objective minds, emptied of their experiences and biases (1994, 16–17).

In choosing to acknowledge one's subjectivity, nonconformist intellectuals make themselves vulnerable to backlash from individuals and institutions that have a stake in the norms of neutrality and objectivity. Many people—including students—associate neutrality and personal detachment with fairness and epistemological legitimacy. The misguided assumption that education is, or can be, perfectly neutral makes it likely that professors who go against the grain to disclose personal experiences, feelings, and perspectives in the classroom will face criticisms for not giving objective consideration to the course material. As we can see, therefore, the choice to be vulnerable involves a willingness to take risks. In hooks's words: "The choice to work against the grain, to challenge the status quo, often has negative consequences" (1994, 203).

Disability studies scholars and instructors can usefully engage bell hooks and other proponents of feminist pedagogy in our classrooms. If we envision teaching itself as a value-laden political practice, then disability disclosure itself becomes an act of political resistance. When we disclose our disabilities, when we publicly acknowledge the particularities of our bodies, we make ourselves vulnerable to backlash. Those who resist and subvert conventional practices may encounter personal and professional challenges. Personally, many professors may be reluctant to share intimate information for fear that students will know too much about them. This can be uncomfortable for those with a deep sense of privacy, and some professors may worry that it will undermine their professionalism in the classroom. In addition, many personal experiences—especially those dealing with disability discrimination and social mistreatment—are painful, and people may have reservations about publically expressing emotions such as anger, sadness, and embarrassment. Similarly, it is nerve-wracking to anticipate how an audience will receive personal narrative: Will they pity you, relate to you, take you seriously, connect your experience to the course material, etc.?[3]

There are professional risks, as well. Many impairments are highly stigmatized, so some people may have legitimate concerns about employment discrimination if they publicly reveal their conditions (for example, those who are HIV-positive, or those who have psycho-emotional impairments or mental illnesses), and these concerns can be intensified for faculty members who are multiply minoritized by race, gender, sexuality, class, or employment status (see Kaul, this volume; Pickens, this volume). In addition, professors teaching courses in disability studies may worry that the turn towards personal narrative will undermine its legitimacy as a "real" and rigorous academic department.

Ultimately, this essay makes the case that vulnerability can be a pedagogical resource, one that is necessary for disability disclosure to be effective. In what follows, I candidly confront some risks around classroom disclosure and propose some ways to mitigate backlash as I invite teachers to practice being vulnerable in the classroom. Drawing from feminist and disability theorists' formulations on pedagogy and epistemology, as well as anonymous feedback from students in a course that I taught on disability theory,[4] I argue that disability disclosure has the potential to: (1) personally empower professors and students alike; (2) enrich course material and provide fertile ground for knowledge production; (3) reveal intra-group differences among people with disabilities as an identity-based group; and, (4) teach students how to communicate across social differences.

Although the central aim of this chapter is to illustrate the emancipatory potential of embracing vulnerability in the classroom, it is important, too, to acknowledge how teachers' social location (i.e., race, gender, sexual orientation) and institutional position (i.e., tenured, graduate student, tenure-track, contingent) influences one's ability to take risks, how the act of disclosure is received by others, and the subsequent likelihood that one will experience significant backlash from students, colleagues, and administrators. Put simply, in a context of social inequality, the risks of disability disclosure are experienced differently (see Samuels, this volume). For instance, as a white, middle-class, cisgender, and heterosexual faculty member teaching among a predominantly white and middle-class student body, I am positioned vis-à-vis disability disclosure in some privileged ways that may not be as readily available or promising to others. For example, even if students were to "punish" me for my somewhat unorthodox teaching methods (e.g., with negative student evaluations), I do not fear losing my job as a result. Hence, the experiences and suggestions that I share here are not intended as a "one size fits all" formula for faculty members' classroom disclosures. Rather, these experiences and suggestions are meant to engage readers in thinking about some possibilities around disclosure as they consider their own classroom practices.

Personal Empowerment

When professors are vulnerable and open enough to share personal experiences, the process of storytelling has the potential to transform instructors and students alike. Of course, I am not the first person to point this out. With respect to personal empowerment, Mossman (2002), a white male English professor, discusses some of his life experiences as a single-leg amputee and provides a powerful example of the first time he wore shorts to class (at the end of a semester), thereby publicly revealing his "disfigurement" to his class. He describes the interaction as follows:

> As I stood before the class that day my disfigurement was no longer hidden by the desk or with pants. . . . I felt their [the students'] confu-

sion and their embarrassment at feeling confused. . . . Difference, abnormality: this was what was being constructed upon me, around me,
through me, and of course I did not necessarily want that construction
to take place; I did not want to be a super-crip, to be heroic or brave
for simply being the professor at the front of the room, for doing my
"normal" job with my "abnormal" body. I needed to take control of my
body, to share in its story, in its social meaning. And so I told a story. I
told the class . . . how my body came to be as it is now . . . the complicated medical history of it. The class listened; I remember saying that
it was all "no big deal." (654–55)

Upon reflection, Mossman argues that through the act of disclosure he was
ultimately able to negotiate difference and normality, claim and achieve inclusion and recognition as "normal," and also undermine disability stereotypes. As
he put it, "[M]y body, when it is placed in situations like that one, demonstrates
that physical abnormality does not equal powerlessness and helplessness, or
heroism and bravery, or anything else necessarily, but rather that disability
equals normality and sameness" (2002, 655). In the end, Mossman's public disclosure of his impairment seemed to provide him a great deal of personal relief,
perhaps because he was freed of the obligation to conform to the pressures of
"compulsory able-bodiedness" (McRuer 2006, 10). Once he no longer had to
keep his physical impairment hidden, he could be himself in class.[5]

Other scholars have focused on the ways in which a professor's decision
to disclose her or his disability affects disabled students' sense of self and their
opportunities to develop mentoring relationships with professors. Kornasky
(2009) describes how her decision to reveal her hearing impairment impacted
her students. As a white woman who has both passed as nondisabled and
openly disclosed her invisible impairment, she writes,

In just the first couple of academic years out of the "able-bodied" closet,
I was approached by more than a dozen students . . . who told me about
their own invisible disabilities and sought me out as an academic mentor. I noticed that students with both visible and invisible disabilities
exhibited a different attitude toward me and about their own identities. . . . These students with disabilities to whom I had disclosed my
disability were more self-assured than my students with disabilities had
been with me when I had passed as nondisabled. They participated more
freely in class discussions and asked more readily and with less self-
consciousness for appropriate disability accommodations.

Kornasky's analysis places students front and center. Professors may shy away from disability disclosure due to uncertainty or fear about potential negative repercussions. However, passing can also deny students with disabilities the opportunity to see people with disabilities succeed in academia. To that end, one of the students from my undergraduate Disability Theory course—who identified as having a learning disability—talked about how the practice of disability disclosure enabled connections between classmates and the professor. Moreover, according to the student, the use of personal narrative "made class feel like I was a part of something," and that they were "not just in class to get a grade."

Yet, despite these examples of disability disclosure leading to personal empowerment and community-building, there is of course no guarantee that empowerment will follow afterwards. It is simply impossible to control how one's story will be received. One semester, I shared a story about being in an extreme state of dependency after surgery on my only hand. My point was to illustrate that human beings live in webs of interdependence and are not as fully independent and self-sufficient as liberal philosophy might suggest. My students, instead, focused intently on the aspect of how my husband tenderly provided care for me, and almost simultaneously let out a collective "Awwww . . . how sweet!" that made me blush. When teachers share personal experiences, they really are putting themselves out there, so to speak. The outcomes of disclosure are unpredictable, and in making them, then, teachers have to cede some measure of control and remain open to the unbidden.

Perhaps one way to mitigate the vulnerabilities that arise from sharing confessional narratives is to establish clear guidelines for confidentiality in class discussions. Many feminist instructors use the initial class session for students to establish collaborative "ground rules" for discussion. One standard rule is that "what we say in here stays in here" so that the classroom is a safe place to talk openly. Instructors with disabilities might adopt this practice and delineate the limits of confidentiality *before* anyone divulges personal information. Such a commitment to confidentiality can then make it possible for people to share disability experiences. As obvious as it may sound, it is also important that instructors and classmates listen actively and attentively to those who choose to disclose their impairments, without interruption. A person cannot possibly feel empowered if their audience does not respectfully take them seriously.

In this vein, "trigger warnings" can be good teaching practices.[6] Occasionally, when teachers and students share stories and life experiences, it can have the unintended consequence of causing mental and emotional distress for those who have experienced similar trauma or social mistreatment. For example, I have been through several painful and stressful surgeries, and when we engage in lengthy class discussions about people with disabilities and their relationship to medical institutions, I occasionally find myself in a tailspin recalling the fear and anxiety that I felt going into the procedures and recovering from them. While I do not want to discourage open and honest communication about difficult and controversial topics, it may be necessary to publicly acknowledge the gravity of some issues, and remind students of ways to practice self-care and let their professors know how they can support them as they navigate such difficult terrain.

Knowledge Production

Beyond contributing to personal empowerment, disability disclosure can enhance and illuminate academic material in several ways. First, disclosure can complement academic research when teachers with disabilities draw from their reservoir of experiences to add a human dimension to abstract concepts. For example, when my undergraduate Disability Theory course discussed disability discrimination within medical institutions, I candidly discussed how doctors exhibited patronizing attitudes toward me when I brought up my plans to start a family ("How do you plan to properly care for a baby with your condition?"). I also talked openly about childhood bullying; the joys of feeling like a part of a vibrant disability culture; how pervasive disability stereotypes impact my sense of self; and the unearned social privileges that I have as a white, middle-class person living with a disability in an advanced industrialized society. When asked to reflect on how sharing and listening to personal narratives impacted their understanding of the course material, one student responded,

> I enjoyed when my classmates and instructor shared their experiences as it pertained to the course material. While listening to others, I can better understand what people go through when they are faced with disability and/or impairment on a daily basis. Hearing other people explain what they have witnessed, lived through, or watched a loved one face gave feeling and emotion to the class and allowed me to have a better understanding of the classroom readings.

Another student added,

> I feel that the personal stories shared by the professor and other students added an element of humanity and realism to the often abstract material in the course. This is because our discussions often directly linked the two and fully explored how real life and the material came together.

Hence, personal experiences can be strategically employed to illuminate and critically analyze the class readings in ways that other resources, including historical facts, statistics, and political and social theories cannot accomplish alone.

 My classes encourage students to think about themselves as junior scholars who are capable of generating their own theories. After all, instructors of record are not the only teachers in the classroom. Students from different walks of life can bring the wisdom of their lived experiences to bear on class discussions, as has long been advocated by feminist proponents of standpoint epistemology (Collins 2000). Standpoint theory holds that all knowledge is constructed in a specific matrix of physical location, history, culture, and interests. For instance, Collins (2000) advocates for the creation of a Black women's standpoint since historically "racial segregation in housing, education, and employment fostered group commonalities that encouraged the formation of a group-based, collective standpoint" (24). Like Collins, I believe that collective dialogue allows people to decipher patterned, structural social phenomena. Further, I see the classroom as a space where instructors and students with disabilities alike can explore and determine the shared conditions in their lives. Although the group "people with disabilities" is diverse—and identities are fluid, plural, and open to revision and contestation—the creation of some shared disability perspectives may be necessary for identity politics to flourish. Thinking about the emancipatory potential of education, bell hooks recognizes the relationship between personal disclosure, standpoint epistemology, and identity politics. In her words,

> Identity politics emerges out of the struggles of oppressed or exploited groups to have a standpoint on which to critique dominant structures, a position that gives purpose and meaning to struggles. Critical pedagogies of liberation respond to these concerns and necessarily embrace experience, confessions and testimony as relevant ways of knowing, as important, vital dimensions of any learning process. (1994, 89)

While people with disabilities do not all share the same experiences, many have been subject to state-mandated institutionalization, encountered discrimination in zoning in public housing, faced limitations on the right to marry and have children, experienced disenfranchisement and exclusion from schools, and more. If we begin from the assumption that all knowledge is constructed in a specific matrix of physical location, history, culture, and interests, therefore, disability disclosure in the classroom can enable people with disabilities to collectively discern how ableism operates and manifests, and how to create strategies for resisting oppression. Likewise, nondisabled students may come to recognize their social privilege and think about what it means to be an ally or take collective responsibility for ableism.

What kinds of hardships might teachers experience when sharing personal experiences in conjunction with the academic subject matter? First, they might experience blowback from unsupportive colleagues. I once heard a colleague say something along the lines of "I'm not into that touchy-feely stuff—I'm a teacher, not a therapist." Other colleagues might not recognize the value of participatory discussion-based learning or be critical because they worry that students lack the skills necessary to facilitate dialogue and manage conflicting perspectives. Finally, I want to acknowledge hooks's contention that "It is not easy to name our pain, to theorize from that location" (1994, 74). Talking openly about injustice can be challenging for those who have been subject to mistreatment, as well as for students who are coming to the realization that they have been unconsciously complicit in structural injustice.

My experience with making disclosures about my disability in the classroom has led me to develop my skill for facilitating productive classroom discussions of difficult topics. For example, I work to keep students focused on connections between personal experiences and course material. I never dismiss them; rather, I see my task as one of helping students forge substantive links between their personal narratives and class material.

Differences within Identity-Based Groups

In addition to encouraging students' interaction with course material, a third potential benefit emerging from making oneself vulnerable through disability disclosure is that of highlighting intra-group differences. While some may be concerned that sharing one's story may run the risk of being "a single story" (Adichie 2009), and should thus be avoided, my experience suggests that personal narratives about one's lived experience do not *neces-*

sarily lead to essentialist thinking. In fact, through conversation with me about my experiences, I hope that students will come to realize that no one facet of our lives is definitive. If I choose to discuss diverse aspects of my personal history, students may understand that my disability does not encapsulate all of me. Moreover, when students report having different lived experiences from each other (or even different interpretations of similar experiences), I can then strategically draw attention to these tensions in an effort to highlight the complex operations of intersectionality.[7] At the most basic level, intersectionality holds that structural social oppressions—such as racism, sexism, heterosexism, classism, and ableism—do not act independently of one another. Rather, these "isms" interrelate, creating a system of oppression that reflects the intersection of multiple forms of discrimination. Thus, shared narratives have the potential to point out that identities are plural, and that a single axis of a person's lived experience cannot be understood in isolation from other salient dimensions.

In order for instructors and students to share personal experience in the classroom without promoting essentialist standpoints, we all must be careful to not overgeneralize from our own particular, situated social positions. In my own stories, then, I sometimes qualify my statements by saying something along the lines of, "I know that my experience and perspective on the issue of X is open to debate, and, in fact, some of the authors we will encounter this semester will contradict and challenge my assertion." One student in my Disability Theory course explicitly acknowledged this tactic in their feedback, writing, "She [the professor] talked about herself, but she was aware that her experience was a part of the larger disability community." I also work to assign readings wherein the central arguments contradict one another in order to dispel the notion that "the disability community" is a monolithic and coherent identity-based group.[8]

Practicing Citizenship

Like hooks, I envision the classroom as a political space, specifically as a microcosm of our wider deliberative democracy. I believe that in courses where students are encouraged to disclose their personal experiences and points of view, they will not only make deeper connections to the substantive course material, but also learn the democratic practice of communicating with others across differences. Being able to adjudicate between competing points of view, including your own, is a skill that is cultivated over time through practice and one that is sorely lacking within American political culture at large. In this way, I suggest that disability disclosure in the classroom does not simply entail the act of sharing one's own experience: it also requires students to actively listen (and listening is not synonymous with hearing) and engage with others.

This vision of democratic deliberation in the classroom is largely informed by the writings of Young (1989; 1997). Young envisions a heterogeneous public where citizens start from their situated positions and attempt to construct a dialogue across differences. Unlike interest group pluralism, which does not require justifying one's interest as compatible with social justice, Young wants citizens to use deliberation to come to decisions that they determine to be more or less just (1989, 267). For Young, social difference is a resource for democratic deliberations because communication across differences leads to expanded understanding and increases the chances that people will transform their position from an initial self-regarding and subjective view to a more broadened understanding of the common good. Unlike political theorists such as Rawls and Habermas, she rejects the idea that we can simply transcend our own particularities and identities in order to think about a political issue from the viewpoint of others. The standpoint of each of us in a particular socio-historical position "makes it impossible to suspend our own positioning" and shed our assumptions when we try to put ourselves in another person's place (1997, 348–49).

In a rare move for most deliberative democrats, Young (1997) explicitly uses the example of disability to support her argument. She examines a survey conducted on behalf of an Oregon Health Plan, which asked able-bodied people to put themselves in the situation of a person with a disability. Because the able-bodied respondents were unable to transcend the particularity of their life experiences, let alone their privilege, the majority of them said that they would "rather be dead" than be wheelchair users or blind. Young notes, however, that the actual statistics of suicide rates among people with disabilities are rather low, and that when you talk with people with disabilities, they usually think their lives are very much worth living. This example bolsters her contention that we cannot adopt another person's viewpoint by simply imagining it. "Generally speaking," she writes, "able-bodied people simply fail to understand the lives and issues of people with disabilities. When asked to put themselves in the position of a person in wheelchair, they do not imagine the point of view of others; rather, they project onto those others their own fears and fantasies about themselves" (1997, 344). Because able-bodied people miss the mark in their estimation of disabled people's lives, Young argues that when those with disabilities are present in deliberations, others can learn to understand important aspects of the social world and make better political decisions. In her words,

> I can listen to a person in a wheelchair explain her feelings about her work, or frustrations she has with transportation access. Her descriptions of her life, and the relation of her physical situation to the social possibilities available to her, will point out aspects of her situation that I would not have thought of without her explanation. In this way I come to an understanding of her point of view. (1997, 355)

Her example suggests that by communicating with people who are open about their lives with disabilities, other citizens are forced to confront their own stigmatized ideas about impairment and also challenge their able-bodied privilege.

Young's democratic theory has had significant implications for my pedagogical practice. Thinking about students as citizens-in-training, I encourage disability disclosure in ways that foster communication across differences since such interactions have the potential to lead to mutual understanding. However, because the outcomes of deliberations cannot be determined in advance, teachers must be vulnerable to the prospect of dealing with conflict and disagreement in the classroom. Some of my colleagues have voiced a deep-seated fear of having to deal with "heated" discussions and disagreements. hooks confronts this fear head-on:

> Fear of losing control in the classroom often leads individual professors to fall into a conventional teaching pattern wherein power is used destructively. It is this fear that leads to collective professorial investment in bourgeois decorum as a means of maintaining a fixed notion of order, of ensuring that the teacher will have absolute authority. Unfortunately, this fear of losing control shapes and informs the professorial pedagogical process to the extent that it acts as a barrier preventing any constructive grappling with issues. (1994, 188)

hooks implies that when instructors forgo open class discussions to avoid potential conflict, they do their students a disservice. Sometimes people have to experience discomfort in order to learn. If students are not given the space and opportunity to challenge one another, they cannot grow.

As mentioned above, such discussions must be shaped and led by instructors to ensure they remain productive rather than harmful, and as fellow participants, instructors can model for students how to talk with those whom they disagree. To establish clear guidelines for civil participation, I include instructions for class discussions in my course syllabi and I reinforce those instructions during contentious class discussions.

When a discussion becomes tense, I often find it helpful to depersonalize the conversation, saying something such as "This conversation reflects wider disagreements within the disability community about whether or not scholars and activists should emphasize or minimize bodily difference." With especially controversial issues that can strike a chord—such as the selective abortion of disabled fetuses—students who feel strongly about the topic at hand can occasionally hijack the discussion. In those relatively rare cases, I usually ask students if we can table the issue and return to the discussion after we have all had some time to reflect on what has already been discussed. Postponing the discussion and allowing students to breathe and collect their thoughts is one way to diffuse tension and ensure a commitment from all participants to the quality of the conversation.

Concluding Remarks

In the end, choosing to embrace an ethos of vulnerability in the classroom by disclosing one's lived experiences with disability is not always easy. It can be emotionally taxing. It can make one susceptible to backlash and criticism. As an unpredictable process, it requires that professors cede some measure of control. Plus, developing the skills necessary to facilitate discussion and channel lived experiences into knowledge production takes a considerable amount of effort and practice. And yet, I argue that in some contexts the rewards outweigh the risks. The classes where I have chosen to be publicly vulnerable have been the most fulfilling and rewarding, albeit the most challenging. In addition, my students have expressed appreciation for my willingness to let them get to know me as a whole person, and to listen to the wisdom that they've gained through their own particular histories. Influenced by bell hooks' commitment to engaged pedagogy, I understand teaching as much more than the depersonalized transmission of objective information. Some version of engaged pedagogy—one that requires us to acknowledge that we are whole, embodied, subjective persons, with particular histories and identities—can generate excitement in the classroom and enable students and teachers to share the joy of learning. ⌋

References

Adichie, Chimamanda Ngozi. 2009. "The Danger of a Single Story." TED talk, accessed August 28, 2015, http://www.ted.com/talks/chimamanda_adichie_the_danger_of_a_single_story?language=en

Berger, Michele Tracy, and Kathleen Guidroz, eds. 2009. *The Intersectional Approach: Transforming the Academy through Race, Class, and Gender.* Chapel Hill: University of North Carolina Press.

Collins, Patricia Hill. 2000. *Black Feminist Thought: Knowledge, Consciousness, and the Politics of Empowerment, Second Edition.* New York and London: Routledge.

Freeman, Elizabeth, et al. 2014. "Trigger Warnings Are Flawed." *Inside Higher Ed.* (May 29), https://www.insidehighered.com/views/2014/05/29/essay-faculty-members-about-why-they-will-not-use-trigger-warnings

Garland-Thomson, Rosemarie. 1997. *Extraordinary Bodies: Figuring Physical Disability in American Culture and Literature.* New York: Columbia University Press.

hooks, bell. 1994. *Teaching to Transgress: Education as the Practice of Freedom.* New York: Routledge.

Johnston, Angus. 2014. "Why I'll Add a Trigger Warning." *Inside Higher Ed.* (May 29), https://www.insidehighered.com/views/2014/05/29/essay-why-professor-adding-trigger-warning-his-syllabus#sthash.3AiFHg3f.dpbs

Kaul, Kate. This volume.

Kerschbaum, Stephanie. 2014. "On Rhetorical Agency and Disclosing Disability in Academic Writing." *Rhetoric Review* 33 (1): 55–71.

Kornasky, Linda. 2009. "Identity Politics and Invisible Disability in the Classroom." *Inside Higher Ed.* (March 17). http://www.insidehighered.com/views/2009/03/17/kornasky

Luke, Carmen. 1996. "Feminist Pedagogy Theory: Reflections on Power and Authority." *Educational Theory* 46 (3): 283–302.

McRuer, Robert. 2006. *Crip Theory: Cultural Signs of Queerness and Disability.* New York: New York University Press.

Mossman, Mark, 2002. "Visible Disability in the College Classroom." *College English* 64 (6): 645–59.

O'Toole, Corbett. 2013. "Disclosing Our Relationships to Disabilities: An Invitation for Disability Studies Scholars." *Disability Studies Quarterly* 33 (2).

Pickens, Therí. This volume.

Samuels, Ellen. 2003. "My Body, My Closet: Invisible Disability and the Limits of Coming-Out Discourse." *GLQ: A Journal of Lesbian and Gay Studies* 9 (1–2): 233–55.

Samuels, Ellen. This volume.

Swain, John, and Colin Cameron. 1999. "Unless Otherwise Stated: Discourses of Labelling and Identity in Coming Out." In *Disability Discourse*. Eds. Mairian Corker and Sally French. Philadelphia: Open University Press.

Young, Iris Marion. 1997. "Asymmetrical Reciprocity: On Moral Respect, Wonder, and Enlarged Thought." *Constellations* 3 (3): 340–63.

Young, Iris Marion. 1989. "Polity and Group Difference: A Critique of the Ideal of Universal Citizenship." *Ethics* 99 (2): 250–74.

Rhetorical Disclosures

The Stakes of Disability Identity in Higher Education

TARA WOOD

In college, students often find themselves negotiating varied emergent identities, and in so doing, they face a myriad of expectations: to be a good friend, to be charismatic and respected, to make their family proud, to be a model student, to be successful. While students with disabilities face these same expectations, they must also continually account for ways of knowing, learning, and being in the world that may differ from those of their fellow students. And unlike their previous experiences in high school, college students may be navigating different kinds of choices about how and when to identify as disabled.

Such identifications of disability often come through stories. Disability studies (DS) scholars such as Siebers (2002) have insisted upon the power of narrative for advancing the lives of disabled people. Siebers argues that while many disability scholars have called for moving beyond first-person accounts of disability experience on the grounds that such narratives only invite pity[1] rather than critical examination of the social and political meanings of disability (50), ultimately, "[h]uman beings make lives together by sharing their stories with each other. There is no other way of being together for our kind" (50). Such storying, however, as Williams (2006) asserts, drawing on Hall (1994), is often subject to the narratives of dominant culture. Consequently, when the identity you want to perform does not cohere with the expected dominant narrative, trouble can ensue (Williams 2006, 5). For instance, if a student does not conform to the archetype privileged and maintained as "normal" by the university, "trouble" may manifest through the complex rhetorical management of disability identity.

In listening to the narratives of students with disabilities who are negotiating this rhetorical terrain, there is much to learn about not only disability and access but also rhetorical agency and the intricacies of identity construction. Understanding how students manage their identities and negotiate disability requires in-depth analysis of processes of disclosure as well as the conditions that invite, coerce, or premeditate revelation of disability. Examining the agentive strategies that students employ when faced with choices about whether or not to identify as disabled can help educators productively consider and purposefully co-construct the conditions and contexts in which disclosure takes place.

In tune with Siebers's (2002) insistence on the political power of narrative, then, to examine how students performed such rhetorical work, I designed a qualitative research project that sought to garner perspectives from students with disabilities about writing and accommodations in college classrooms. During the 2012–13 academic year, I conducted semi-structured interviews with thirty-five students with disabilities at a large Midwestern university. My initial study design called for interviews with twenty students with registered disabilities who were currently enrolled at the university and taking composition courses. This sample selection process was purposive, or "based on the assumption that the investigator wants to discover, understand, and gain insight and therefore just select a sample from which the most can be learned" (Merriam 2009, 77). Patton (2002) writes that "the logic and power of purposive sampling lies in selecting *information-rich* cases for study in depth. Information-rich cases are those from which one can learn a great deal about issues of central importance to the purpose of the inquiry, thus the term *purposeful* sampling" (230, emphasis in original). While there are many types of purposive sampling, I used a combination of three types: maximum variation purposive sampling, convenience purposive sampling, and on-going purposive sampling. Glaser and Strauss (1967) first identified maximum variation sampling as ideal for grounded theory research because data could be more grounded with "widely varying instances of the phenomenon" (Merriam 2009, 79). In this case, widely varying meant ensuring that participants had a range of different disabilities. Convenience sampling occurs when researchers base sample selection decisions on issues such as time, money, and/or location. Over the course of the study, my sample size changed: I initially wanted to conduct twenty interviews, but later increased my sample size to thirty-five participants in order to reach a broader range of experiences and perspectives (e.g., electing to interview both students who were and who were not registered with the disability services office).

My recruitment process began in the fall 2012 semester when I approached the director of disability services, asking that she send out my recruitment flyer to an email list of enrolled students registered with campus disability services. During this initial recruitment period, I had numerous responses but only a small handful of interviews. Thus, to increase my study population, I offered participants compensation, and after some resistance from the disability services office around disseminating information about my study, I sent recruitment materials to the entire student body at the university.

Thirty-five students (both undergraduate and graduate) from a wide range of disciplines participated in the study. Their reported disabilities ranged from mental disabilities such as post-traumatic stress disorder (PTSD), bipolar, or obsessive-compulsive disorder to physical disabilities such as Friedreich's Ataxia and Usher Syndrome. Some experienced chronic illnesses such as migraines or HIV, while others reported learning and cognitive disabilities, such as dysgraphia or ADD. Participants' ages ranged from 19–52; nineteen participants were women, while sixteen were men. Fifty-six percent of student participants were white, 21 percent were American Indian, 8 percent were African-American, 8 percent were Asian, and 7 percent were Hispanic. Sixty-three percent were registered with campus disabilities services, 31 percent were not, and 6 percent were registered with state disability rehabilitation services.

I conducted semi-structured interviews, using twenty-four baseline questions with a variety of purposes (ranging from background questions to questions about their values and feelings about writing and accommodations). Most interviews lasted around one hour, and some took over two hours. I audio-recorded the interviews and transcribed them myself shortly after each interview. I began my analysis with a process of "initial coding" (Saldana 2013, 100) to allow trends to emerge as organically as possible and then practiced axial coding as I developed larger categories to arrange the data (209).

The stories and insights shared in my conversations with the participants in this study enable both a purposeful visibility and critical examination of what their experiences may suggest about how disability is positioned in college classrooms. With this analysis, I ask about how and why students disclose and what they gain or lose when they make disclosure choices, and I explore the conditions that shape their decision-making in order to enrich understanding of the rhetorical negotiations of disability identity in higher education. Ultimately, I argue that in order to understand the stakes of disclosure for disabled students, we must listen to and learn from the stories they have to tell.

Disability Identity: Rhetorical Agency, Stigma, and Patterns of Resistance

It's nothing new to point out that a dominant discourse in the experiences of disability identity in higher education (or anywhere, for that matter) is stigma (Goffman 1963). However, a significant critique of the way stigma is often portrayed is that it fails to consider the agency of disabled people, often portraying them as victims of negative perceptions or evaluations (Brune 2014). Yet, the relevance of stigma theories to disability studies remains important because "the study of stigma and empowerment as mutually exclusive" ignores the ways in which the two are deeply intertwined, even "complimentary" (Brune 2014). In their interviews, students conveyed complex orientations toward disability and stigma, and although many of their narratives reflect their experiences with stigmatized identities that are both constructed by and imposed upon them, they also reveal key moments of resistance and rhetorical agency.

Through these students' narratives, it becomes clear that the very notion of disability "self" is widely contested. Stigma emerged in students' discourse as a primary mediating factor in their interactions with others, and many students shared strategies for negotiating stigmatizing social and political structures (that included, but certainly were not limited to, disability). To illustrate how students actively resisted disability stigma, I draw on theories of rhetorical agency forwarded by Kerschbaum (2014) and Cooper (2011). Building on Cooper's (2011) definition of rhetorical agency as "an emergent property of embodied individuals" (421), Kerschbaum suggests that agency should be considered interactionally and as shaped by the readiness and responsivity of particular agents and audiences. While Kerschbaum (2014) focuses primarily on disability *self*-disclosure, it is nevertheless vital to consider the ways that selves are often contested terrain. Collectively, the student narratives shared here reflect diverse approaches to disability identity, including adoption of dominant narratives, embracement of disability identity, and resistance to disability identity. In the following subsections, I share some student narratives, using these examples to suggest that disabled students actively negotiate their disability identities and, further, that the choices they make illuminate an active tension between medical models of disability and embodied experience, the collision of oppressive structural forces, and the

importance of community and connection for cultivating positive identification with disability.

Resistance to Disability Identity

Many of the students who participated in my study resisted identifying with
disability or being defined by their disabilities. Some might interpret this
resistance to disability identity as a desire for the norm, but I believe it may
be more useful to understand that resistance in terms of an active navigation
of the conflicting messages students receive about disability. Consider the
stories Diane and Gavin shared. Diane said that her therapist advised her
against openly advertising her identity as someone with Tourette's, and that
she liked this advice because "Tourette's isn't really me . . . I feel like myself
as a person is more than my disabilities, and I shouldn't be defined by my disabilities." Though Diane disassociated Tourette's from her identity, she also
vividly narrated her way of describing disability and claimed she'd been using
this description from a young age. She explained, "I always notice it. It's like
the best way to describe it is try and keep your eyes open without blinking . . .
if you try and keep your eyes open without blinking, you're gonna eventually
blink and then you look around and you notice, did anyone notice me blink?
It's always there. It's always nagging at me." Although Diane mentioned several times that she doesn't want disability to define her, her metaphor for her
experience with Tourette's nevertheless reflects the profound impact of disability on her embodied experience.

While Diane expressed a desire to be understood as more than her disabilities, Gavin explained that he "combats" and "survives" his disability.
When I asked him if he considered disability to be a large part of his identity,
he told me:

> No, I don't allow it to become a portion of my identity. It's like any-
> thing else in life. It's a problem. It's a problem like, being an engineer,
> you think analytically about things so I'm more of the type of person
> who would rather identify any problem or any bump in my life and
> do my best to overcome that. My identity is not defined by whatever
> diagnosis I've currently been prescribed. I don't allow it to because if
> I did, I'd just be more depressed of a person than I already have been.

Later, however, Gavin expressed complete faith in the diagnoses offered up
to him, saying, "I do trust the doctors . . . they're the ones who are much

more educated and much more intelligent on the subject." This seeming contradiction—resistance to the medical label and complete faith in the expertise of his medical team—illuminates the vicissitudes of disability identity, especially for those students who are experiencing recent or changing diagnoses. The significance of both Diane and Gavin's resistance to disability identity is that they are very much in the (unfolding and unstable) process of interpreting variant rhetorics of disability, and the tensions they express reveal that their conceptions of disability are interactionally constructed.

Just as Gavin and Diane negotiate the various messages they receive about disability, two student-veterans who participated in the study, Chesty and Mike, both expressed the impact of stigma on their educational experiences. Both drew on stigma to explain their decision not to disclose mental disability. Chesty spoke at length about the negative impact of his disabilities. Yet, on campus, all he says about those disabilities is that he has "physical impairments," offering no additional details, and he never discloses his mental disabilities. I asked why he doesn't talk with his instructors about his mental disabilities, and he explained, "The anxiety, I don't want to put them off. I don't want them to be weirded out. I think that with PTSD, veterans have gotten a really bad rap as far as that goes, so I don't want them to be nervous." Mike, another student-veteran, also said that he would disclose some of his physical disabilities but not his mental disabilities, explaining that to do so is "too personal. It's a mental health problem, and I don't want people to look at me like I'm crazy or that I'm subnormal."

Two widely available identity constructions for veterans are the Homeric hero and the ticking time bomb (Weigal and Miller 2011). Weigal and Miller note that the stigma and fear associated with the time bomb can be intensified when paired with traditional notions of masculinity that are heavily engrained in military discourse, while the returning hero is treated as if he should be able to overcome any trauma he experienced. Both Chesty and Mike noted that the ticking time bomb archetype mediates their disclosure practices: Chesty doesn't want to make his teachers nervous; Mike doesn't want people to think he's crazy. Neither man seems willing to occupy an identity that contradicts positive military identity (the returning hero). Or perhaps another way to understand their resistance to disclosing is as a strategic rhetorical choice. Each man recognizes the risks involved with disclosure of mental disability and manages that risk through concealment. In contrast to the above examples, Kerschbaum (2014) analyzes the disability disclosure of memoirist Georgina Kleege, pointing out that Kleege's self-identification as "blind" operates as strategic resistance to the stigma of blindness. Can

Chesty and Mike's lack of disclosure also be considered strategic? Does the decision to withhold assert rhetorical agency? Yergeau (2015) theorizes such possibilities, asking, "Rather than refuting disability disclosures, what might it look like instead to orientate ourselves as attracted to disclosures, or even attracted to the refutation of disclosures?" (7). She goes on to argue that, "It is easy, tidy, and convenient to dismiss the diagnostic gaze as an example of disabled passivity" (8). When Chesty and Mike refuse to voice their identity as mentally disabled, they eliminate potential consequences from the rhetorical field; consequently, they are enacting agency in regards to the circumstances of their own discursive interactions. Their experiences also raise questions regarding the impetus for disclosure of mental disabilities in the first place. That is to say, when is it useful to disclose a mental disability in a classroom? What purpose does it serve? Scholars such as Valeras (2010) have examined the choices people with hidden disabilities make regarding when (and when not) to disclose and have found that many individuals learn various strategies of disclosure, including passing, strategic self-disclosure, and impression management; points I'll address in greater detail later in the essay.

Structural Forces Collide: Negotiating Multi-Dimensional Stigma

Students' narratives offered many examples that illuminated Goffman's (1963) assertion that stigma is produced in personal exchanges. The fear of being ostracized, of being labeled as "remedial" or "dumb," and the fear of isolation were all manifest in the production of stigma in these encounters. Marxist geographer Gleeson (1999), however, has critiqued Goffman's focus on the personal encounter for obscuring attention to the sociopolitical structures that support the manifestation of stigma. It is not that Goffman would deny that identities are embedded in social and political structures but, rather, that his choice to emphasize the personal occludes certain interpretations of disability experience. In the following three examples, I show how the production of stigma is often mediated by the collision of multiple structural forces of oppression.

Jake traced the impact of stigma to his early-childhood educational experiences. He said that he knew he was a "really smart kid," but he was being treated like he was slow "because one aspect of his academics, which was basically just speed reading" proved difficult for him. He followed up by saying, "And so I thought I was dumb . . . I couldn't stand having these remedial classes. I couldn't stand being this kid who's struggling." He also talked about the stigma associated with separation from "normal" kids, saying, "Being pulled out of the normal classroom to go to a special classroom, even young children still understand that special equals different and different is a stigma." As a result of Jake's elementary experience, he elects not to disclose his disability in college even though doing so prevents access to accommodations.

 Jake's disability identity is clearly impacted by the stigmatized intersections between being "special" and being "disabled." While remediation may be an obvious contributing factor to disability stigma, other students' narratives raised additional structural forces of oppression. Blair, who referred to her disability as a "problem" several times throughout our interview, talked about the interconnected, double-impact of stigma that she experiences as both an individual with a disability and as a female student in the hard sciences. Blair said, "I don't want people to identify me by my disability because I'm in [pre-med]; it's a really hard major and there's already a stigma of being a girl. And it's still really hard and I don't want people to think I'm not as smart as everyone else. And then if I identify with my disability, people will be like, 'Oh she's not as smart as everyone,' but that's just not true at all." Greg only disclosed being HIV positive to one teacher during his eleven years of studying in higher education. He disclosed to this one teacher because she revealed to the class that her son had HIV. Greg said, "It was just nice to have somebody understand where I was at. Because that is still such a stigma in society. It's just not something that I want everybody to know about. And most people don't know." When I asked why he thinks the stigma persists, he said, "because it's still mainly associated with gay men. That's it right there."

In the cases above, various structural forces, including remedial education, special education curricula, sexism, and homophobia intersected with students' experience of disability and their negotiation of a disability identity. This version of stigma, framed through multiple oppressive structural forces, doesn't neatly map onto the version of stigma production that Goffman (1963) identifies. For example, Jake's decision to avoid disclosure in college is deeply connected to his experiences in remediation at a young age. These early experiences shaped his later decisions. As Kerschbaum puts it, "Over time, individuals learn ways of managing disability discourses, motivated by their past experiences as well as by their short- and long-term goals for identity construction and social interaction" (2014, 63). Thus, we cannot continue to wonder why college students do not always take advantage of disability accommodations available to them without also interrogating the sociopolitical systems of stigma they have experienced alongside the intersectional impact of multiple systems of stigma. Greg and Blair's reflections on the multiple stigmas they face demonstrate the multidimensionality of the dominant discourses that both Williams (2006) and Hall (1994) describe. These intersections inform the performance (or non-performance) of identity as both Greg and Blair actively manage stigma associated with femaleness, queerness, and disability.

Connection and Community: Embracing Disability Identity

There were many moments in my interviews in which students discussed the impact and import of their interactions with other disabled people. Significantly, these reports of connection and community often coincided with positive conceptions of disability or, at the very least, comfort with disability identity. George, an avid blogger, reported that interacting with other disabled people offers a "comforting feeling" because of the realization that "there are other people out there who have these same issues." He said, "I have the ability to help them, and usually when I converse with individuals with OCD or depression or any other disorder, I usually learn stuff too. And so it's kind of a two-way street in a sense." Hilary reported that she is very open about her disability and jumps at the chance to write about her experience with Bipolar Disorder (BD). She said, "I'm pretty open about it because I hate the stigma of it." She shared several narratives about how she gains satisfaction from connecting with others, including her active contributions to a Reddit subgroup for people with BD. She explained, "I post on there a lot to help people who have just been diagnosed. Because I remember how terrible that was . . . I went through a period of great shame about it. I felt like, 'Oh I'm a freak. I can't have a normal relationship.' And I think if people have that shame, they won't talk about it, but if you realize it's not a big deal, it's like diabetes: you go get treated." Hilary's rhetorical agency emerges interactionally via her expression of comfort, community, and acceptance. She actively writes about her disability, she interacts with others who share her disability, and this connection might be understood as her way of reducing stigma via the establishment of shared disability community.

Veronica also emphasized the importance of interacting with other disabled people, speaking at length about a deeply profound connection with a friend who shared her same learning disability (LD). She said:

> We have an incredible memory for things . . . I think knowing other people with disabilities is helpful for people, and I don't know if that necessarily happens on a large campus like this or if it happens in

high school. But I think it's helpful just because you see what different kinds there are, and also if you have something very similar, you can discuss it and you can say, 'Oh ok, I realize that this is that learning difference coming into play and somebody else understands what I'm going through.' . . . It was nice to know that someone was using the same mechanisms that I was using.

Not only does Veronica develop the same positive import that Hilary describes, she also experiences validation of her LD as difference, potentially even positive difference, and is able to confidently assert her strategies for learning. George, Hilary, and Veronica all point out the positive impact that interaction with other disabled people has had on their lives, their feelings of self-worth, and their ability to help others.

While students shared numerous examples of ways that they constructed positive disability identities, such identities are nevertheless shaped by broader cultural narratives and structural forces. Identity scholar Lin (2008) argues, "Although people who find themselves in subordinate positions can attempt to construct positive identities for themselves in their struggles to gain recognition, it is often the dominant regimes of the powerful that dictate the identity game to them on the basis of a rigged and stacked text" (1). These dominant regimes—the normate narrative, the able-bodied collective—were present within many students' narratives; yet, there were also moments when students actively navigated the tension between their lived experiences and the rhetorical pressure of the norm, as well as moments when they cunningly negotiated the multi-dimensionality of various oppressive structural forces such as sexism and homophobia.[2] Perhaps most importantly, students were able to construct positive conceptions of their disability identity where they forged connections based on interdependence and validation. In the following sections, I tease out some of the specific strategies of disclosure that students employ as they make choices about when and how to openly acknowledge their disability.

Disability & Disclosure: Rhetorical Strategies for Impression Management

In her introduction to *Problematizing Identity: Everyday Struggles in Language, Culture, and Education*, Lin (2008) writes, "For different subjects (or social actors) located in differential socioeconomic and sociopolitical positions, the notion of identity is double-edged and is a weapon with risks and dangers (and often with far greater risks and dangers for subordinated groups)" (2). Disabled people are a subordinated group, but students with disabilities are doubly subordinated: on one hand, their disability itself implies a type of subordinated body, and on the other hand—as students— they are subordinate to the authority of the teacher. The stakes of disclosure are fraught with risk, and students employ various and complex measures to manage the identities they reveal to their instructors. In this section, I begin by framing impression management as risk management for students with disabilities and then discuss two agentive strategies that were prominent in my study: strategic genericism and selective disclosure.

Risk Management, Rhetoricity, and Responsivity

Sociologists Miall and Herman (1994) define impression management as "self-presentation and/or public display of identities created through the management of personal information" (208). Students with disabilities employ diverse and complex tactics for managing the components of their identity that they regard (or that others consider) as connected to disability. Though we might characterize all students (disabled and nondisabled alike) as consistently managing the impressions they put forward, students with disabilities face an added layer of risk due to the entrenchment of disability in frameworks of ableism and stigma. Disclosure of disability operates as a type of *risk management*. By risk management, I refer to the assessment and prioritization of risk in a given context. Some of the risks that students with disabilities may face upon disclosure include stigma, judgment, denial of access, and/or exposure to discriminatory and hurtful rhetorics of ableism. In response to these risks, two noticeable strategies of disclosure emerged from my interview data. Both of these strategies are modes of risk management; modes that demonstrate the sophisticated and complex rhetorical agency of disabled students as they make decisions about how to present themselves.

One of the most compelling narratives of disclosure shared in this study came from Tyler, an art student. Tyler's disclosure narrative not only elucidates the significance of perceived response in the disclosure act but also the complex variables at play in a given moment of identity management for disabled students. She first said, "I'm still trying to figure out how to communicate about [disability] with certain people," and then went on to describe a multifaceted experience of disclosing to two different professors:

It's kind of an interesting situation. There are two professors who are dating. So I told the girl professor. Just 'cause I don't think she's a very emotional person, but I still think that she'd be more empathetic than a male professor who can be really cynical. I think he's one of my favorite professors, but if I were to start tearing up in the middle of this conversation, I would feel really uncomfortable, so I told the female professor. And part of it was because I realized that no one in the art school knew about this condition whereas my entire family knows, all my closest friends know, people at my workplace know, so I was wondering if art has to do with the rest of my life, why am I not telling these people about it? So I sat down and talked with [her] about it, and she was really encouraging and supportive of it and wanted me to pursue artwork that explored my feelings or reactions to the disability. And so I did create a couple of pieces that were responses to the everyday [experience of disability]. So I think she most likely would have communicated that with [him], which I was kinda hoping would happen just so I wouldn't have to tell him. . . . And I think just in the sense that he like has a better understanding of where my questions are coming from.

I asked, "So with the female, it was less a decision about something you needed practically in the class and more about your art community at [this university] and them knowing where you're coming from?" and Tyler answered:

Just to have someone else understand. Especially last semester. I've been dating someone for about six months and so with that I've been wondering, 'Okay what would marriage look like? Is this person willing to continue dating me and potentially marry me knowing there's that risk of me becoming blind or deaf? And we've had that conversation many times, and he's been incredibly encouraging, supportive, and just surprisingly willing, and so I was just thinking about it a lot last semester and become really upset about it and cry or something and I don't know just be unsure about what I was gonna do so it was just a big part of my thought process last year. So I think I just wanted to have this dialogue within my artwork about it, and then I didn't want to just announce to the class, 'This is what it's about.' I kind of wanted to talk to my professor about it and see what she thought about that. . . . You're creating something and then other people are going to say I like that or I hate that. And it would be hard if you do that too soon. It's deeply personal. . . . It's an emotional thing.

Tyler's narrative reveals many of the complexities of the disclosure process. Tyler highlights the differences in her choices for disclosure among different faculty, suggesting that personality type and gender played a role in her selection process for determining a safe disclosure recipient. She also reveals how her own personal relationships impacted the choices she made about disclosure in the college setting, and she seems concerned with how her exploration of disability in her own personal expression, her artwork, might be perceived by her peers. The impression she wants to make seems positioned between her desire to be authentic to her own experiences and her concern about how those experiences will (or will not) be appreciated and understood by her professors, her peers, her partner, even herself.

As did Tyler, others students weighed their disclosure choices on their anticipated response from teachers and administrators. April, for example, expressed resistance to disclosing on the grounds that teachers might judge her for not electing to use campus disability services. She said, "I should tell them, but at the same time I feel like I'm gonna get scolded for not going to the disability center. I feel like they're not going to respect that I'm telling them, very unofficial. So I try not to tell them unless I feel closer to them." For April, trusting her professors not to judge her choices is paramount to her decision to disclose. George reported that he discloses to teachers in order to make certain they don't think he is cheating on exams when he uses a coping technique that involves mouthing words to himself.

While April and George both manage risk in ways that prevent unfair judgment, Tom's approach to disclosure as risk management is a means of ensuring access for himself. He said, "They have to know. It's like helping myself by telling them. If I try to pass as normal and not tell my professor, that's really hurting myself . . . I guess it doesn't matter if they accept me or not. It is what it is. I'm not trying to be their friend." The experiences shared by April, George, Tyler, and Tom all demonstrate ways that students assess the risks of disclosure, and, as Tom shows, how they factor in the connections between disclosure and access to accommodations.

Strategies of Disclosure: Strategic Genericism and Selective Disclosure

Rhetorics of self-advocacy dominate much of the discourse on disclosure, but this focus obscures the reality of ableism and instead places a burden on the individual student (see Torkelson and Gussell 2011). A more useful approach to theorizing disclosure requires acknowledgement and appreciation for the rhetoricity of disabled students, particularly in terms of the strategies they employ as they disclose a disability. I turn now to discuss two such strategies: strategic genericism and selective disclosure. These strategies should be understood as agentive rhetorics of risk management employed as part of students' assessment of the rhetorical situation and of the perceived responsivity of various audiences. To begin, one prominent strategy reported by many study participants involves revealing their status as disabled yet resisting a specific revelation of their *type* of disability; I refer to this tactic as *strategic genericism*. Amber reported that she uses the generic disability services email to disclose that she has a disability but generally avoids specifying what type of disability she has. When I asked her why, she said, "I don't think they need to know, I guess. I don't want them to treat me differently. . . . Everybody thinks that people with Bipolar are crazy." Andy reported that he will disclose if he thinks he might use accommodations but that typically he just uses the generic form because he doesn't "feel like there's any more to be said." Greg said that when he has to miss class, he provides doctor's notes and reports illness but does not reveal HIV as the cause. For Andy, his motivation comes out of questioning the purpose of revealing his specific disability while for Amber and Greg, this strategy seems to be a self-protective measure.

Leah also reported that she enacts strategic genericism in practices of disclosure, explaining:

> I feel that sharing the specific disabilities I have with a professor is sharing things that can be easily judged one way or the other. Other disabilities are accepted by society as legitimate and thus, a professor can't react badly to it. Migraines and depression, I feel, are things that general society might not automatically deem a disability. It might take having a conversation with someone like me, who has been so significantly affected by them, for a sway towards disability to happen. By not describing my disability, the professor doesn't have the opportunity to judge whether it is legitimate or not.

Leah's resistance to specifying her disability indicates her savvy understanding of social attitudes toward her particular type of disability. She points out that many might regard her disability as not quite a disability; both migraines and depression are invoked so often they have become "commonplace" experiences and may not be interpreted as a disability experienced by a minority. Leah's observation draws attention to the ways in which degree of disability impacts disclosure. In her case, she suspects that people may regard her as *not disabled enough* to merit accommodations; therefore, she employs strategic genericism as a self-protective measure to ensure that she is accommodated, rather than scrutinized, by her professors (see Yergeau 2015).

A second strategy used by disabled students in their disclosing process is the practice of *selective disclosure*, revealing some disabilities while concealing others. James reported that he felt more comfortable telling teachers about ADD and less comfortable disclosing OCD and Tourette's, even though the latter two disabilities more substantially impact his classroom experience. Lillie expressed that she will disclose her LD to professors but that she does not disclose her depression because "learning disabilities tend to be accepted, and I almost feel like depression isn't even a problem." Here, Lillie echoes Leah's comment about commonplace attitudes about depression. Chesty and Mike, the student-veterans, also report practicing selective disclosure, readily volunteering information about their physical, but not mental, disabilities. Diane, like several of the students in this study, has multiple disabilities, but she usually only discloses the Tourette's (her only "visible" disability), and only that when she perceives the course as "strenuous."

Disability scholars such as Valeras (2010) have pointed out that, "[w]hether passing is deliberate or not, maintaining an able-bodied public persona requires copious amounts of energy." Practices of selective disclosure reflect many of the larger dynamics of disability identity, including distinctions between visible and invisible disabilities, the politics of passing, and hierarchies between physical and mental disabilities. For those with both visible *and* invisible disabilities, they may have different choices when visibility forces disability onto the rhetorical field, making them differently susceptible to risk and judgement and leading to a different set of rhetorical choices. For those with both mental *and* physical disabilities, the stigma of being mentally ill, "crazy," or dangerous often leads them to feel that it is far too risky to fully own that identity on campus. As Price (2011) has argued, the rhetoricity of the "mad" subject runs contrary to what Wallace (2006) has dubbed the "presumption of normativity" upon which the entire academic enterprise seems predicated (Price 2011, 45). The practice of selective disclosure demonstrates that disabled students are acutely attuned to the attitudinal, social, and even political barriers they may face if they openly identify as mentally disabled.

A Sway toward Disability

The complexities of disclosure for disabled students are not reducible to an email sent to instructors from disability services. To appreciate this complexity, teachers need a deep level of understanding and respect for the stakes of disclosure and should attempt to construct conditions that invite—but don't coerce—revelation of disability. Price warns that "mere awareness is not enough" (2011, 45), and I'd add that moving beyond awareness requires not only appreciation and analysis of student rhetorical strategies but also an active engagement with how instructors, administrators, and staff might also position themselves as purposefully responsive agents. The rhetorical complexities of disclosure reveal a great deal about current attitudes toward disability, about the ways in which agency is indeed emergent and interactional within rhetorical situations, and about the rhetorical acumen of students with disabilities in their practices of identity management and in their endeavors for access.

References

Brune, Jeffrey A. 2014. "Reflections on the Fiftieth Anniversary of Erving Goffman's *Stigma*." *Disability Studies Quarterly* 34 (1).

Cooper, Marilyn. 2011. "Rhetorical Agency as Emergent and Enacted." *College Composition and Communication* 62 (3): 420–49.

Dolmage, Jay. 2014. *Disability Rhetoric*. Syracuse: Syracuse University Press.

Glaser, Barney, and Anselm Strauss. 1967. *The Discovery of Grounded Theory*. Chicago, IL.

Gleeson, Brendan. 1999. *Geographies of Disability*. London: Routledge.

Goffman, Erving. 1963. *Stigma: Notes on the Management of a Spoiled Identity*. New York: Simon & Schuster.

Hall, Stuart. 1994. "Cultural Identity and Diaspora." In *Colonial Discourse and Postcolonial Theory*. Eds. Patrick Williams and Laura Chrisman. New York: Columbia University Press, 392–403.

Kerschbaum, Stephanie. 2014. "On Rhetorical Agency and Disclosing Disability in Academic Writing." *Rhetoric Review* 33 (1): 55–71.

Lin, Angel M. Y. 2008. "The Identity Game and Discursive Struggles of Everyday Life: An Introduction." In *Problematizing Identity: Everyday Struggles in Language, Culture, and Education*, edited by Angel M. Y. Lin. New York: Routledge. 1–10.

Longmore, Paul. 2013. "'Heaven's Special Child': The Making of Poster Children." In *The Disability Studies Reader*. 4th ed. Ed. Lennard J. Davis. New York: Routledge, 34–41.

Merriam, Sharan B. 2009. Qualitative Research: A Guide to Design and Implementation. San Francisco, CA: Jossey Bass.

Miall, Charlene E. and Nancy J. Herman. 1994. "Generic Processes of Impression Management: Two Case Studies of Physical and Mental Disability." In *Symbolic Interaction: An Introduction to Social Psychology*, eds. Nancy J. Herman and Larry T. Reynolds. Dix Hills, NY: General Hall., 208–23.

Patton, M. Q. 2002. *Qualitative Research and Evaluation Methods*. 3rd ed. Thousand Oaks, CA: Sage Publications.

Price, Margaret. 2011. *Mad at School: Rhetorics of Mental Disability and Academic Life*. Ann Arbor: University of Michigan Press.

Saldana, Johnny. 2013. *The Coding Manual for Qualitative Researchers*. 2nd ed. Los Angeles: Sage Publications.

Shapiro, Joseph. 1994. *No Pity: People with Disabilities Forging a New Civil Rights Movement*. New York: Three Rivers Press.

Siebers, Tobin. 2002. "Tender Organs, Narcissism, and Identity Politics." In *Disability Studies: Enabling the Humanities*. Eds. Sharon L. Snyder, Brenda Jo Brueggemann, and Rosemarie Garland-Thomson. New York: Modern Language Association, 40–55.

Torkelson, Ruth, and Lori Gussel. 2011. "Disclosure and Self-Advocacy Regarding Disability-related Needs: Strategies to Maximize Integration in Postsecondary Education." *Journal of Counseling and Development* 74 (4): 352–57.

Valeras, Aimee Burke. 2010. "'We Don't Have a Box': Understanding Hidden Disability Identity Utilizing Narrative Research Methodology." *Disability Studies Quarterly* 30 (3/4).

Walters, Shannon. 2014. *Rhetorical Touch: Disability, Identification, Haptics*. Columbia: University of South Carolina Press.

Weigal, Bekah Hawrot and Lisa Detweiler Miller. 2011. "Post-Traumatic and the Returning Veteran: The Rhetorical and Narrative Challenges." *Open Words: Access and English Studies* 5 (1): 29–37.

Wallace, David L. 2006. "Transcending Normativity: Difference Issues in 'College English.'" *College English* 68 (5): 502–30.

Williams, Bronwyn T., ed. 2006. *Identity Papers: Literacy and Power in Higher Education*. Logan, UT: Utah State University Press.

Yergeau, Melanie. 2015. "Autistext: On the Politics of Non-Disclosure." Paper presented at the Conference on College Composition and Communication, Tampa, FL.

II

Intersectionality

Bodyminds Like Ours

An Autoethnographic Analysis of Graduate School, Disability, and the Politics of Disclosure

ANGELA M. CARTER

R. TINA CATANIA

SAM SCHMITT

AMANDA SWENSON

"I don't understand, you write such smart papers . . . I worry this 'accommodation' would make your peers uncomfortable, can't you do without it? . . . Why are you taking so few classes? . . . I wish I could take my time like you do . . . Although we have your records, we need further documentation of your disability to provide the accommodations you are requesting . . . Haven't you spent years dealing with this? Why is it still such a big deal? . . . 'Everyone's disabled when it rains. You can't drive to that part of campus without a permit' . . . I get tired all the time, too! . . . We all get depressed sometimes . . . Have you tried acupuncture? . . . The committee is sorry to inform you that your grant application was denied because your 'time-to-degree' process does not meet the required standards. . . . Disabled people receive too many benefits . . . People with your disability don't go to graduate school; I think you need to consider a more realistic career path . . ."

These are just a few of the many micro (and macro) aggressions that we, as disabled graduate students, experience daily in the academy.[1] The culture of academia presumes that the bodyminds (Price 2015) best suited for academia are those that demonstrate discipline, restraint, productivity, and autonomy. Too often, disabled, neurodivergent, and chronically ill bodies are framed as unproductive, impaired, dependent, disorderly and, therefore, of little intellectual or productive value. Graduate students with disabilities, therefore, encounter significant barriers to participation. Not quite "novice" and not quite "scholar," disabled graduate students must navigate a complex web of power. The connections among academic norms and rituals; institutional policies; hierarchies of race, nation, class, gender, and sexuality; and the corporeality of our bodies present circumstances that are distinct from the struggles of disabled undergraduate students or disabled faculty members. In this chapter, we argue that the convergence of white capitalist academic institutions and the discourse of able-bodyminds as good, productive, disciplined, and capable promote the exclusion and erasure of graduate students with disabilities in academia. Together, we discuss this precarious positioning within academia; the politics of disability disclosure in critical and justice-based fields of inquiry; how concepts of passing and performing disability intersect with other aspects of our identities (race, class, gender, sexuality, nation); and the contours of "crip life" as scholars-in-training. We narrate our experiences facing and resisting barriers meant to exclude our bodyminds from academia—an institution created and structured around the ideal, productive body that is ideologically predetermined for white, cisgender, heterosexual, able-bodied males.

Through mutual exchange and "risking the personal" (Keating 2000, 2), we build our collective wisdom and offer visions of change that not only increase accessibility and inclusion for graduate students with disabilities but promote holistic transformation. Keating (2007, 125–26) argues "Blame and guilt are not useful but accountability is." We share our experiences as an effort to shift toward mutual accountability and change. Through our vulnerability and transparency, we invite you into our experiences and set aside shame and guilt so that, together, we can envision futures that are inclusive and accessible for all.

> ANGELA: In our first brainstorming session, we identified five deeply embedded components of ableism within the academy: ideology, bureaucracy, physicality, temporality, and sociality. Acknowledging these features of academic ableism is incredibly significant because people often think of ableism in terms of individual (in)actions or attitudes; but as with other forms of oppression, ableism is built into the foundation of academia. Can we begin our discussion by expanding on these ideas?
>
> SAM: Ideologically, graduate students represent "the best and brightest" in their field. The myth of meritocracy ignores structural inequalities that allow some to succeed at the direct expense of others and

inherently assumes not just a bodymind that is *capable* but one that is superior. This "superior" bodymind could never be a disabled bodymind because disability always already serves as the other. Disabled graduate students constitute a paradox that academia is trying to assimilate—either through erasing our disabilities in order to rightfully include us as *able* or by using our disabilities as justification for excluding us as *unable*. The issue and focus is, of course, our bodyminds and not the structures, practices, or policies of the academy. Moreover, graduate students exist in a liminal space within the academy; we are classified as students *and* as university employees/staff. We're a category that blends/exceeds the employee/student binary; thus, the resources, accommodations, and support we need are often hard to acquire or do not exist.

AMANDA: And when people think of ableist structures, they immediately think of physically accessible doors and buildings. These accommodations, or lack thereof, are certainly important ways our experiences on campus are constrained. When we point to the physical ableism of the structural hierarchy imposed in graduate school, we are also signifying the kind of physicality needed to maintain the "proper" graduate student timetable. Our bodyminds cannot work forty hours a week, let alone the sixty our "good" graduate student peers do. We cannot take as many classes, attend as many meetings, or read/write as fast as is expected. We physically cannot bear the toll of this labor and are told repeatedly that this is a failure inherent in our bodyminds. This, of course, coincides with the temporality of graduate education, which is, in our current neoliberal moment, continuously speeding up. There are "time-to-degree" benchmarks we inevitably miss and funding opportunities tied to these markers. Graduate students are expected to progress through programs at a timely rate and through each milestone in a particular way. This usually leaves disabled graduate students behind, because we simply cannot work in this way.

Relatedly, so much of academia involves social connections. These networks are typically built through traveling to conferences, but can be as simple as going out with your cohort or attending dinner events with visiting scholars. For disabled graduate students, it can be very difficult, if not impossible, to keep up with our daily lives and attend these "off the clock" engagements. Conference travel is particularly strenuous on our bodyminds, meaning post-panel dinners or late-night networking is rare. We often miss out on the kinds of connections built between our peers and with potential mentors. Disabled graduate students feel isolated, misunderstood, unsupported, and without recourse—regardless of our specific academic location or the encouragement we have from our advisors.

TINA: This speaks to our history. We have never met each other "physically," and have only communicated through online venues. Someone said their colleagues were surprised we were writing a group paper having never met in person. This, too, highlights our experience of academia as ableist. For most, networking, collaborative research, and writing, are acts that happen in person. Here, our disabilities intersect with our class (making the funding of travel difficult); sexuality and gender (the bodily labor of reproduction, for example); and cultural norms (notions of extended family who might also need care—not only are we supposed to be able-bodied and put academia first, but our families should also be able-bodied and not require our care). For so many reasons, our first virtual meeting was a moment not only for networking and beginning collaborative writing but also one of building community. Doing academic work in this nontraditional way, with people we "don't know," is one way we are thinking about academia differently and in a way that works better for our bodyminds.

SAM: What has been most surprising to me has been the kinds of ableism I've experienced within Feminist/Women's Studies. I struggle with the field, particularly as a person who is chronically ill, neurodivergent, queer, and trans. I feel excited to work in a department where there is an equal emphasis on the study of "disciplines"/"disciplinization" as there is on dynamics of power/oppression/privilege and so forth. Still, I feel academic feminism has a ways to go before we're living up to our expressed commitment to disability, in both practice and curriculum. While the field's social justice orientation acknowledges ability status as one vector of power, I sometimes get the feeling that "disability" is tagged on at the end (much like the B or T in LGBT).

ANGELA: Right, people know they should be attentive to disability, but that doesn't always translate to action. I routinely get the feeling of "oh yeah, that's important but we're still fighting other fights, so we'll come back to disability later." Folks are often unaware how their ableism manifests in their scholarship and academic work. When I try to call attention to this, I'm told that it "wasn't their intention" and everyone is "still learning" to think about disability. This situates me as the "insider," there to explain how ableism and dis/ability are working in that moment.

AMANDA: We often become the voice of information for our and all disabilities, which we simply cannot do—that in itself acts as a potential silencing of other bodyminds and an act of violence on these bodyminds that are continuously marginalized through their misrepresentation. Yet, we are also continuously called forth to speak for bodies that we cannot speak for—I know I've often had to say, "I can't speak for that narrative" or "I'm literally not qualified"—which then silences us when we finally can speak for our own bodies.

SAM: I would also like to consider the consequences of the Cartesian bodymindspirit split in social justice scholarship. So much academic work is framed as solely an *intellectual* endeavor, relegated to the mind. Like indigenous and women of color, people with disabilities critique academic intellectualism that attempts to transcend the body and advocate that the (disabled, queer, brown/black) body is a valid onto-epistemological location (see for example Moraga and Anzaldúa 1981, Moss and Dyck 2002). Moreover, self-care is often encouraged but not always feasible for graduate students. Lorde's assertion that self-care is a radical act becomes stripped of its transformational qualities when we merely *think about* "self-care" but are not actually allowed to *do* acts of care (1988, 131).

AMANDA: Panels and speakers at my university who talk about self-care always put the onus on the graduate students to step forth and take action: see a therapist, go to yoga and stop the pattern that "you" bring onto "yourself." I find that my University conflates the individual with the entire system: "we're all tired" (Keating 2007, 24–26). Therefore, no one ought to "stand out," no one ought to push and test these boundaries. Self-care becomes this tricky place where the graduate student has to work within a rigid, designated space.

SAM: I've been to workshops and panels where "self-care" is represented in either/or terms—described as "relaxation" or "leisure"—implying that the opposite of self-care is production and activity. While these panels have, no doubt, produced important questions, definitions of self-care that emphasize *leisure* and *idleness* make me wary because they approximate capitalist notions of production. This conversation reminds me of Betcher's critique (2007, 6–10) of "wholeness" in western cultures where brokenness is interpreted as a sign of pathology, motivating people toward "wholeness." "Broken" and socially unacceptable bodyminds like ours inherently contradict the notion that bodies should be "whole" and, therefore, tuned for maximum efficiency and productivity.

AMANDA: This points toward the "incurable" disabled bodymind, or the bodymind that is not the demarcated disabled body. Disability Studies theorizes this body as the supercrip (for example, Clare 1999)—we are currently discussing and pushing back against this construct—which is pushing so hard against the overarching machine: the academy. Often these bodyminds are thought of as courageous for even going to grad school, better yet if they work in Disability Studies. However, if these individuals push too hard against the academy, the academy will often remind us of our social and hierarchal place. As long as we are Foucauldian docile bodies, the machine is okay with us.

TINA: While *some* disciplines recognize the need for self-care, what that means for the disabled bodymind requires even more bodily labor for us. There's a lack of recognition by the academy, and those who inhabit it, that our bodyminds must *always* do more work and that for us, self-care means something very different than it might mean for others the academy also marginalizes.

Speaking specifically about my discipline, I had conflated the radical praxis of a few with the field as a whole. A qualitative methods class I took revealed to me how deeply embedded ableism is in geography. In that class, I was inspired to write about fieldwork and research for disabled students in geography, but when I started researching, I found nothing. There were articles theorizing disability, sure, but not much about actually "doing" research while disabled. It was as if my body, and bodies like mine, had not been considered.

So, it seems that geography has yet to really deal with the fact that disabled bodyminds wish to do more than obtain a bachelor's degree. And, as is the case with almost all academic departments, graduate student and faculty requirements are conceived of in ways that automatically preclude the disabled body. Funding packages are not reconceptualized for students who need reduced course loads. Research funding is not thought through for those whose bodyminds will not be the ones driving, travelling, standing. Most advisors don't think about advising students that don't "fit the mold" *unless* they encounter a disabled student. And so the disabled student, aside from learning new ways of thinking, new literatures, and planning research, is also trying to "teach" the advisor, the department, the discipline about disability. And all that extra work is not factored into "productive" time. This means that while I was once a staunch disciplinarian, fiercely identifying as a geographer above all else—today I see I cannot be a geographer. I cannot belong to any one discipline, because they were *all* formed and created without the inclusion of disabled bodyminds. Some try harder than others to add and stir us in, but I can't be stirred into a structure that is predicated on a body I do not have. So I see myself as interdisciplinary. Intersectional. Feminist. Geographer. Anthropologist- and Sociologist-adjacent. Just like we often have to cobble together our accommodations, which we can never disentangle, which cannot *but* intersect with our other aspects of our identities, we have to cobble together our disciplines.

SAM: Tina's discussion of methods reminds me of many women of color theorists who have to "make a way out of no way" when there weren't methods that acknowledged the wisdom of their communities (Phillips 2006, xxvii). While clearly women of colors' insights are manifested from their specific race-class-gender lenses, there are important areas of commonality, specifically, where people with disabilities have had to assert their experience as oppressed people as a valid form of authority.

ANGELA: This year, my university surveyed graduate students about their experiences. Questions specifically asked how students felt about the ways faculty/administration/peers treated them based on race, class, gender, sexuality, ethnicity, and citizenship. But not a single question asked about ableism or disability. It was as if the disabled graduate student, or ableism, simply couldn't exist. Relatedly, it's the twenty-fifth anniversary of the ADA, which is often credited with "opening the doors" of higher education for disabled people. What has been your experience, with asking for, and receiving, accommodations through your university's Office of Disability Services (ODS)?

AMANDA: I no longer go to ODS. They're incredibly kind, but for the most part, they deal with undergraduates, which is not what I need. I go straight to my professors who have given me extensions and have (often) been gracious.

ANGELA: Right, ODS doesn't seem to understand the needs of graduate students. During my second year, I asked ODS if the 1–3 day extension for papers could be adjusted. I explained that while this works for undergraduates, it doesn't accommodate a graduate student's workloads. I was assured this accommodation was "set up to work for everyone." After an hour-long conversation, ODS agreed to "work on the language" of my accommodation letter, encouraging professors to grant me extended time. A week later, I was informed that if I needed more than 1–3 days, I had to get further testing to quantify my disability. At that point, I decided to figure it out myself. From then on, I met with the professors—outed myself as disabled—and talked about my need for extended time. If the professor wasn't willing to work with me, I simply could not take their class. These are exactly the kinds of invasive conversations and interactions that ODS is supposed to handle. Now that I am out of coursework, ODS can do even less for me because none of the accommodations they offer make sense with preliminary exams or dissertation work.

SAM: A friend at another university has multiple, chronic illnesses and her colleagues frequently imply that she is "the golden child" because she receives extensions when she needs them. I'm frustrated because they don't understand that extensions aren't a reward or prize. Personally, I decided against pursuing official accommodations with ODS. I barely have the financial means to pay for my basic medical care, let alone the additional medical costs incurred by having it officially documented for my university. I've disclosed my ability status and have generally been met with understanding; however, there seems to be a culture of silence regarding disability among graduate students.

TINA: Clearly extensions means we: a) do not manage our time wisely and are, therefore, b) not a good "fit" for academia, and c) get special treatment we do not deserve. (For more on how other marginalized groups, such as women of color, negotiate hegemonic practices of the academy, see Garrison-Wade et al. 2011 and Gutiérrez y Muhs, Niemann, González, and Harris 2012). In general, my experiences can be summed up as follows. Institutionally, asking for and receiving accommodations, has been a failure. Particular individuals in ODS, the university, and professors, are kind and helpful. What bothers me about accommodations is that they are individualized. Classes, programs, and TA responsibilities are not designed with accessibility in mind. Just like the university, which was created by and for rich, white, men in a racist-sexist-hetero-patriarchal society; women, people of color, people with disabilities, and so on, have been "added in." They try to add us in and stir us into their already ableist-sexist-racist structures to make some sort of "diversity" soup. But why can't classes be designed to be accessible from the start? We were never conceived of as belonging; we were never meant to be citizens of the university. So it is no wonder that we hit walls and continually encounter the limits of disability offices and "reasonable" accommodations.

ANGELA: This struggle speaks to my next question. Disability disclosure has impacted every aspect of my graduate experience—from disclosing to my department that I needed to take medical leave, to professors each semester asking for accommodations, to colleagues/peers when they ask why my path doesn't match theirs. Disclosing never ends. And now, as an instructor, I disclose to my students. I do this as a political act of resistance and solidarity, to stand with other disabled students and to challenge the myths surrounding disability. I went from never wanting to disclose and feeling really horrible when I had to, to now feeling like it is imperative to my survival and my politics—even if I often still hesitate before doing so. How has disclosing your disability impacted your experience as a graduate student?

TINA: I agree, it is "imperative to my survival and my politics" to disclose. And yet, sometimes the work of it all—not just disclosing, but then working to obtain what you need—is a job unto itself. Dealing with individuals has its upside. Helpful and friendly staff and professors make my heart smile. But what's harder to talk about are those people who don't seem to get it. They don't get the extra work we have to do. They don't get that asking for accommodations is *reasonable* and not special treatment. They don't get that their policies—from funding, to time to completion of various "benchmarks"—cannot fit neatly onto our bodies. And I think the worst part of disclosing is being *forced* to disclose. And we are forced to disclose in ways/details we do not want to share because for some, describing something based on our lived experience is *still* not enough.

In a recent grad meeting, in which I participated virtually, we discussed the creation of shared online space for graduate documents. One student advocated a particular platform that my disability makes difficult to use. I voiced two reasons for going with another platform, one of which was accessibility. I was then asked, "What do you mean by accessibility? It's certified by some association for the blind so it's accessible." This white, able-bodied man's question required me to reveal the specificities of my medical history. My word, that it was inaccessible, was not enough. But it's more than individuals; we have to think of the entire university as disabling. As Kuusisto says, "The academy disables itself. Failed architectures and insufficiency of imagination always speak the tacit unspoken phrase: 'your body is a problem'" (Kuusisto 2015, par. 6). It's not just administration. It's not just the buildings. It's not just the policies. It's not just some individuals. Thankfully there are some understanding professors who put their "critical/social justice theory" into practice through action. But there are also those who force us to disclose, who question our experiences of ableism and accessibility simply because they are not identical to their own experiences, or to their notion of what accessibility and disability are "supposed" to look like.

SAM: I am sad and frustrated that you were coerced to disclose. I'm thinking about the politics of authenticity here. It seems that this person needed to know that you had an "authentic" reason for switching to more accessible technology. That leads me to think about how bodies get coded as more (or less) authentically disabled where "authenticity" is defined by the able-bodied gaze (Jones 2013).

AMANDA: It seems like disability and disabled-identifying bodyminds have to render themselves through this very narrow lens that is always preceded by the able-bodied gaze, which always privileges the able-bodied transcription of the disabled narrative, identity, body, etc. Brueggemann states that she purposely claims a deconstructed, precarious identity since it calls attention not only to the disability (which incites dialogue) but to her ability to claim autonomy and agency (Brueggemann and Moddelmog 2002, 316).

Theoretically, I like to think of the disabled body as continuously "becoming," especially in relation to identity (Butler 1990, 33). How will we reconfigure our identities in relation to our disabilities, especially since disabilities are not fixed? The concepts of passing and coming out really challenge how I feel about identity, especially misconceptions about the construction of identity through coming out as disabled. This is one area where I perform my disability. I went through a brief period of time where I was very open about being disabled, mainly because I never knew when my disability would present itself so I would prepare other people—if I exposed the disability, then other people wouldn't be so alarmed when my disability exposed itself. However, grad students and professors alike were really taken aback by my medical-like frankness. Some wanted to coddle me. Then there are those who reacted very aggressively toward me, silencing me. Suddenly thrust into this polar vortex of rapidly shifting identities where I had to accommodate myself toward others' inabilities to see me, I was really frustrated, anxious, and depressed. So I stopped disclosing. It was important for me to think about this shifting identity because, as Simi Linton (1998, 21) says, passing can engender anxiety. However, disclosing can produce a different type of anxiety. Before, I wouldn't take my medication in public; now I am more open about it, letting other people assume what they want. After an EEG, I will go to a coffee shop to reward myself and I won't wash the glue out of my hair. Little things like that slowly, but inconspicuously, drift attention away from able-bodiedness.

TINA: Your points about identity, Amanda, bring us to the concept of intersectionality. For me, my disability cannot be disentangled from other axes of difference and power that simultaneously work to oppress and privilege me. Upon returning from medical leave, I needed to use a wheelchair. My privilege as a married woman with a husband who happened to be on sabbatical allowed me to take classes I otherwise could not—I needed him to drive me, to get into rooms and open the doors not built for my chair, doors I cannot open for automatic buttons apparently are too expensive to install. (I was told it was because of fire codes, which, upon checking, turned out to be false).

Moreover, I experience the dual-bind of race/nationality and ability: the invisibility of my race/immigrant status and the hyper-visibility of my disability, as well as my family's immigrant cultural norms and ideas about ability. I benefit from white privilege despite not identifying as white growing up because of my immigrant background and culture. (Ahmed 2014 suggests that students of color with disabilities are even more depleted by the academy.) My sister and I were the first in our family to graduate college, and my disability necessarily intersects with the immigrant work ethic and need to do what was denied to my mother. As a girl, my mother was allowed to complete more education than her brothers (the fifth grade). She desired to continue further, however, but her gender precluded it. At the same time, I struggle with my family's immigrant cultural norms about disability. Some wish I didn't have to disclose and see me using a chair as sad, as demonstrating my illness. They do not see it as an empowering aide that actually gives me *more* mobility. A picture of me attending class in a wheelchair on Facebook causes transnational reverberations from family in my home country. Questions. Pity. Concern. Until I can explain, the wheelchair, and hence the photo, signifies disability instead of successful independence.

ANGELA: I'm quick to "come out" as a queer, working-class femme, but I always seem to pause before coming out as disabled. I don't think it's as simple as internalized ableism, but I'm not sure why I hesitate. (For a recent discussion of disability studies, internalized ableism, and coming out "crip," see Talley 2013). Becoming disabled has strengthened my identity as a working-class person, complicated my identity as a queer, and taught me how to better understand my white privilege. Since becoming disabled, I better understand how capitalism shapes our bodies—marking us as usable/unusable and disregarding us when/if labor cannot be extracted. I was raised by a single mom living paycheck to paycheck, so living without a safety net is not new to me. My understanding, though, of how able-bodiedness is in its own way a social safety net has completely shifted my understanding of socioeconomic oppression. Like many working-poor, my identity was constructed on "working-hard." Now I understand more clearly how social institutions and systems are structured so that individual "hard work" doesn't make much of a difference—it's your ability to claim membership within, and gain privileges from, your race, class, gender, citizenship status, and having an able-body. Under capitalism, it's a kind of twisted privilege to be considered worthy of exploitable labor; I never would have known or thought that to be true until I became disabled.

With my disability, participating in the queer community is harder. Staying out late, being at shows or clubs, or even going to Pride impacts my bodymind, and I soon decided these activities weren't "worth it." As a result, I've felt disconnected and alienated from my community. I recently connected with a neuro-queer community and these spaces help me think about how my disability—neurodivergence—queers me (Finley 2010). This helps me understand how my sexuality/gender intersects with my disability. Conversely, my whiteness facilitates passing as able-bodied. I am presumed to be competent and knowledgeable and "belonging" in academia. No one has ever *overtly* accused me of "milking the system" or "playing the disability card," because I am assumed to be "working my hardest" thanks to white privilege. Studies show that students of color are tracked out of education, often through "special education," and rarely get to college, let alone graduate (Ferri and Connor 2005; Wagner, Newman, Cameto, Garza, and Levine 2005). My able-bodied whiteness helped get me to college, and even after becoming disabled that same whiteness helps me stay in graduate school.

SAM: I struggle with identity-based language to describe myself because I am limited by the language I choose and the politics of identity. (Should I refer to myself as "disabled" or not? Am I allowed to use that word?) I move among terms as needed to help people understand my experiences, but I could describe myself as a white, working-class, transmasculine, queer, neurodivergent person with a chronic illness. I'm realizing more and more that my disabilities are eclipsed as my gender expression approximates a white masculine norm. Whiteness and masculinity are coded as expressions of confidence, intelligence, and capability in Western culture. The more I approximate this ideal, the more invisible my disability seems to become. While not intentional, I get asked to lecture on gender-related issues more than any other area of my research/activism. I love lecturing on issues pertinent to transgender studies, but I sometimes feel tokenized and that it contributes to the invisibility of my disabilities.

My gender identity makes it difficult for me to access scholarships and grants targeted to scholars in my field. Trans folks frequently do not qualify for scholarships geared toward women, or students doing research in feminist/women's studies (e.g., AAUW 2015) because there is an assumption that the grantees would automatically be cisgender women. Thus, I've had to be creative when it comes to finding money which means that I have to strategically use "supercrip" narratives to my advantage, omit my gender identity, and allow my feminine legal name to carry my application through.

ANGELA: I'm intrigued, Sam, by your discussion of using the supercrip narrative, and how those narratives intersect with other identities. I've certainly done this too, and it makes my heart hurt every time. I hate that it often feels like the only option available—play into the narratives that oppress us to survive. This ties into the idea of passing. . . . As if disability is something you can just "get together" and then it doesn't impact you anymore. The problem, of course, is our bodyminds, not academia.

SAM: It's true, I disclose now to lend authority to my experiences, usually drawing from medical authority as a form of "verification." I often feel that my subjective experience is not enough. Thus, I have to draw on other sources of authentication, but I risk reproducing harmful psycho-medical models of neurodivergence and disability. We all seem to navigate a dangerous web of truth/truths to survive.

ANGELA: Speaking of survival, can we talk a bit about funding? The limited years of graduate student funding is a barrier that causes me serious distress. My department does everything it can to fund folks, but with each new semester past the guaranteed years, there is the renewed chance they won't be able to cobble together funding or a teaching position. Are there other barriers, or issues, that we haven't talked about yet that anyone would like to discuss?

TINA: Funding is definitely an obstacle. Part of the problem, as Angela alludes, is that funding is not thought of through the lens of accommodations, nor does it include the complexities of health care. Just like we often have to fight for accommodations, it seems we are always fighting for funding, regardless of our university.

SAM: My barriers include not only structural issues but lack of insight. The people that know about my ability status often seem to lack a fundamental awareness of what it means to be a person with chronic and mental "illnesses" (Wendell 2001). I prefer to teach face-to-face because it adds much needed structure and socializing to my life. However, teaching face-to-face takes up most of my "spoons" (Miserandino 2003). Paired with my visible queer/transness, I grapple with transphobia on a daily basis, which expends energy in ways that able-bodied, cisgender, neurotypical people do not face. When I teach, my physical body acts as a bridge for inviting students to shift toward critical consciousness, and I often need to pull up the drawbridge for the rest of the day (Anzaldúa 1990, 147–48). My colleagues will go back to their offices and work more, but I can't do that. When I teach online, I can get depressed because online work promotes social isolation. There has to be some middle-ground where I can work effectively, but I haven't been able to find that middle-ground yet. I think there is room to really delve into our consciousnesses and assess what (if any) assumptions we—scholars and academics—might hold about the lives and bodies of graduate students with disabilities. However, I feel I've been extended accommodations *already* and that I should have been able to "catch up" or "get over" whatever was preventing me from working at the expected pace. I had to tell my dissertation committee that I was so ill last semester that I made very little progress on my dissertation. It felt shameful to admit. Generally, I get the sense that not only are graduate students going through some "rite of passage," but that graduate students have not "earned" time away from our work like accomplished scholars who can reduce obligations that might interfere with their research.

ANGELA: The one thing that frustrates me most is the response I get from folks when I talk about life as a disabled graduate student. I've been told to "seriously consider the implications of forging a politics from a wounded identity." I talk about disability because I need us to "imagine otherwise," and then work to build that reality. I say *need* here not want, because academia is in a particular moment of possibility—every day there is more talk about how the status quo is unsustainable. The precariousness of graduate school for disabled people must be a part of this conversation.

We invite scholars to join us in reimagining graduate education for bodyminds like ours. This begins by examining the regimes of truth that guide our work in the academy and how these "truths" contribute to the exclusion and exploitation of disabled graduate students and other marginalized people. How can we think about "professional development" differently? How can graduate programs help students with disabilities prepare for academic futures that actively incorporate our lived realities?

First, graduate programs should consider how their politics, structures, and rituals impact disabled students. Academics should honestly assess how they participate in these systems and work with people with disabilities to increase our participation, to value different ways of thinking and being. Academia should not "accommodate" the individual but, rather, redesign programs to be inclusive from their inception. The concept of "progress" in graduate education must be one of the first things to change. University structures are rooted in progress narratives. The expectation that graduate students should engage in multiple physically, spiritually, and psychically demanding academic activities such as teaching, research, professional development, writing, networking, funding, and job searching is not a sustainable way of life for *anyone*. However, these expectations disproportionately impact students with disabilities. Practically, this means allowing flexibility in "time to completion" and recognizing that graduate students should not be considered financial burdens on departments because they require more funding. Equal funding timelines for all does not lead to equality or social justice. Departments and programs cannot see disabled graduate students as financial burdens if we value critical theory and destabilizing capitalism and other oppressive structures.

Next, graduate programs and professional organizations should provide support for professional development for disabled grad students. Establishing travel funding specifically for working-class, disabled scholars/graduate students would bolster our scholarship and participation. Organizations and conference committees can livestream, and use communication access real-time translation (CART) and American Sign Language (ASL) in some, if not all, of the sessions, as well as allow virtual presentations and participation.

Programs should illustrate a commitment to disability in course offerings, programming, and pedagogical instruction. Training should be offered for faculty, staff, and students to understand disability as a social justice issue. Some ways to incorporate disability may include workshops like "dismantling ableism" or "unpacking my ableist knapsack" to facilitate greater understanding of ableism in the academy. Scholars should reframe their disciplinary "canons" by examining canonical works through the lens of disability. With excavation, scholars may recognize that disability already exists in various disciplines, helping rupture preconceived notions about the existence of disability in academia. Likewise, programs, events, and classes should be held in buildings that are physically accessible—buildings with doors that stay open and can be opened by someone in a wheelchair or someone with fatigue; gender-neutral and physically accessible bathrooms; classrooms with easily movable furniture; adjustable lighting; and "access copies." Whenever possible, programs should be livestreamed, with CART and ASL translation or, at least, recorded.

Lastly, faculty should also develop a strong working relationship with ODS—one that goes above and beyond knowing they exist. All instructors, including TAs, should be taught how to develop accessible classes and access measures as a part of teaching *before* a student has to ask for an accommodation. It should be widely understood that teaching in an accessible way is a necessary component of inclusive, equitable education. With this, ODS should be reimagined in order to better meet the needs of graduate students. As our experiences have demonstrated, accommodations on an individual basis do not sufficiently destabilize structural ableism or reduce inequality. Thus, graduate student accommodations must be collectively revised and shared. Moreover, how to obtain them should not be part of the "unwritten" rules of academia.

We hope that our collective discussion can be a starting point for reimagining the university in a way that includes disabled bodyminds. We have posed questions that require deeper thought, and discussion, by all in academia. We have also offered concrete changes that departments and ODS can take to include bodyminds like ours. But also, we have written together to challenge the isolation that we have all felt as disabled grad students. We write together—volunteering our time, energy, and spoons—to collectivize. Finding one another, and writing together, has been our collective first step to challenging and transforming the structures that disable us.

References

AAUW. 2015. "Local Scholarships." http://www.aauw.org/what-we-do/educational-funding-and-awards/local-scholarships/

Ahmed, Sara. 2014. *Willful Subjects.* Durham, North Carolina: Duke University Press.

Anzaldúa, Gloria. 1990. "Bridge, Sandbar, Drawbridge, Island: Lesbians of Color Haciendo Alianzas." In *Bridges of Power: Women's Multicultural Alliances*, edited by Lisa Diane Albrecht and Rose M. Brewer. Philadelphia, PA: New Society Publishers.

Betcher, Sharon V. 2007. *Spirit and the Politics of Disablement*. Minneapolis: Fortress Press.

Brueggemann, Brenda and Debra A. Moddelmog. 2002. "Coming-Out Pedagogy: Risking Identity in Language and Literature Classrooms." *Pedagogy* 2(3): 311–35. doi:10.1215/15314200-2-3-311

Butler, Judith. 1990. *Gender Trouble: Feminism and the Subversion of Identity*. New York: Routledge.

Clare, Eli. 1999. *Exile and Pride: Disability, Queerness, and Liberation*, 1st ed. Cambridge, MA: South End Press.

Ferri, Beth A. and David J. Connor. 2005. "In the Shadow of Brown: Special Education and Overrepresentation of Students of Color." *Remedial and Special Education* 26(2): 93–100. doi:10.1177/07419325050260020401

Finley, Klint. 2010, January 29. "Interview with Neurodiversity Advocate Kassiane." *Technoccult*. http://technoccult.net/archives/2010/01/29/interview-with-neurodiversity-advocate-kassiane

Garrison-Wade, Dorothy F. and Gregory A. Diggs, Diane Estrada, and Rene Galindo. "Lift Every Voice and Sing: Faculty of Color Face the Challenges of the Tenure Track." *The Urban Review* 44(1): 90–112. doi:10.1007/s11256-011-0182-1

Gutiérrez y Muhs, Gabriella and Yolanda Flores Niemann, Carmen G. González, and Angela P. Harris. 2012. *Presumed Incompetent: The Intersections of Race and Class for Women in Academia*. Boulder, CO: University Press of Colorado.

Jones, Meadow. 2013, November 25. "The Able-ist Gaze: Imagining Malingering." *The Feminist Wire*. http://www.thefeministwire.com/2013/11/the-able-ist-gaze-imagining-malingering/

Keating, Ana Louise. 2000. "Risking the Personal: An Introduction." In *Interviews = Entrevistas*, edited by Gloria Anzaldúa and Ana Louise Keating. New York: Routledge.

Keating, Ana Louise. 2007. *Teaching Transformation: Transcultural Classroom Dialogues*, 1st ed. New York: Palgrave Macmillan.

Kuusisto, Stephen. 2015. "Disabling the Academy." *Planet of the Blind*. http://www.stephenkuusisto.com/uncategorized/disabling-the-academy

Linton, Simi. (1998). *Claiming Disability: Knowledge and Identity*. New York: New York University Press.

Lorde, Audre. 1988. *A Burst of Light: Essays*. Ithaca, NY: Firebrand Books.

Miserandino, Christine. 2003. "The Spoon Theory." *But You Don't Look Sick*. http://www.butyoudontlooksick.com/articles/written-by-christine/the-spoon-theory/

Moraga, Cherríe and Gloria Anzaldúa. 1981. *This Bridge Called My Back: Writings by Radical Women of Color*. 1st ed. Watertown, MA: Persephone Press.

Moss, Pamela and Isabel Dyck. 2002. *Women, Body, Illness*. Lanham, MD: Rowman & Littlefield.

Phillips, Layli. 2006. "Introduction: Womanism: On Its Own," in *The Womanist Reader*, edited by Layli Phillips. New York: Routledge.

Price, Margaret. 2015. "The Bodymind Problem and the Possibilities of Pain," *Hypatia* 30.1.

Talley, Heather Laine. 2013, November 26. "Afterword: The Disability Forum." *The Feminist Wire*. http://www.thefeministwire.com/2013/11/afterword-the-disability-forum/

Wagner, Mary and Lynn Newman, Renée Cameto, Nicolle Garza, and Phyllis Levine. 2005. *After High School: A First Look at the Postschool Experiences of Youth with Disabilities: A Report from the National Longitudinal Transition Study-2 (NLTS2)*. Menlo Park, California: Office of Special Education Programs, U.S. Department of Education. http://www.nlts2.org/reports/2005_04/ nlts2_report_2005_04_complete.pdf

Wendell, Susan. 2001. "Unhealthy Disabled: Treating Chronic Illnesses as Disabilities." *Hypatia* 16(4): 17–33.

Complicating "Coming Out"

Disclosing Disability, Gender, and Sexuality in Higher Education

RYAN A. MILLER

RICHMOND D. WYNN

KRISTINE W. WEBB

"The depression, my own sexual identity, any just regular problems I'm having in my day—[I] put forward this front that's a very positive one and so I tend to highlight my competency as a student and a positive personality," explained Marie, an undergraduate student. "The things I like, being happy, and silly, and jokey . . . those other identities fall to the background to a large extent." Within a student organization, she recalled working to overcome perceptions by others that she was unintelligent, thanks to her blonde hair and bubbly personality. She had discovered ways to manage the stigma that accompanied some of her identities by highlighting her competence and selectively disclosing her identities, processes that required significant time and energy. Marie referred to managing her identities as a complex process "that I'm not sure I've figured out yet."

Marie's experience of selective disclosure of disability and sexuality offers one depiction of the disclosure processes utilized by self-identified lesbian, gay, bisexual, transgender, and queer (LGBTQ) students with disabilities in higher education. This chapter provides a complex portrayal of the contextual and strategic disclosure processes as enacted by undergraduate and graduate students who self-identify as LGBTQ and with a disability based upon a study conducted at two public universities in the Southern United States.

The chapter first situates the study within the literature related to disclosure of disabilities and LGBTQ identities, and then presents an overview of the study's methods. Findings related to students' contextual, strategic, avoided, and comparative disclosure processes are presented and discussed.

Queer/Disability Disclosure

Depictions of "coming out of the closet," the phrase often associated with openly identifying as LGBTQ, have been utilized, expanded, and critiqued by disability studies scholars and queer theorists (McRuer 2006; Olney and Brockelman 2003; Samuels 2003; Shakespeare 1999; Sherry 2004). However, comparisons and analogies of disclosure experiences often construct disability and LGBTQ identity as mutually exclusive and may marginalize the perspectives of LGBTQ people with disabilities, along with erasing the presence of additional intersecting experiences of race, class, and other identities.

College students with disabilities may be particularly vulnerable because they experience challenges that are related to stigma and discrimination by people in their environments (Kranke, Jackson, Taylor, Anderson-Frye, and Floersch 2013). Gill's (1997) significant work on disability identity development identified four types of integration, including "'coming out' (integrating how we feel with how we present ourselves)" (39). In fact, Collins and Mowbray (2005) reported that stigma and fear of disclosure were among the biggest barriers to college students with disabilities. Identity development literature pertaining to LGBTQ students has likewise considered the role of disclosure. The heavily cited Cass (1979) model of "homosexual identity formation" (219) relies heavily upon disclosure of a gay identity, with some element of disclosure present in four of the six stages proposed in the model. Later models, though breaking from linearity, still emphasized disclosure to various degrees (D'Augelli 1994; Fassinger 1998). As a result of harassment (potential or actual), many LGBTQ students may not disclose their identity to others (Rankin 2005).

In higher education, LGBTQ students with disabilities "too often have been viewed dichotomously and disconnected, and rarely distinctively" (Harley, Nowak, Gassaway, and Savage 2002, 535). The single participant in Henry, Fuerth, and Figliozzi's (2010) study, a gay undergraduate with a physical disability, reported less discrimination due to his sexual orientation (conceived as invisible) than related to his disability, which was highly visible. Despite several theoretical and empirical works related to disability and LGBTQ identities, additional research is needed to consider the disclosure processes related to disability and sexuality undertaken by undergraduate and graduate students. This chapter aims to make a contribution toward fulfilling that need.

Methods

This qualitative study is grounded in critical and postmodern epistemologies that question existing power relations and standardized social identity categories and attempt to deconstruct dominant discourses (Lather 1991; Tierney and Rhoads 1993). Specifically, the study utilized situational analysis, a postmodern extension of grounded theory (Clarke 2005). Situational analysis is designed to generate "thick analysis" (Clarke 2005, 29) of the research problem rather than generate theory, as in traditional grounded theory. This chapter presents results related to disclosure of identities from a larger study concerned with how students conceptualize their multiple, intersecting social identities. Using situational analysis allowed the researchers to remain open to multiple, nonlinear, and seemingly contradictory approaches that students employed in disclosing their multiple identities, as evidenced by the four overlapping thematic findings presented in this chapter.

The study took place at two public universities in the Southern United States: a large, research-intensive university (University 1) and a mid-size state university (University 2). Disability and LGBTQ resource centers, and course offerings related to disability and LGBTQ identities were in place at both universities. The researchers utilized a common interview protocol at each institution but allowed for flexibility in the interview process and for participants' areas of interest to emerge. The study was approved separately by the Institutional Review Board at each institution.

Study participants included twenty-five students from University 1 and six students from University 2. Table 1 provides an overview of the participants. The researchers used purposive sampling techniques (Jones, Torres, and Arminio 2014) to recruit students satisfying particular criteria that would yield rich information: (1) present enrollment as an undergraduate or graduate student at University 1 or 2; (2) at least eighteen years of age; (3) self-identification as LGBTQ; and (4) self-identification with a disability of any kind. In accordance with this study's epistemological and methodological approach, we did not place restrictions on participation such as particular disability diagnoses or clinical labels. We recruited participants through email networks and social media postings via student affairs offices, disability and LGBTQ resource offices, and academic programs. Potential participants were asked to contact a member of the research team to discuss the study further and arrange time for a one-on-one interview lasting from one to three hours. About a third of the participants opted to have follow-up interviews to continue discussing their experiences. During data analysis, pseudonyms were assigned to all participants to protect confidentiality.

Semi-structured, in-depth interviews with participants offered the benefits of both a basic structure, through a pilot-tested interview protocol, as well as flexibility to allow students' perspectives to emerge (Jones et al. 2014; Legard, Keegan, and Ward 2003). All interviews were audio recorded and transcribed for analysis. We shared the transcripts with participants for verification and also gave each participant the opportunity to follow up with feedback about the study. Grounded theory coding methods, including first cycle (initial, in vivo, and process) coding and second cycle (focused and axial), coding were utilized (Charmaz 2006; Saldaña 2009). In vivo and process codes were identified within each interview transcript, while eighty-seven initial codes were identified across all cases and were then transformed into six focused codes and two axial codes. Initial codes related to disability and LGBTQ disclosure were reexamined in order to identify the four thematic findings presented in this chapter.

A multiplicity of backgrounds, identities, and perspectives on the team strengthened the study. The three primary researchers included: a white, queer male student affairs administrator who does not presently have a disability; an African American, gay male assistant professor and program director who does not presently have a disability; and a female white professor who has ADD and depression who identifies as heterosexual. We shared information about the study and about ourselves as researchers during each interview. All team members participated in all phases of the research, from design to analysis and writing. The researchers kept in frequent contact through telephone meetings, in which we reflected frequently on our positionalities and our own influence on the study (Jones et al. 2014). The findings presented in this chapter are the result of unanimous agreement among research team members.

In accordance with the study's critical and postmodern lenses, we sought to achieve catalytic validity with our participants (Lather 1991). A catalytic standard of validity seeks to engage participants in a research process that will raise consciousness and promote future action toward social change. Anecdotal feedback we have received from the participants attesting to the benefits of participating in the interview (i.e., increased self-awareness, mo-

Table 1. Overview of participants and identities disclosed during interviews

Pseudonym	University	Classification	Disabilities	LGBTQ identities
Abby	1	Graduate	Narcolepsy	Queer
Adrianna	1	Graduate	Addiction, anxiety, depression, eating disorders, OCD, PTSD	Bisexual
Aurora	1	Undergraduate	Anxiety, depression, neurodivergent	Non-binary/transgender, polyamorous, queer
Brad	2	Undergraduate	Asperger's, bipolar disorder, dyslexia, dysgraphia, processing disorder	Asexual, biromantic, transgender
Carlo	1	Undergraduate	ADHD	Gay
Christopher	1	Graduate	ADHD, dyslexia	Gay
Dani	1	Graduate	Visual disabilities	Gay
Desi	1	Undergraduate	ADHD, anxiety, Asperger's, depression	Demisexual, queer, transgender
Diego	1	Graduate	Anxiety, depression, narcolepsy	Gay, queer
Elijah	1	Graduate	Bipolar disorder	Gay
Ella	1	Undergraduate	Anxiety, depression, hard of hearing	Queer, transgender
Emily	2	Undergraduate	Autism spectrum disorder	Transgender
Eva	1	Undergraduate	Anxiety, depression, eating disorder, PTSD	Bisexual
Haley	1	Graduate	Depression, pregnancy	Queer
Jackie	1	Undergraduate	Anxiety, autoimmune disease, brain malformation, depression	Asexual, quoiromantic
Jason	2	Graduate	ADHD, bipolar disorder, generalized anxiety disorder, visual disabilities	Transgender
Kristen	1	Graduate	Anxiety, depression	Bisexual, queer
Lauren	2	Graduate	Hard of hearing	Bisexual
Lorenzo	2	Undergraduate	Autism spectrum disorder	Androphile, queer
Madison	1	Graduate	Autism spectrum disorder, mental health	Queer

Table 1.—*Continued*

Pseudonym	University	Classification	Disabilities	LGBTQ identities
Maria	1	Undergraduate	Anxiety, depression, PTSD	Genderqueer, queer
Marie	1	Undergraduate	Anxiety, depression	Lesbian
Miranda	1	Graduate	Anxiety, autism spectrum disorder, Lyme disease, neuromuscular condition, OCD	Asexual, panromantic, queer
Rodney	1	Graduate	ADHD, depression, heart condition	Gay
Sandy	1	Undergraduate	Anxiety, depression, OCD, sensory processing disorder	Lesbian, queer
Sebastian	1	Graduate	Lyme disease	Gay, queer
Shannon	1	Undergraduate	Anxiety, depression, frequent injuries/ temporary disabilities	Bisexual
Stan	2	Undergraduate	Autism spectrum disorder	Bisexual, transgender
Taylor	1	Undergraduate	Anxiety, depression, PTSD	Non-binary/trans, pansexual, polyamorous, queer
Will	1	Undergraduate	Asperger's	Gay
Zachary	1	Undergraduate	Tourette's syndrome	Gay, queer

tivation to explore queer/disability identities further) suggests that we have had some success in this regard.

Findings

The remainder of this chapter presents thematic findings related to disclosure of identities from the study. We address students' decisions to disclose contextually, disclose strategically, avoid disclosure, and compare processes of queer/disability disclosure. The types of identity disclosure as well as the motivation for disclosing are not represented as mutually exclusive in students' narratives, but emerged in an overlapping manner and represents intersectionality and salience of identity.

Disclosing Contextually

Students described their disability and LGBTQ identities and processes of disclosure and perception management as shifting depending upon the campus context or situation, and in relation to academics, as contingent upon particular faculty members, peers, and classroom spaces. Identity disclosure and performance shifted and evolved in context. Students described a complex process of appraising the situation before determining whether, when, and how to disclose particular social identities on campus.

Students in this study thought college faculty were undereducated about disabilities and thus they felt stigmatized by their professors. Many students seemed to adopt a situational, wait-and-see attitude before disclosing either their disability or LGBTQ identities. These beliefs were apparent from Lauren, a female graduate student who identifies as bisexual and hard of hearing:

> I would ask previous professors what their experiences were [with] my current professors to see if that was something I should be aware of. And I did have a professor, you know, say, "I would hold off unless you absolutely need to give that letter just because this professor may treat you differently." And I held off and I'm glad I did because I saw that treatment be very skewed toward another student who had a disability in my class.

The same student discussed the contextual manner in which she discloses her LGTBQ identity but she appears to be less stigmatized: "Well, usually in a social setting the fact that I am LGBT, that comes up naturally because I am very proud to talk about my partner and things like that."

The context or environment in which students were involved may play into how they identify. Lorenzo, a male undergraduate who has autism spectrum disorder (ASD) explained this scenario.

> I usually use two terms—I actually shuffle between two terms with regard to my sexuality—it really depends who I am talking to. With regards to my sexuality, I identify as a queer individual in the sense of queer as an umbrella term for all LGBT people, but I also identify specifically when I am talking to other queer individuals as an androphile.

Some college students who have disabilities may experience functional limitations or lags in development that can make the transition to adulthood difficult and could ultimately affect their self-sufficiency, independent living (Leavey 2005), and abilities to identify contextual opportunities to disclose either LGBTQ or disability identities. Lorenzo reported, "That's why it's quite common, I think, for people to be on the autism spectrum, for example, a-gender or gender-neutral identified because they never picked up gender socialization when they were younger. They're just neutral or they don't really consider themselves to be a gendered person." Lorenzo elaborated on this idea:

> I acknowledge that when I was younger, and this was largely as the result of having Asperger's Syndrome, I wasn't perfectly socialized into the gender of being a male when I was younger and my parents never really sweated it. It wasn't until I got secondary sex characteristics and people started to really acknowledge me, especially within the LGTB community, that people started to regard me as a masculine person that I started to hold on to the idea of being masculine.

Stan, a male undergraduate student who identifies as transgender and bisexual, and has ASD and anxiety disorder, expressed his progression with his identities. He appears to have developed an earlier sense of his LGBTQ identity; however, he may have experienced difficulty deciding in which contexts he should disclose.

> When you're a child and you're trans, there isn't really any angst or anything going on, you're fairly happy about it. You're a few pills away from being where you want to be, that's not bad. But then your parents respond to it and your friends respond to it and it instills this level of self-loathing. That's the suicide rate right there: where you're beaten up and told that you're confused and stuff.

Thus, for Stan, initial disclosures of transgender identity may lead to significant backlash and fuel self-doubt.

Most participants described their disclosure decisions as dependent on context; for example, assessing whether they had formed a close relationship with someone. Sebastian described trying to come out as gay in a "natural way": "What I mean by that is if someone says, 'Do you have a girlfriend or something?' I'll just correct them and be like, 'I don't date girls, but no I'm single.'" Kristen acknowledged that relationships could change substantially depending upon disclosure decisions and that it was thus necessary to evaluate likely reactions from others ahead of time. Similarly, Marie went through a process of deciding whether a relationship was important:

> I need to have a relationship with that person. If this is someone I'm only going to see in class twice every week and not going to have much of a relationship with, there's no point for me in taking that risk and bringing it up. But if it's someone I'm seeing a lot that I have a friendship with, to some extent I do want them to know, because it impacts so much of the way I interact with people, both of these things. I want to be able to say, "Hey, I'm going on a date," and be able to have a conversation about that, or, "Hey, I had a really shitty day yesterday," and have a conversation about that.

Marie placed a significant value on building trust within the context of a relationship before she would be willing to disclose her identities. Though many participants based disclosure decisions on context, some participants generally preferred to disclose their identities. Jackie skewed toward disclosing when possible:

> I guess the people that I'm friends with that I start a relationship with, then I immediately give up the information. . . . But I think just the way I was raised, I don't see a fault in myself. Like I don't see that it's a bad thing that I should hide. It's a shitty thing that I have to deal with, but I'm dealing with it and it's affecting who I am. I'm like, "Yeah, I got an autoimmune disease and a brain malformation."

By contrast, Madison felt no need to disclose if the situation did not arise or she did not see it as relevant: "Basically, the way I work for all things is if it comes up, I'll talk about it, but a lot of things just don't come up." Madison offered the example of sharing an office with another graduate student who wondered why she received exam accommodations. Explaining that such conversations did not always go well, she tended not to disclose if she did not find it relevant.

Disclosing Strategically

Students assessed particular contexts and situations, as described in the previous section, and faced decisions around whether and how to disclose identities. Disclosure of LGBTQ and disability identities was linked to strategic and political decisions of acting to educate others and serve as an embodied representative of a particular identity group. Identity performance in the classroom, particularly informing others, came with consequences, such as burnout and disengagement. Participants also highlighted the ways in which they performed particular social identities at various times and spaces (Butler 1993).

Contextual disclosures of identities could become strategic disclosures that participants used to accomplish certain goals. Ella described her approach in class as one of "strategic outness" in sharing her trans identity and going through a number of questions about the utility of coming out in the moment to achieve goals of advocacy and visibility. Diego also shared that when leading a student group or meeting with administrators, he carefully considered when he needed to "put a face" on an identity such as disability or queerness so that he could advocate most effectively. Passing also figured into strategic disclosure. For example, Abby described herself as "not visibly disabled, so I am [a] lot more selective about who I talk to about that." The notion of disclosing strategically depends, in large part, on one's ability to either pass or not feel the need to disclose.

Everyday disclosures of being queer were important to Kristen for political reasons:

> I think being a member of the LGBT community is very important to me. I try to make a point, depending on the circumstances or who I am talking to, of self-identifying, just telling people about my sexual orientation and my identities. Mostly because I want people to be aware that this isn't just a heteronormative society. Not everyone walking around is obviously attracted to the opposite sex and it's not all cookie-cutter.

Strategic disclosure applied not only to goals related to visibility and awareness but also related to personal risks and benefits. In trying to assess others' reactions ahead of time, Marie weighed the costs and benefits of disclosure:

> For me, it's always trying to judge beforehand, "What is this person's reaction going to be?" The anxiety can make it really hard to share that with people, because running through your head you're like, "Oh, no! What if they freak out? What if they say something really nasty?" All of these things. But it's just trying to suss out, "Have they said things before that make it sound like they'd be OK with this?" Obviously,

it's a lot easier to talk about these things with someone who is also affected by them.

Lauren described how she decided whether or not to disclose when she knew she would have required interaction with her peers in class.

At the undergraduate level when we were in a class, and we were supposed to share about ourselves on this drawing, and there was a guy in the class that did something about him and his partner and the other students' response to it was extremely disrespectful, like, one girl who said, "I'm sorry I can't listen to this," and started quoting Bible verses and stuff like that. That's when I knew that me being who I was—I had to change my answers on some of my things because I didn't want to be affiliated with that, because I was going to have to work with these people for the next four months.

Both Marie and Lauren sought to assure themselves there would be a positive reaction if they came out or they would avoid disclosure if they anticipated hostility.

Avoiding Disclosure

A few participants said they sought to avoid disclosure whenever possible. Ella talked about being outed as trans against her will or inadvertently. For example, the university used Ella's legal name when she first became a student, but she eventually was able to correct it, which she appreciated. Rodney's unintentional disclosure came as a result of using Facebook as an undergraduate when it was new and marking that he preferred men on his profile without the understanding that family might find out. He still avoided disclosure when he thought it was unnecessary, such as in conversation if someone saw his wedding ring and assumed he was married to a woman. For Rodney, seeking to avoid unnecessary disclosure characterized not only his queer identity but also his multiracial identity.

Diego also avoided what he referred to as the "coming out ritual" but eventually discovered that opting out of the process could lead to unanticipated consequences.

[Refusing to come out as gay] led to confusion with one of my very best friends, who thought that I was like horribly in the closet and needed to go see a therapist. It's like, no, I just don't want to share that. I thought when I came here, very deliberately that I was just going to keep a professional identity. Then I realized, probably my second or third year, that that's only possible to an extent unless I want to be happy and normal—to not think of this place as hell.

Brad described how he avoided disclosure of his transgender identity in an attempt to benefit from participating in a religious group on campus; a resource he believed would help him develop his spiritual identity.

They have groups which are well intended but like they are gender seg-regated and . . . a lot of people knew me before I even came out to myself as transgender so they all knew me by my girl name. They saw me as a girl; they refuse like to acknowledge that I could be anything differ-ent. They had me and my partner join groups—which was fine for my partner, not so much for me, because they made me join the girls group and I did not want to. I ended up joining mostly because I was like well I can probably still get things out of it and I hadn't even come out to them at all, so they still didn't have any reason to think I should be in a guys' group and I've since stopped going to those groups.

Adrianna preferred to avoid disclosure unless necessary and had in mind a particular image from which she wanted to distance herself, saying, "I don't want to be the political queer. I don't want to be 'the gay student,' I don't want that identity. I don't mind it. But I'd rather be the intellectual who has interesting things to say." For some students, avoiding active disclosure of sexuality and disability was preferred.

Natalie, a transgender female who identifies with autism spectrum dis-orders and several other disabilities, found safe places although she hadn't disclosed either a disability or LGBT identity.

The only place that I can say was effective for me was our high school Latin classes and Latin Club, which at the time, again I was not iden-tifying myself in any way. The Latin Club there and the Latin classes tended to attract most of the people with queer identities. It was a safe place to be and to exist.

Although Stan did not formally disclose to his classmates during his years in high school, he did not deny or negate his LGBT identity:

Being a queer person in modern schools, I learned to duck when I heard somebody say "faggot," you know? I'd hear it shouted across a field and then I'd see a filled coke bottle land in the dirt because they were calling me "faggot" and throwing stuff at me. There's nobody to talk to about that shit, you know? I didn't have anybody to go to. So, you're just by yourself.

Thus, participants explained a variety of reasons they occasionally or routinely avoided disclosing disability and/or LGBTQ identities.

Comparing Queer/Disability Disclosure

Lastly, participants compared processes and circumstances for coming out as queer or disabled. Sebastian humorously compared the ritualized queer coming out story with disability:

It always comes up in a moment. It's never this thing, or I need to sit them down and like, "Tonight's the night." I make a special dinner and hope it goes really smoothly. I'm going to tell them I have Lyme disease. It's always contextual. It's always what should be said in the moment.

This comparison seemed to illustrate Sebastian's preferred approach for disclosure to be an ordinary, everyday act, around both having Lyme disease and being gay. Desi described both disclosure processes as contextual: "With individuals that I don't really know, I don't really mention it. I don't feel like it's something that they need to know unless it's in the context of doing something for a student organization or it's in the context of talking about social justice with them." Desi often linked disclosure decisions to opportunities to educate others about marginalized communities, and he found it important to share his identities in those situations.

Jackie disclosed her sexuality less readily than disability because she viewed her asexual identity as operating in the background and being less salient overall, explaining that she had "other stuff to worry about." Similarly, Madison described disclosures of sexuality as less prominent since she was not looking for a relationship. Disability disclosures, on the other hand, became more important: "Right now, the disability ones tend to be the most, just because they affect me more than other ones. As I said, the queer identity is kind of on the back burner and I'm not really dating anyone. I'm not actively looking for relationships, so it's not as relevant." Madison felt disability more actively shaped her daily experience, and thus she disclosed disability more often.

Lauren was raised in a family immersed in Deaf culture. She relayed the following story about her mother's ideas about her LGBTQ identity:

> I do think it is interesting to note that not only am I hard of hearing, I grew up as a CODA, which is a child of a deaf adult; which that itself is another community. They are a group of people that do not have that disability but grew up in that community. It's interesting. I know my mom thinks that I started liking girls because of being CODA, which I guess there is a high percentage of CODA who are identifying with LGBT. I told my mom it had nothing to do with that.

Family dynamics could present challenges around disclosure. Eva contrasted her experience of going through mental health struggles with disclosing her sexuality:

> In our family, all you need is more familial support. Therapy is like a way to trap you, something like that. It just wasn't a super positive view. Even though, some people needed it. Stuff like that. That stigma still scares me and freaks me out sometimes, which is why I'm more hesitant to tell people that I'm struggling emotionally or something like that, versus being open about my sexuality because apparently, now it's somewhat cool to be gay, which is true to an extent.

Stan, an undergraduate student, attempted to seek support from an LGBT group but didn't find the assistance he wanted.

> I went into the gay youth help thingy center and it was political. It had sort of that angry atmosphere that I just . . . and it was cliquish and so I just thought about going to some of the meetings that they have, but I mean I have anxiety problems and going to something like that alone: that's not great.

For Stan, venturing into an LGBT-identified space triggered his anxiety and could necessitate additional disclosures. Another student, Adrianna, was forthcoming about her sexuality but private about her experiences with addiction and eating disorders due to stigma. Dani contrasted her experiences of disclosing sexuality readily with being more cautious around disability.

> I normally only talk about my disability if I trust someone. I would say that is not necessarily true with my sexuality. I don't know how much that is because of my current context, where I feel like in school in general I will not get a negative reaction to having a same-sex partner. I don't know what kind of reaction I'll get to having a disability. But I find that for the most part people already know. If they don't, they're not paying attention. I think disability is harder. Partially because, it's funny, I don't want to be seen as different. I don't want to be seen as less able in an academic way. I think that there are few people who would see my sexuality as making me less academically able. They're just not related in the same way.

Dani viewed potential reactions to disclosure of disability and sexuality as fundamentally different. Sexuality could often be disclosed readily, while disability required a more cautious evaluation of context and relationships.

Brad compared disclosure of his disability and gender identities particularly in academic settings. He described a history of traumatic experiences related to being targeted because of his disabilities, yet he was comfortable disclosing his disability in class, but not his gender identity:

> In middle school, I couldn't read as fast as them. I was extremely socially awkward and there was a point I was in special ed. I was made fun of all the time and they beat me up on numerous occasions. . . . Teachers dismissed it as that's just how kids are. Now, in classroom settings like I know that my teachers by law have to follow my accommodations and so I don't get too worried about that, but like I am absolutely terrified of telling my teachers my preferred name and preferred pronouns.

Despite the difficulty he faced in the past related to his disabilities, Brad believed that current legal protections allow for easier disclosure of his disability identity in academic settings while the lack of protections related to gender identity inhibited him from disclosing that aspect of himself.

Conclusions

Students' descriptions of their decisions to disclose their identities contextually illustrate the complexity of identity management. In this chapter, we described four intersecting approaches to disclosure of queer/disability identities that students described employing in their higher education experiences: disclosing contextually, disclosing strategically, avoiding disclosure, and comparing queer/disability disclosure. These processes were fluid and evolving, as students described times when they might avoid disclosure and other circumstances when they deemed it important to disclose their identities and thus start an educational conversation or carve out a comfortable environment for themselves. The findings from this study affirm and extend Jason Orne's (2011, 2013) work on strategic (LGBTQ) outness and identity management to incorporate disability and intersectional queer/disabled experiences. For example, Orne (2013) highlighted that "queer people can use alternative identifications to fine-tune the management of their identity," a concept that this study extends to disability and queer/disability identity intersections, as participants in this study employed various identity labels contextually. Further, this work suggests that an uncritical celebration of a linear process of "coming out" regardless of context or circumstances should continue to be reconsidered (Klein, Holtby, Cook, and Travers 2015). Instead of viewing "coming out" as the pinnacle of identity development, it is important to understand the nuanced disclosure decision making that individuals invoke as a way of managing the benefits and risks of disclosure and as a way of reinforcing their own agency.

Several questions emerged from this study that clearly warrant further investigation. Previous research indicated the type of disability impacted whether students with disabilities completed college degrees (Pingry O'Neill, Markward, and French 2012). Future work ought to explore whether and how type of disability also affects the timing of LGBTQ or disability disclosure. Several students with ASD participated in the current study and many indicated they disclosed their LGBTQ identities after their disabilities were diagnosed, suggesting an area for future exploration. We also wonder about the relationship between disclosure of LGBTQ identities and mental health/psychological disabilities. Mental health issues among LGBTQ young adults are well documented in the literature (i.e., Heck, Flentji, and Cochran 2011; Wyatt and Oswalt 2014); however, given the number of participants who disclosed mental health disabilities such as anxiety or depression, questions arise about the bearing these disclosure have on students' mental health and orientations toward disclosure processes.

In this study, disclosure decisions needed to be made in large part because most students identified with disabilities considered invisible or hidden. Likewise, some participants judged themselves as able to pass for cisgender/heterosexual and thus not always assumed to identify as LGBTQ. Contextual disclosure decisions balanced students' goals such as benefiting themselves or others, or disclosing strategically to accomplish activist, educational, or political ends. Many discussed the importance of having a relationship with someone, such as a friend or family member, or having a potential relationship, such as an academic advisor or research colleague, before disclosing. Comparisons were made between disclosing queer and disability identities, with students generally exhibiting a less involved process in deciding to disclose queerness as opposed to disability, which sometimes warranted careful calculations, particularly in contexts such as employment and teaching. Some students tended to avoid disclosure altogether when possible to avoid stigma or lamented that, at times, they were inadvertently outed.

Ideally, these findings will contribute to an enhanced awareness among educators, administrators, and policymakers. Much existing literature on students with disabilities and LGBTQ students in higher education suggests, by omission, that the two groups are mutually exclusive (Harley et al. 2002). As educators begin to recognize the reality of students' multiple identities, they must understand that the experiences of LGBTQ students with disabilities will not necessarily mirror that of heterosexual/cisgender students with disabilities or LGBTQ students without disabilities. This chapter suggests that students may draw strength from the ability to holistically consider their experiences related to multiple identities, but that they may also be subject to more stigma and discrimination than their peers as they continually consider whether and how to disclose disability and LGBTQ identities in higher education. Students carefully take in information about the climate in each classroom and campus and, in turn, decide whether and how to disclose their identities. This suggests that educators must be attuned to improving both active (e.g., interrupting hateful comments in class) and passive (e.g., providing visual and textual representations of diverse identities) components of educational spaces so that all students feel valued and free to disclose their identities if they so choose. Students who feel valued and know that their voices matter are more likely to remain engaged in all aspects of academic life. This reinforces their engagement and resilience and leads to overall personal and professional success (Hill and Wang 2015; Owen and Dunne 2013; Thomas and Hanson 2014).

References

Butler, Judith. 1993. *Bodies That Matter*. New York: Routledge.

Cass, Vivienne C. 1979. "Homosexual Identity Formation: A Theoretical Model." *Journal of Homosexuality* 4 (3): 219–35. doi:10.1300/j082v04n03_01

Charmaz, Kathy. 2006. *Constructing Grounded Theory: A Practical Guide through Qualitative Analysis*. Thousand Oaks, CA: Sage.

Clarke, Adele E. 2005. *Situational Analysis: Grounded Theory after the Postmodern Turn*. Thousand Oaks, CA: Sage.

Collins, Mary Elizabeth, and Carol T. Mowbray. 2005. "Higher Education and Psychiatric Disabilities: National Survey of Campus Disability Services." *American Journal of Orthopsychiatry* 75: 304–15. doi:10.1037/0002–9432.75.2.304

D'Augelli, Anthony R. 1994. "Identity Development and Sexual Orientation: Toward a Model of Lesbian, Gay, and Bisexual Development." In *Human Diversity: Perspectives on People in Context*, edited by Edison J. Trickett, Roderick J. Watts, and Dina Birman, 312–33. San Francisco: Jossey Bass.

Fassinger, Ruth E. 1998. "Lesbian, Gay, and Bisexual Identity and Student Development Theory." In *Working with Lesbian, Gay, Bisexual, and Transgender College Students: A Handbook for Faculty and Administrators*, edited by Ronni L. Sanlo, 13–22. Westport, CT: Greenwood Press.

Gill, Carol J. "Four Types of Integration in Disability Identity Development." *Journal of Vocational Rehabilitation* 9, no. 1 (1997): 39–46.

Harley, Debra A., Theresa Nowak, Linda J. Gassaway, and Todd A. Savage. 2002. "Lesbian, Gay, Bisexual and Transgender College Students with Disabilities: A Look at Multiple Cultural Minorities." *Psychology in the Schools* 39 (5): 525–38. doi:10.1002/pits.10052

Heck, Nicholas C., Annesa Flentje, and Bryan N. Cochran. 2011. "Offsetting Risks: High School Gay-Straight Alliances and Lesbian, Gay Bisexual, and Transgender (LGBT) Youth." *School Psychology Quarterly* 26 (2): 161–74. doi:10.1037/a0023226

Henry, Wilma J., Katherine Fuerth, and Jennifer Figliozzi. 2010. "Gay with a Disability: A College Student's Multiple Cultural Journey." *College Student Journal* 44 (2): 377–88.

Hill, Nancy E., and Ming-Te Wang. 2015. "From Middle School to College: Developing Aspirations, Promoting Engagement, and Indirect Pathways from Parenting to Post High School Enrollment." *Developmental Psychology* 51 (2): 224–35. doi:10.1037/a0038367

Jones, Susan R., Vasti Torres, and Jan Arminio. 2014. *Negotiating the Complexities of Qualitative Research in Higher Education*. 2nd ed. New York: Routledge.

Klein, Kate, Alix Holtby, Katie Cook, and Robb Travers. 2015. "Complicating the Coming out Narrative: Becoming Oneself in a Heterosexist and Cissexist

World." *Journal of Homosexuality* 62 (3): 297–326. doi:10.1080/00918369.2014.9 70829

Kranke, Derrick, Sarah E. Jackson, Debbie A. Taylor, Eileen Anderson-Frye, and Jerry Floersch. 2013. "College Student Disclosure of Non-apparent Disabilities to Receive Classroom Accommodations." *Journal of Postsecondary Education and Disability* 26 (1): 35–51.

Lather, Patti. 1991. *Getting Smart: Feminist Research and Pedagogy with/in the Postmodern.* New York: Routledge.

Leavey, JoAnn Elizabeth. 2005. "Youth Experiences of Living with Mental Health Problems: Emergence, Loss Adaptation and Recovery." *Canadian Journal of Community Mental Health,* 24 (2): 109–26. doi:10.7870/cjcmh-2005-0018

Legard, Robin, Jill Keegan, and Kit Ward. 2003. "In-depth Interviews." In *Qualitative Research Practice: A Guide for Social Science Students and Researchers,* edited by Jane Ritchie and Jane Lewis, 138–69. London: Sage.

McRuer, Robert. 2006. *Crip Theory: Cultural Signs of Queerness and Disability.* New York: New York University Press.

Olney, Marjorie F., and Karin F. Brockelman. 2003. "Out of the Disability Closet: Strategic Use of Perception Management by Select University Students with Disabilities." *Disability & Society,* 18: 35–50. doi:10.1080/ 713662200

Orne, Jason. 2011. "'You Will Always Have to "Out" Yourself': Reconsidering Coming Out through Strategic Outness." *Sexualities* 14 (6): 681–703. doi:10.1177/1363460711420462

Orne, Jason. 2013. "Queers in the Line of Fire: Goffman's Stigma Revisited." *The Sociological Quarterly* 54 (2): 229–53. doi:10.1111/tsq.12001

Owen, Derfel, and Elizabeth Dunne. 2013. *The Student Engagement Handbook: Practice in Higher Education.* United Kingdom: Emerald.

Pingry O'Neill, Laura N., Martha J. Markward, and Joshua P. French. 2012. "Predictors of Graduation among College Students with Disabilities." *Journal of Postsecondary Education & Disability* 25 (1): 21–36.

Rankin, Susan R. 2005. "Campus Climates for Sexual Minorities." *New Directions for Student Services* 2005 (111): 17–23. doi:10.1002/ss.170

Saldaña, Johnny. 2009. *The Coding Manual for Qualitative Researchers.* London: Sage.

Samuels, Ellen. 2003. "My Body, My Closet: Invisible Disability and the Limits of Coming-Out Discourse." *GLQ: A Journal of Lesbian and Gay Studies* 9 (1–2): 233–55. doi:10.1215/10642684-9-1-2-233

Shakespeare, Tom. 1999. "Coming Out and Coming Home." *International Journal of Sexuality and Gender Studies* 4 (1): 39–51. doi:10.1023/a:1023202424014

Sherry, Mark. 2004. "Overlaps and Contradictions between Queer Theory and Disability Studies." *Disability & Society* 19 (7): 769–83. doi:10.1080/0968759042000284231

Thomas, Gail B., and Janet Hanson. 2014. "Developing Social Integration to Enhance Student Retention and Success in Higher Education; The GROW@BU Initiative." *Widening Participation & Lifelong Learning 16* (3): 58–70. doi:10.5456/wpll.16.3.58

Tierney, William, and Robert Rhoads. 1993. "Postmodernism and Critical Theory in Higher Education: Implications for Research and Practice." In *Higher Education: Handbook of Theory and Research* (vol. 9), edited by John C. Smart, 308–43. New York: Agathon Press.

Wyatt, Tammy, and Sara Oswalt. 2014. "Sexual Behaviors of College Freshmen and the Need for University-Based Education." *College Student Journal* 48 (4): 603–13.

Students with Disabilities
in Higher Education

Welfare, Stigma Management, and Disclosure

KATHERINE D. SEELMAN

In college, Sam used Supplemental Security Income (SSI) and Medicaid for income and health services and supports. He transitioned through school with a goal of full employment after graduation. Sam did not feel comfortable disclosing his disability or his use of SSI, which is often referred to as welfare. Does the use of SSI, even as an income support during college, add to the burden of disability stigma and complicate disclosure? If so, what educational and social policy strategies might help alleviate this burden for college students? Very few scholars have published about the impact of the SSI benefit on a student's identity, student willingness to disclose, or public attitudes about SSI and students with disabilities. While many students with disabilities will function within a university context of mainstream norms and a human services context of Social Security programs, there is scant literature examining these intersecting student experiences. The purpose of this chapter is to explore the role of stigma at the intersection of disability and public welfare, such as SSI, and consider implications for social policy and higher education practice.

Supplemental Security Income and Postsecondary Students

SSI is a program administered within the U.S. Social Security Administration. SSI provides a uniform federal income floor while optional state programs supplement that floor (U.S. Social Security Administration 2015). The SSI program makes cash assistance payments to aged, blind, and disabled persons (including children), who have limited income and resources. The federal government funds SSI from general tax revenues. In 2014, the federal benefit rate for SSI was $721 per month for a qualified person. Students on SSI are eligible for Earned-Income Exclusions. For 2014, the amount of earnings that will have no effect on eligibility or benefits for SSI beneficiaries who are students is $7,060 a year. Assuming little or no other income, students with disabilities receiving SSI are poor.

In some states, those who are SSI beneficiaries may be automatically eligible for Medicaid; an SSI application is also an application for Medicaid. In other states, potential beneficiaries must apply for and establish eligibility for Medicaid with another agency. Medicaid is administered by states within a framework of federal guidelines. The Medicaid program is funded jointly by states and the federal government. States may opt to pay for services such as personal attendants and assistive technology. Perhaps nothing tries a family's or a student's patience more than the process of deciphering the obscure requirements for eligibility to Social Security benefits or attempting to analyze a complex table about supports provided by a higher education institution.

At the University of Pittsburgh in 2012, students organized Students for Disability Advocacy (SDA). A number of SDA members were receiving SSI (Lalwani 2012). They tended to adopt a pragmatic approach about their use of SSI, viewing it as a bridge to careers, paying taxes, and avoiding poverty. But programs such as SSI may themselves create barriers for these students. A number of SDA students are or will be candidates for prestigious income stipends and awards but will also require personal attendant services (PAS) in order to get out of bed in the morning. SSI is the gateway to Medicaid and Medicaid is the public payer of Personal Attendant Services. SSI has income eligibility limits that will bar acceptance of some prestigious academic awards.

Professionals who have responsibilities for supporting these students on campus, such as mentors and counselors, also bear some responsibility for becoming familiar with these data, programs, and policies. Just how many students are enrolled in higher education and what is known about their disabilities, race, and economic status? These questions are not easily answered because of scant availability and quality of data.

Stigma at the Intersections of SSI, Disability, Postsecondary Education, and Employment

As increasing numbers of students with disabilities enroll in postsecondary education, there is an increasing presence on campus of students receiving SSI and other social security benefits. A 2004 study by Berry, Conway, and Chang showed that recipients of Social Security Disability Insurance (SSDI) and Supplemental Security Income (SSI) programs represented 8.3 percent of all undergraduates with disabilities or 125,000 students. Of these students, 57 percent or 71,000 received SSDI benefits, 36 percent were SSI beneficiaries and 7 percent or 8,000 received both. The study suggested that race of students with disabilities intersected with disability and poverty in the SSI program. A recent study (Raue and Lewis 2011) showed growing enrollment of students with disabilities in postsecondary degree-granting institutions. These institutions reported enrolling approximately 707,000 students with disabilities in the twelve-month 2008–09 academic year, with about half of these students reported enrolled in public two-year institutions. Approximately 11 percent of the institutions responding to the study provided disability benefits counseling, including Supplemental Security Income (SSI), Social Security Disability Income (SSDI), Medicare, and Medicaid.

The profile of students with disabilities in higher education is changing in ways that have further implications for students' disclosures. In 2009, the U.S. Government Accountability Office (GAO) issued a report entitled *Higher Education and Disability* (United States Government Accountability Office 2009). As table 2 shows, students reported having a range of disabilities, but the distribution of disability types has changed from 2000 to 2008. For example, the proportion of students that reported having attention deficit disorder had increased from 7 to 19 percent. Overall, the largest group of students with disabilities is those with mental and cognitive disabilities.

The meanings students themselves give to disability, decisions about disclosure, and stigma management have been captured in a number of narrative and descriptive studies (Fuller, Healey, Bradley, and Hall 2004; Hutcheon and Wolbring 2012; Jacklin 2011; Kranke, Jackson, Taylor, Anderson-Frye, and Floersch 2013). Students who are perceived as having less severe disabilities may be stigmatized because of the special treatment they receive, which is not available to nondisabled students (Porter 2015). Students with invisible disability moving into the job market may not disclose for fear of becoming less competitive if their disabilities are disclosed.

Further, accounts of stigma-related commentary about welfare recipients have been reported by the popular press. In an article in the *Pittsburgh Post-Gazette* (Giammarise 2013), a Pennsylvania state legislator commented about a proposed name change from Department of Welfare to Department of Human Services. He opined: "Why in the world would we want to rename the Department of Public Welfare? . . . I think there should be a stigmatism for being on welfare. . . . You should not be satisfied with living off the fruit of your neighbor's labor." Nonetheless, the name was changed to the Department of Human Services, in part due to strong advocacy by the Pennsylvania disability community. Deborah Stone (1984), a social policy analyst, argued that disability carries a heavy load of meaning by serving as a welfare category used by the state to reconcile tensions between two different distributive principles, work and aid. In turn, and with seeming sarcasm, Stone noted those "privileged" by being categorized as disabled are subject to handicap and stigma.

Conceptualizing Stigma at the Intersection

A relevant and rich body of interdisciplinary disability studies scholarship about stigma exists in the social sciences, public policy, and the humanities, which is helpful in understanding the potential impact on disabled students of aid programs. These approaches and concepts routinely locate the problem of stigma at both the individual and social systems levels. Scholarly works by Goffman (1963); Stone (1984); Garland Thomson (1997); and Schur, Kruse,

Table 2. (GAO Table 7) **Percentage of distribution of main type of disability among postsecondary (undergraduate) students with disabilities, 2000, 2004, and 2008 percentage**

Main Type of Disability	2000	2004	2008
Mental, emotional or psychiatric condition/ depression	17.1	22.4	24.3
Attention deficit disorder	6.7	11.6	19.1
Orthopedic or mobility impairment	29.0	24.8	15.1
Other	13.2	5.8	15.0
Specific learning, dyslexia	5.0	7.7	8.9
Hearing impairment or problem	15.1	17.3	5.8
Blindness or visual impairment	5.2	3.7	2.7
Speech or language impairment	.03	.05	0.7
Brain injury	1.2	1.0	1.7
Developmental disability	0.6	0.6	0.7

and Blank (2013) have produced concepts and other analytic tools useful in conceptualizing and analyzing stigma, including intersectionality of disability with poverty and race.

Stigma and Social Acceptance

In a classic study, sociologist Erving Goffman, who is not associated with disability studies but rather with social psychology, described the relationship of stigma to social acceptance of people with disabilities, racial minorities, and those who are poor, as well as the relationship between stigma and internalized oppression. In his seminal work, *Stigma*, Goffman (1963) provides the reader with a definition of stigma and an introduction to the social assumptions that lead to categorizing a person as ordinary or categorizing a person as different.

Attributes of the ordinary person are adopted by society as social normative expectations that distinguish the ordinary person from the person who is different. The "different" person may be viewed as stigmatic if he or she has one or more types of stigma. Goffman posits three types of stigma. They are: (a) abominations of the body, which are various physical deformities; (b) blemishes of individual character, including mental disorders and unemployment, and (c) tribal stigma, such as race and religion. The stigmatized person is perceived as having a virtual identity that corresponds with one or more of the types of stigma. His or her virtual identity may contrast with his or her actual identity. Stigma occurs when a person has an attribute that is deeply discrediting. Goffman describes the stigmatized individual as disqualified from social acceptance. He then distinguishes between the discredited and the discreditable individual. The discredited individual possesses an attribute that is already known by others, while the discreditable individual has an attribute that is unknown. This situation, of course, resembles that of the student with either a visible disability or a hidden disability.

Stigma generates issues for the individual in the presence of so-called normals. The discredited individual is not sure about how normal people will identify and view him. The discredited individual has a visible disability so he or she must devise a stigma management strategy to handle the tensions generated by being unsure of social acceptance. If the individual is discreditable, hiding his disability, he or she may attempt to control information so as to mask the stigmatic attribute. He or she may employ passing as a stigma management strategy.

Cultural Perspective

In *Extraordinary Bodies*, Rosemarie Garland Thomson (1997) approaches the development of stigma by associating disability with a representation system akin to race and gender. Her central questions involve clarification of how cultural representation attaches meaning to the physical differences we term disability. Decidedly feminist in approach, she supplements her analysis of the cultural representation of disability and the intersection of body and culture using Goffman's explanation of stigma. While Goffman understands disability as a stigmatic attribute enshrined in social norms, Garland Thomson locates disability as an attribute embedded in culture. She views disability as corporeal deviance, which is a property, not of the body but as a product of cultural rules. Goffman describes the normal individual, the ordinary person, and sometime refers to them as "normals" and Garland Thomson introduces the term "normate"—a composite identity of individuals who do not have stigmatized identifiers. She deconstructs perspectives on body properties as individual attributes and reconstructs them as products of cultural rules about bodies. She questions why differences within social groups are not simply perceived without assigning negative value attributed to disability. Chiding Goffman for his inattention to justice issues, Garland Thomson forcefully asserts that stigma theory reminds us that the problems involve inequalities, negative attitudes, misrepresentations, and institutional practices that result in the process of stigmatization.

The *Disabled State*

Political scientist Deborah Stone forcefully argued that the social status of people with disabilities is related to technical decisions within bureaucracies, informed by political pressures and public consensus about redistribution policy. Stone's *The Disabled State* (1984) begins with a quote by Alexis De Tocqueville, a great chronicler of U.S. democracy. De Tocqueville reminds us: "Nothing is as difficult as the nuances which separate unmerited misfortune from an adversity produced by vice. . . ." Stone carries forward De Tocqueville's insight as she analyzes the meaning of disability stigma in public programs from which human service systems are built and implemented and on which so many people with disabilities depend. She locates the perpetuation of disability stigma, which she views as mostly unmerited, in government disability policy and administration.

Her central question is: What is the meaning of expansion of disability programs in advanced industrial societies? Like Goffman, Stone is interested in categorization of disability. While Goffman defined stigma and the categorization of the attributes of stigma and its impact on social identity, Stone is interested in the administrative category of disability used in social programs and its impact on perceptions of disabled individuals. She notes that governments ascribe a highly flexible meaning to disability so that it can be used to give coherence to their activities related to two major public resource redistribution principles: work and aid. On the one hand, she recognizes that social meaning of work is positive, deeply embedded in Western values such as the Protestant Ethic. On the other, she joins many other social commentators in recognizing that the social meaning of aid is often negative, associated with inability, laziness, and dishonesty (Blumkin, Margalioth, and Sadka 2008). Recipients of social aid are often people with disabilities, including students. To apply Goffman's term, they are discredited or discreditable people.

Stone notes that the administrative category of disability creates a political privilege in the form of social aid and exemptions from certain obligations of citizenship but entails handicaps, social stigma, dependence, isolation, and economic disadvantage. For Stone, the growth of social programs perpetuates stigma. Disability programs are overloaded with clients whose health has been impacted by industrial and other environmental pollutants. Health costs for these individuals are mainly absorbed by the public sector often in the form of taxes that pay for social programs.

Stone seeks to refute the various stereotypes associated with those receiving social aid, such as inability, laziness, and dishonesty. She observes that common wisdom blames the user of social aid, who is generally assumed to be seeking to maximize his well-being—an argument derived from classical liberal theory. Stone argues that the flexibility of the administrative category of disability provides moral, medical, and clinical opportunities to expand. Various interests over time have manipulated the disability category in social programs to their advantage—such as legislators bowing to the demand of constituencies by adding additional conditions and diseases. As a result, the numbers of people on social programs and their costs have dramatically increased. Stone explains that program expansion has unbalanced the relationship among public resources allocated to make profit, resources committed to worker wages, and resources committed to taxes. She notes that society and governments have options. For example, they can choose to redistribute responsibility for health impacts to employers (toxic substances and environmentally caused illness, workers' injuries) and to workers through requirements of health maintenance.

Socioeconomic Exclusion

Lisa Schur, a political scientist; Douglas Kruse, an economist; and Peter Blanck, a lawyer and social scientist, apply a broad sweep of economic, social, and political analysis to inclusion and exclusion of people with disabilities in their 2013 book, *People with Disabilities: Sidelined or Mainstreamed*. They provide the reader with a highly readable dose of reality and sobering evidence about the intersection of disability with race and poverty. Their approach to stigma and disability is a reminder of its cross-cultural universality. They also describe the barriers stigma generates for individuals as a result of attitudes and the structure of the socioeconomic system.

In their analysis of economic, social, and political inclusion of people with disabilities, Schur, Kruse, and Blank explore models of discrimination within an employment context and the impact of stigma on opportunities such as employment. Moving across methodological approaches, they use facts and figures, narrative, and the results of qualitative interviews with U.S. disability leaders to provide a sweeping description of inclusion and exclusion of people with disabilities in social, economic, and political life, globally but mainly in the U.S.

They, too, recognize stigma as a universal phenomenon. Schur et al. are insightful in suggesting that people with disabilities may face greater stigma in societies based on individualistic values that emphasize independence and self-reliance as well as in cultures where disability is viewed as a character defect or punishment for transgressions committed by oneself, relatives, and ancestors. Influenced by Goffman and various models of discrimination, the authors express concern about the general lack of interest in economic problems faced by people with disabilities in the U.S. Their data translates into a moving narrative of social exclusion as a composite of a U.S. disability population characterized by low to no employment, low paying jobs, and impoverished recipients of SSI. They point out that, as a proportion of the population, fewer marry and many live alone.

On the positive side, universal design and assistive technology, more accessible transportation, and other environmental changes have vastly improved the lives of people with disabilities. The authors devote considerable attention to deinstitutionalization, community-based services and supports, and independent living as examples of positive trends. But, the message of the need for economic transformation is pervasive. One of their interviewees, Andy Imparato, a leader in the disability movement, was quoted as saying:

> I don't think we've prioritized building wealth and . . . human capital, . . . and I think because of that, to a large degree, we are being supported by a federally driven infrastructure that expects us to be poor and expects us to be outside the labor force and punishes us when we get too successful. (225)

Discussion

Does the use of SSI, even as an income support during college, add to the burden of disability stigma? Findings from Goffman, Stone, Thomson Garland, and Schur et al. suggest that students with disabilities are likely to be further burdened when they have additional non-normative differences related to race and receiving public aid in contrast to working. The intensity of stigma may vary by disability and demographics. Some types of disability, such as mental and cognitive disability, may be less acceptable and thus vulnerable to more intensive discrimination. For these students, disclosure may be particularly problematic.

Stigma is a phenomenon that apparently exists at the individual and social system levels as the individual internalizes social norms. Operationalizing Goffman's constructs of virtual social identity and actual social identity, students may experience the stress of not being able to predict the disposition and arrangement of acceptance in a social situation such as a university class. Are they perceived as less valuable—and more costly—because of their physical attributes, their psychosocial characteristics, and economic status? Do they lack moral character? Are they lazy? For Goffman, social norms serve as independent variables that determine who is or who is not socially acceptable. Goffman views social norms as determinants of social identity. His work has powerful explanatory value for educators concerned with students with disabilities. His concept of passing is evident in the behavior of students with hidden disabilities. Students may manage stigma by nondisclosure or lack of involvement with other students with disabilities in the face of perceived discrimination, including that exhibited by employers discussed in Schur et al. They may trade-off disclosure for maximizing employment opportunities.

Unlike Goffman, Garland Thomson, Stone, and Schur et al. are associated with the field of disability studies, which, in turn, is highly sensitive to values associated with social justice, fairness, and human rights. Garland Thomson is critical of Goffman's value neutrality. He practices value neutral social analysis as he explains stigma. He does not comment on underlying valuation of human beings based on differences that can lead to discrimination, negative attitudes, misrepresentations, and institutional practices that characterize the process of stigmatization. Her ethical concerns are closer to Deborah Stone's emphasis on justice and the power of government in distribution of resources and to Schur et al. who integrate human rights into their analysis. Garland Thomson's commentary on assigning value to differences in body properties has been influential in refocusing the unit of analysis away from the individual to culture. Students with disabilities are immersed in popular culture, which values the "perfect body." Her work is reminiscent of the policy arguments that led to change in the term for mental retardation perceived as pejorative, which is now referred to as intellectual disability.

Conclusion

This brings us to the second question posed at the beginning of this chapter. What educational and social policy strategies might help alleviate the burden resulting from the often multiple stigmatic categories for college students? Like Garland Thomson, Schur et al. emphasize values, citing human rights, and lay out models of discrimination in practice. But the quote from Imparato strikes at the heart of the problem. At its core, it identifies a forbidden topic suggested in the introduction of this chapter, poverty, use of public aid, and disability. Current models of disability—medical, social, or other—are insufficient to explain the situation of people with disability. An economic factor is missing. Stone is a natural ally of Imparato, with her big picture holistic framework. She understands that too many problems are incorporated into the disability definition in social programs. She also understands that increases in the cost of social programs impact on public support for them and on public perception of disability. Stone argues that some disability-related economic costs are externalized but could be internalized in the price of products and fines and distributed at the source of the problem, which is often industry, rather than welfare, programs. Social programs, and in particular the category of disability, carry too heavy a burden in paying for these costs.

Scholars have addressed the role of stigma in the design of welfare programs (Stuber and Kronebusch 2004; Blumkin et al. 2008) and recommended public policy strategies to relieve the stigma associated with welfare. However, improved data on the demographics of students with disabilities could drive more enlightened higher education policy formation. Social psychology research in stigma and discrimination related to racial segregation and gender discrimination have been used in court cases as varied as *Brown v. Board of Education of Topeka, Kansas* and sexual abuse in the workplace. Data can fuel cases of discrimination in higher education among our students with disabilities. The *Americans with Disabilities Act* provides protection for an individual who is regarded or treated as if he or she has a disability. But, what of those with hidden disabilities? Perhaps those who are scholars as well as those who serve as university administrators, faculty advisors and mentors to these students can provide more leadership and advocacy in their respective roles and settings. Then again, perhaps poverty has replaced sex as the hot rail of forbidden topics for those involved and no one will provide this vital service.

What strategies might relieve the stigma associated with the intersection of disability, poverty and race in higher education? Stigma is present in social norms; within the cultural fabric, and on the individual, social and public policy levels. Because stigma is composed of so many determining factors, a holistic approach is appropriate. Higher education has institutional biases at the policy and practice levels. Therefore, culture of diversity initiatives might begin at the executive level and include not only protected classes such as race but the intersection of these classes with disability and poverty. These initiatives educate and operationalize support for students, faculty and staff who are disabled, of varied races and ethnicities and with limited resources. The initiatives are only effective if commitments to them are represented in budgets, policies and procedures, accessibility of the built-in information and communications environments, cultural events, personnel, hiring, financial support and counseling. Because students with mental and cognitive disabilities are increasing in numbers on the campuses, commitments are adapted to their profile. Accommodations involve availability of twenty-four-hour services and supports. They involve knowledgeable and sensitive mentors, counselors, peer groups, and advocacy rights training, which is so vital to their success.

On the one hand, the United States values individualism and hard work as well as enjoying the apparent comfort derived from sameness in appearance and recognized behaviors. On the other, the individual student with disability may not meet these accommodation needs and norms and therefore, become victimized by stigma. His or her adjustment to campus life and academic performance may indeed require self-management, but self-management, which is informed by peers, mentors, and counselors, who can interact with her in an appropriate and meaningful way in a process that nurtures self-confidence and success.

References

Berry, Hugh, Megan Conway, and Kelly Chang. 2004. "Social Security and Undergraduates with Disabilities: An Analysis of the National Postsecondary Student Aid Survey." *Information Brief* 3 (4). National Center on Secondary Education and Transition. http://www.ncset.org/publications/info/NCSETInfoBrief_3.4.pdf

Blumkin, Tomer, Yoram Margalioth and Efraim Sadka. 2008. "The Role of Stigma in the Design of Welfare Programs." *CESIFO Working Paper* no. 2305. http://www.ssc.wisc.edu/econ/workshop/stigma_Feb_22.pdf

Fuller, Mary, Mick Healey, Andrew Bradley, and Tim Hall. 2004. "Barriers to Learning: A Systematic Study of the Experience of Disabled Students in One University." *Studies in Higher Education* 29 (3): 303–18. doi:10.1080/0307507041 0001682592

Garland Thomson, Rosemarie. 1997. *Extraordinary Bodies: Figuring Physical Disability in American Culture and Literature*. New York: Columbia University Press.

Giammarise, Kate. 2013, July 2. "Pa. Welfare Dept. to Change Name to Human Services, But Slowly: Bad Connotations Spurred Push to Relabel Agency." *Pittsburgh Post-Gazette*. http://www.post-gazette.com/stories/local/state/pa-welfare-dept-to-change-name-to-human-services-but-slowly-693943/#ixzz2Xtb47ie4

Goffman, Erving. 1963. *Stigma: Notes on the Management of Spoiled Identity*. New York: Simon & Schuster.

Hutcheon, Emily, and Gregor Wolbring. 2012. "Voices of 'Disabled' Post-Secondary Students: Examining Higher Education 'Disability' Policy Using an Ableism Lens." *Journal of Diversity in Higher Education* 5 (1): 39–49. doi:10.1037/a0027002

Jacklin, Angela. 2011. "To Be or Not to Be a 'Disabled Student' in Higher Education: The Case of a Postgraduate 'Non-declaring' (Disabled) Student." *Journal of Research in Special Educational Needs* 11 (2): 99–106. doi:10.1111/j.1471-3802.2010.01157.x

Kranke, Derrick, Sarah E. Jackson, Debbie A. Taylor, Eileen Anderson-Frye, and Jerry Floersch. 2013. "College Student Disclosure of Non-Apparent Disabilities to Receive Classroom Accommodations." *Journal of Postsecondary Education and Disability* 26 (1): 35–51.

Lalwani, Nikita. 2012, June 24. "Income Limits Restrict Services for Pennsylvania's Disabled Students: The Physically Challenged Often Must Choose Between Benefits and School Funds." *Pittsburgh Post-Gazette*. http://www.post-gazette.com/news/state/2012/06/24/

Income-limits-restrict-services-for-Pennsylvania-s-disabled-students/stories/201206240239

Porter, Nicole B. 2015, January 20. "Special Treatment Stigma after the ADA Amendments Act" *Pepperdine Law Review*, forthcoming. University of Toledo Legal Studies Research Paper. doi:10.2139/ssrn.2552854

Raue, Kimberley, and Laurie Lewis. 2011. *Students with Disabilities at Degree-Granting Postsecondary Institutions.* (NCES 2011–018). U.S. Department of Education, National Center for Education Statistics. Washington, DC: U.S. Government Printing Office. http://nces.ed.gov/pubs2011/2011018.pdf

Rauterkus, Erik, and Catherine Palmer. 2014. "The Hearing Aid Effect in 2013." *Journal of the American Academy of Audiology* 25: 893–903. doi:10.3766/jaaa.25.9.10

Schur, Lisa, Douglas Kruse, and Peter Blanck. 2013. *People with Disabilities: Sidelined or Mainstreamed?* New York: Cambridge University Press.

Shelton, J. Nicole, Jan Marie Alegre, and Deborah Son. 2010. "Social Stigma and Disadvantage: Current Themes and Future Prospects." *Journal of Social Issues* 66 (3): 618–33. doi:10.1111/j.1540–4560.2010.01666.x

Stone, Deborah. (1984). *The Disabled State.* Philadelphia: Temple University Press.

Stuber, Jennifer, and Karl Kronebusch. (2004). "Stigma and Other Determinants of Participation in TANF and Medicaid." *Journal of Policy Analysis and Management* 23 (3): 509–30. doi:10.1002/pam.20024

U. S. Government Accountability Office. 2009. *Higher Education and Disability: Education Needs a Coordinated Approach to Improve Its Assistance to Schools in Supporting Students.* http://www.gao.gov/assets/300/297433.pdf

U. S. Social Security Administration. 2015. *Red Book.* http://www.socialsecurity.gov/redbook/eng/ssi-only-employment-supports.htm

Wallhagen, M.I. (n.d.). *Hearing Loss: Impact, Policy Implications and Future Directions.* http://ncpssmfoundation.org/Portals/0/hearing-loss.pdf

"Overcoming" in Disability Studies and African American Culture

Implications for Higher Education

WENDY S. HARBOUR

ROSALIE BOONE

ELAINE BOURNE HEATH

SISLENA G. LEDBETTER

"What do you mean by "overcoming"? This question arose in a staff meeting for the HBCU Disability Consortium project last year,[1] after several project staff members used the term "overcoming" to describe how students were dealing with disability-related access problems or negative attitudes of others. The HBCU Disability Consortium project, funded through a grant by the U.S. Department of Education,[2] established a consortium among disability services providers at Historically Black Colleges and Universities (HBCUs) and conducted research on culturally relevant practices for disability services and pedagogy. Questions about the meaning of overcoming as it relates to HBCUs and disability studies came from the first author of this chapter, a white disability studies professor and former disability services provider at a predominantly white institution (PWI). She disliked the word "overcoming" because of her disability studies background and experiences as a culturally Deaf and disabled woman. This intrigued other project staff, who felt they were using a positive term to describe students' persistence in the face of various challenges. What emerged from the following discussion was a rich, cross-cultural and interdisciplinary conversation that we share here, with hope that others will join our dialogue.

In the field of disability studies, the term "overcoming" tends to have a distinctly negative connotation that is consistent with a long history of pathological views of disability. For members of HBCUs and many African Americans, the term is a positive one that brings to mind the Civil Rights Movement. This article looks at how disability studies and African American culture use the term "overcoming," supplemented with our own anecdotal experiences and a review of relevant research with African American college students who have disabilities. After suggesting ways to reconcile disparate views of the term "overcoming," we generate a series of recommendations and considerations that can be implemented in higher education to address racism and ableism on campuses. Our aim is to create additional education and dialogue around race and disability, to frame these topics as critical topics for student development, and to minimize barriers and obstacles that students with disabilities and African American students may need to surmount or overcome.

Critical Race Theory and Disability Studies

African Americans and the Black community[3] have good reason to be cautious about disability conversations and disability studies. Baynton (2001) has noted that this is, in fact, not just a characteristic of African Americans or Black people; most racial and ethnic groups try to distance themselves from disability. A common basis for this is that many have experienced discrimination due to the assumptions of others that their skin color, religious beliefs, gender, race, or class render them physically, emotionally, or intellectually inferior, sick, weak, or disabled (Baynton 2001). In the case of African Americans, the construct of disability was used historically to justify slavery, to the point where medical professionals suggested that slaves would be prone to mental and physical disabilities if they were set free or treated as the equals of whites (Baynton 2001). People with developmental disabilities ("morons") were even considered evidence of how whiteness could be racially "tainted" as different races mixed (Dolmage 2014, 102). Since the abolition of slavery, there has been a long history of racism, segregation, and over-representation of African Americans in special education systems predominantly run by white, nondisabled educators. This is particularly true for students labeled as emotionally or behaviorally disturbed, learning disabled, or intellectually disabled (Connor, 2008; Harry and Klinger 2006; Losen and Orfield 2002; Skiba, Poloni-Staudinger, Gallini, Simmons, and Feggins-Azzis 2006). Discussing disability as a medical condition has also been problematic. African

Americans have been denied access to health care (see, e.g., NAACP 2015), and have been abused and exploited by medical researchers, as illustrated by examples such as the infamous Tuskegee experiments (CDC 2013) and the case of Henrietta Lacks, whose cells were stolen by medical researchers (Skloot 2011).

But it is also true that the field of disability studies has been slow to connect with critical race theorists and African American studies. One reason for this lack of connection may be white privilege in a white-dominated field. Black writer and educator Chris Bell famously suggested that the field should actually refer to itself as "White Disability Studies" (2006, 275). Bell maintained that the entire field, operating from the privileged position of its dominant constituents (i.e., white academics at PWIs) tends to unintentionally "whitewash disability history, ontology, and phenomenology" (2006, 275). Other disability studies researchers have suggested that if the field were scrutinized by African Americans, even foundational models and theories may need to change, because African Americans have different views of and experiences with institutional and political systems (see, e.g., Mollow 2006). When the areas of race and disability have been investigated together, they have often been set up as distinct and static categories or hierarchies (Ferri 2010). There is very little work regarding the ways that race or ethnicity interact with disability or how, perhaps, they even oppress each other in society and in the academy (e.g., James and Wu 2006; Taylor 2015; Tettenborn 2006), although this is changing with the emergence of works by authors like Therí Pickens (2014), Ellen Samuels (2014), and Cynthia Wu (2012). Authors have also started exploring race in the context of Deaf studies and American Sign Language (see, e.g., McCaskill, Lucas, Bayley, and Hill 2011).

At the same time, the field of African American studies has also often reduced disability to its most ableist stereotypes (Bell 2011). For example, critical race theory (CRT) has traditionally avoided the topic of disability due to its association with racism, deviance, medicine, and a lack of intelligence (Watts and Erevelles 2004), although more authors are exploring intersections between the two fields (see, e.g., Annamma, Connor, and Ferri 2012). If the field views disability as a negative condition and legitimate grounds for discrimination, inequities are exacerbated for people with disabilities—especially those who are African American (Banks and Hughes 2013; Baynton 2001).

However, concern about the implications of addressing disability is not unique to African American studies and critical race theory—it is a widespread problem in higher education. Scholars, researchers, and administrators in higher education may view disability as an individual problem to be accommodated, rather than a campus diversity issue involving ableism (see, e.g., Linton 1998; Mollow 2006; Price 2011; Taylor 2011). This negative orientation toward disability can contribute to the assumption that normalization or overcoming is indeed the best option for people with disabilities (Banks and Hughes 2013; Linton 1998). Individual African Americans with disabilities who want to reflect critically on their experiences may face a "web of intra-cultural prejudice," where models and information about disability are consistently negative or built on outdated stereotypes (Banks and Hughes 2013, 377).

In fact, disability studies, African American studies, and critical race studies each reject biomedical determinism and look for ways disability and race are socially constructed (Ferri 2010; Watts and Erevelles 2004). With origins in a Civil Rights Movement social justice framework, each uses narratives and first-person accounts to illustrate racism or ableism (Ferri 2010; Watts and Erevelles 2004).

Furthermore, disability studies scholars and African American studies scholars share histories that intersect at many points, albeit from different orientations. For example, historically, both African Americans and disabled people have been exploited by "entertainment" venues (e.g., freak shows, circuses) that portrayed them as exotic or fearful oddities (e.g., Adams 2001; James and Wu 2006; Samuels 2014). Both groups have been victimized by eugenics movements and ongoing efforts to control their reproduction (e.g., James and Wu 2006; Skloot 2011). Both groups face high rates of incarceration (e.g., Ben-Moshe, Chapman, and Carey 2014; Moore 2015; Treatment Advocacy Center 2014). As discussed above, both groups struggle with access to public education, and in the well-known case of *Brown vs. the Board of Education*, attorneys saw this connection, arguing that federal interference with segregation of African American children could also lead to integration of Native Americans, girls, and disabled children (Tushnet 1994). In recent years, police violence against both groups has started to gain media attention and the focus of both communities (e.g., Cokley 2015; Heideman 2014; Jeserich and Moore 2013).

Bell has called for "representational detective work" (2011, 1)—a willingness to delve into representations of disability and Blackness, even when they are hidden from plain view, with no assumptions that one must be sacrificed in order to investigate the other. Likewise, Ferri (2010) has recommended looking critically at conflicts of interest, power differentials, and other aspects of race and disability as first steps in addressing concerns or questions. Scholars in African American studies, critical race theory, and disability studies have also recently begun to inform each other's work (e.g., Annamma et al. 2012; Dolmage 2014; James and Wu 2006; Pickens 2014; Samuels 2014; Taylor 2015; Tettenborn 2006; Wu 2012). By examining "overcoming"—a term that holds deep and complex meanings for disability studies scholars and African Americans—this chapter seeks to do some of the critical detective work advised by Bell (2011) and Ferri (2010).

"Overcoming": Divergent Views

Disability Studies and "Overcoming" as Oppression

Disability studies scholar Simi Linton wrote about negative aspects of overcoming in her book *Claiming Disability: Knowledge and Identity*, saying that "both passing and overcoming take their toll" (1998, 21). The term may simply mean that someone with a disability has overcome ableism and stigma in order to succeed, but most of the time, it means someone had the will and desire to overcome disability itself. Overcoming is then perceived as a "triumph" (19)—all the problems associated with the disability no longer exist. It also implies that the individual is able to "pass" as nondisabled (i.e., normal) because s/he has successfully overcome what makes him/her different (19). Linton emphasizes that this expectation of overcoming exacts a high price because the individual with a disability must constantly strive to be something that is impossible to achieve (i.e., nondisabled) and meet a socially constructed standard that does not exist (i.e., normal). If individuals do not "overcome," their mental or physical state is blamed rather than ableism, society, politics, or access barriers.

Disability studies has a foundation in the medical and sociopolitical models of disability. The medical model, as it is traditionally described, assumes that a disability is inherently problematic for the individual; it must be cured, fixed, or normalized (usually by a professional). The traditional sociopolitical (i.e., social) models of disability assume that people with disabilities may have impairments of some kind, but disability is a social construct like gender or race. Because the construct of disability is subject to changes based on contexts, theorists in disability studies have been able to critique those constructions and the discourse around them (e.g., Asch 2001; Devlieger, Rusch, and Pfeiffer 2003; Linton 1998; Siebers 2008; Taylor 2011).

In the sociopolitical models, overcoming brings to mind images of Tiny Tim or other "supercrips" who seem to do the impossible (e.g., a blind man climbing Mt. Everest, a Deaf musician, a marathoner who is an amputee) (Shapiro 1993). Within Deaf culture, overcoming deafness is associated with oralism, cochlear implants, and the marginalization of American Sign Language and Deafhood (e.g., Lang 2003; Valente, Bahan, and Bauman 2011). Thus, overcoming means buying into society's ableist definitions of normality and internalizing the attitude that disability is a problem to be conquered.

The difficulty with associating any word or phrase with medical or social models of disability is that this association ignores the complex, multi-layered and culturally-bound meanings that may exist for diverse cultural groups, including African Americans (Bell 2006; 2007; 2011). Indeed, critiques of the medical and social models have noted that separating out the medical and physical experience of disability (e.g., as impairment, a condition, or illness) from sociopolitical experiences of disability are artificial (see, e.g., Gabel and Peters 2004; Owens 2015; Shakespeare and Watson 2002). This is especially critical in discussions of disability and race, since both are embodied physical and mental experiences, defined by Pickens as the "tangible, sensory living from which humans make sense of their world" (2014, 1). Identities of being ill, disabled, Black, or African American may all be fluid and are highly individualized experiences (Owens 2015; Shakespeare and Watson, 2002). The models are slowly evolving to acknowledge this fluidity on individual, cultural, and societal levels (Owens 2015). Relevant to this chapter's analysis of "overcoming," expanded definitions of the models also allow resistance to ableism and racism (among other forms of oppression) that may play out on different levels as well (Gabel and Peters, 2004). This leads to our discussion of how African American culture defines "overcoming," and its implications for individuals, groups, and resistance, as well.

African American Studies and Overcoming
as Liberation from Oppression

The most iconic representation of overcoming in African American culture is the song "We Shall Overcome," which is virtually synonymous with the Civil Rights Movement. The Library of Congress describes the song's lyrics as "some of the most influential words in the English language" (Library of Congress, n.d., n.p.). The song originated as a work song sung by slaves in the fields, but by the 1960's, the Student Non-Violent Coordinating Committee was using it, stimulating its evolution as the defining anthem of the Civil Rights Movement (Adams 2013).

We shall overcome, We shall overcome, We shall overcome some day.
CHORUS: Oh, deep in my heart, I do believe, We shall overcome some day.
The Lord will see us through, The Lord will see us through, The Lord will see us through some day (CHORUS)
We're on to victory, We're on to victory, We're on to victory some day (CHORUS)
We'll walk hand in hand, We'll walk hand in hand, We'll walk hand in hand some day (CHORUS)
We are not afraid, We are not afraid, We are not afraid, today (CHORUS)
The truth shall make us free, The truth shall make us free, The truth shall make us free some day (CHORUS)
We shall live in peace, We shall live in peace, We shall live in peace some day (CHORUS)

The words of "We Shall Overcome" emphasize that overcoming is connected to salvation, community, freedom, and peace. After the 1963 March on Washington, even absent the music, the phrase "We Shall Overcome" took on a life of its own. In a Memphis speech shortly before his death, Dr. Martin Luther King, Jr. described the song's power this way (as quoted in Adams 2013, n.p.):

> There's a little song that we sing in our movement down in the South . . . You know, I've joined hands so often with students and others behind jail singing it: "We Shall Overcome." Sometimes we've had tears in our eyes when we joined together to sing it, but we still decided to sing it: "We Shall Overcome." Oh, before this victory's won, some will have to get thrown in jail some more, but we shall overcome.

"Overcoming" in the context of the African American pursuit of equality implies a community of individuals united against all odds. They know there will be more struggling and hard times ahead, but they will prevail. The phrase "we shall overcome" implicitly requires each individual to testify and believe the words. Thus, the concept of overcoming encapsulates a major philosophical orientation of African Americans; it connotes freedom, tenacity, struggle, and survival, not only in African American culture but also in education (also see, e.g., Adams 2013; Banks and Hughes 2013; Library of Congress n.d.; Moore and Neal 2006; Nichols and Tanksley 2004; Wallace, Moore, Wilson, and Hart 2012).

On one hand, overcoming can be highly problematic if African Americans adopt the belief that disability can be overcome. Yet disability studies scholars who refuse to use the term "overcoming" ignore the historical and cultural implications for African Americans. To reconcile these seemingly incongruent points of view, we look at how HBCUs teach overcoming and implications for PWIs.

"Overcoming" in Higher Education: HBCUs and African American Students with Disabilities

The HBCU Disability Consortium has operated in concurrence with several researchers who have suggested that HBCUs are important places to learn about disability, African American culture, and Blackness (Davis 2006; Haughton 1993; Kynard and Eddy 2009; Ruffins 2008). There are currently one hundred HBCUs in the United States (NCES, n.d.). These institutions of higher education, which first emerged after the Civil War, were set up to serve as bastions of African American knowledge and culture. Although HBCUs have always included students from other racial and ethnic groups, students at these schools continue to be predominantly African American or Black (Cantey, Bland, Mack, and Joy-Davis 2013; Jewell 2002; NCES n.d.). HBCUs are well-known for producing African Americans with advanced degrees in a variety of fields, including engineering and law (Cantey et al. 2013; Jewell 2002). As a result of their history, HBCUs care deeply about African American identity formation, values cultivation, academic achievement, and leadership development (Arroyo and Gasman 2014; Cantey et al. 2013; Jewell 2002). These intertwine and intersect with lessons about overcoming.

HBCUs teach students explicit and implicit messages about overcoming obstacles and the odds against Black people, as well as becoming strong in order to survive, succeed, and dismantle racism in society (see, e.g., Nichols and Tanksley 2004; Shaw 2006). The concept of "overcoming" pervades the narrative describing the mission and role of HBCUs. For example, in 2014, U.S. President Barack Obama described HBCUs as campuses founded to be "beacon[s] of hope" for African Americans as institutions that wage "war against illiteracy and ignorance" and forge "pathways to help students overcome barriers to equal opportunity" (Obama 2014, n.p.). Likewise, the President of Howard University, Dr. Wayne Frederick, has declared that, "we must overcome those barriers" of racism (Rosen 2015, n.p.). Students, as well, perceive the role of the HBCU as developing and supporting their ability to "overcome." For instance, a participant in a study of African American male students with disabilities noted that he was learning to "overcome race" [*sic*] at the HBCU he attended (Banks and Hughes, 2013, 373).

Self-improvement and the creation of social change are "inseparable" in the worldview and culture of HBCUs (Shaw 2006, 93). Helping students to overcome is critical to the self-improvement and social change objectives of HBCUs; it constitutes an essential focus of processes via which HBCUs prepare college students for their roles in the African American community and society.

Despite this, it is difficult to find literature focused explicitly on the concept of "overcoming" at HBCUs. Given our work within HBCUs, we (the authors) suspect that this may be because the concept is so integral to the HBCU and African American experience. Once the authors initiated conversations about overcoming, team members were able to think of many anecdotal stories illustrating how the concept is operationalized within the culture of HBCUs. When the authors and other project staff shared their stories with the HBCU Disability Consortium advisory board, they agreed this was their shared experiences at HBCUs as well.

For example, project members noted that when HBCUs lack sufficient resources of one kind or another, faculty, staff, and students are expected to be stoic and creative, finding ways to prevail over any problems and learn something from the experience. The team observed that even HBCUs with adequate resources expect the college experience to involve developmental, personal, and academic struggles that helped students learn to overcome, although no one could remember explicit discussions about this—it is simply a part of campus culture.

African American fraternities and sororities have received negative media attention for hazing rituals (Hughey and Hernandez 2012), but some members of the HBCU Disability Consortium raised the possibility that hazing rituals were also connected to the idea of proving one's ability to overcome obstacles through struggle and sacrifice. (For discussion of hazing and initiation rituals, see, e.g., Hughey and Hernandez 2012; Jones 2000). Greek organizations, therefore, foster a sense of pride that graduates from African American fraternities and sororities are self-assured, well-equipped for leadership roles in society and confident of their ability to overcome anything.

We were mystified when we found virtually no research or commentary explicitly addressing overcoming in these contexts. During our discussion with the consortium advisory board, one board member—a school counselor—noted that she discusses overcoming with her students after connecting it to ideas of resilience. Although some interesting work exists related to models of resiliency in Black students with disabilities (e.g., Jones 2010, Williamson 2007), the term "resiliency" has a medical and clinical aspect that does not resonate as a major touchstone of African American history and culture.

We found that research about postsecondary African American students with disabilities is also scarce. Two studies of African American women in higher education (Caesar-Richardson 2012; Nichols and Tanksley 2004) discussed how students believed that overcoming, strength, and succeeding in spite of odds were important in combating experiences of sexism and racism, with peers and in the campus climate. Caesar-Richardson (2012) listed terms students may use instead of "overcoming" or "strength," including "bearing up" (95), "getting over it" (122), "staying silent" (123),"dealing with it" (133), or "handling it" (133). In both studies, students longed for mentors who could help them navigate their communities and their emerging understandings of themselves as both strong and vulnerable (Caesar-Richardson 2012; Nichols and Tanksley 2004).

Studies by Petersen (2009), Banks and Hughes (2013), and Banks (2014) showed how African American college students with disabilities wrestle with identities as both African Americans and people with disabilities. Inadequate information about disability services and accommodations can hamper students even further (Banks 2014). As students begin to develop a critical consciousness about race and disability, they also struggle to make sense of their experiences with racism, ableism, and sexism (Petersen 2009), but this can also have devastating consequences. As men in Banks' study (2014) learned about disability services, they frequently refused to use them, uncertain about whether it was okay to ask for help or whether it would negatively affect how others viewed their masculinity.

Banks and Hughes (2013) used a framework from W. E. B. DuBois (368) to describe the students' struggle as a "double consciousness." The male students in their research were perceived as pathological troublemakers because they were Black men. They were simultaneously perceived as not being intellectual enough because they had disabilities. Their research participants felt supported by HBCUs in their racial and intellectual development (Banks and Hughes 2013; Jewell 2002), but disability was perceived as yet another obstacle to overcome individually and collectively. A disability services director at the HBCU (a nondisabled African American male) told them about other African Americans with disabilities and mentored them toward academic excellence. After students learned more about disability, working hard and achieving in the face of obstacles (i.e., overcoming) then became a form of resistance. They also began connecting their disability-related resistance to the broader Civil Rights Movement. One student said, "If they [civil rights workers] can do it, I can do it" (376) and another identified Dr. Martin Luther King, Jr. as a personal hero because Dr. King could be an inspiration and help him "overcome stereotypes of racial and disability discrimination" (376).

Like these students, we will attempt to reconcile disabled and African American interpretations of "overcoming" while honoring both communities and their histories. In the next section, we explore possible connections between the two perspectives. We also look at positive consequences of a more nuanced and flexible definition of the term.

Reconciling Definitions of Overcoming

As a model for our work on "overcoming," we reference Èva Tettenborn's work on the concept of "melancholia" in contemporary African American literature (2006). Although melancholy is viewed as an emotional disability or mental illness, the medical and psychiatric definitions are not synonymous with how "melancholia" is defined in African American literature. There the term is used to describe a "mental attachment and yearning for a lost object" (103–5) and a process of grieving and mourning. Tettenborn carefully challenges assumptions about whether melancholy is a disability, without implying that disability is an inherently negative label that should be avoided. Further, she describes melancholy in African American literature as a source of political power that resists dominant versions of memory and history. Melancholy imagines what else might be lost and the power of that loss, even if there is no official record. It affirms and asserts that the person/self experiencing melancholy exists and is worthy of expressing loss. It also affirms that the "lost object" exists, whether it is an actual object, person, place, a memory, or a way of being (107). Furthermore, melancholy manifests as both an individual and a communal phenomenon "transgressive, powerful, and political potential" (118). Likewise, we ask our readers to consider the potential of "overcoming."

However, like "melancholy," the term is not uniformly positive and powerful. Caesar-Richardson's research (2012) focused on African American women with disabilities at a PWI who also had mental and emotional health concerns. Her participants believed that strength and being able to handle or overcome problems demonstrated ability and competence in academia, combatted discrimination, and connected the women to roles in the Black community as caregivers and matriarchs. However, they also admitted that this strength made any perceived weakness or vulnerability a liability. Admitting to any kind of depression, anxiety, or stress was a luxury for wealthy white people, and they described the unwillingness to talk about this as "spirit-murdering silence" (119). In handling micro-aggressions, outright discriminations, and the low expectations of others, the women in this study often assumed problems existed in their own personal failings or lack of skills and knowledge. Only upon reflection did they begin to locate problems in peers, faculty, or the campus. This was reinforced when they received implicit and explicit messages that strength and capability in academia is equated with professionalism and academic ability (for further discussion, also see Price 2011). Being strong meant being self-reliant, self-sacrificing, and self-silenced, but institutional racism and sexism still caused stress, illness, and isolation. Students who were able to link to the disability community, find ways of incorporating disability into a sense of self, or find systems of support were better able to deconstruct the ways the disability, Black, and campus communities were validating or marginalizing their experiences.

Perhaps this is where higher education can reconcile disability studies and African American views of overcoming. The first step for both groups is simply to acknowledge that the term is laden with layers of complex meanings and can only be defined in context. Higher education is a valuable place to begin deconstructing this term and others (like "melancholy"). If PWIs follow the lead of HBCUs, campuses can be places having deep conversations about systemic oppression and ways to address it—not as mere intellectual exercises or theory but as a student development issue and a way to graduate competent leaders.

In a more flexible reflexive definition of "overcoming," the main consideration is the object of overcoming. When "overcoming" indicates resistance, social justice, community, culture, and rights, then it automatically defines oppression and injustice as that which must be overcome. Then the word is powerful for anyone, regardless of race, ethnicity, or disability. In higher education, a careful analysis of discourse around overcoming may also trigger self-reflection about individuals and their identities. This type of dialogue may be especially helpful for students trying to learn about the intersections of their identity. As Audre Lorde noted in 1984, there can be incredible power (and greater ability to overcome) when individual labels, beliefs, and identities become an integrated whole:

> I find that I am constantly being encouraged to pluck out some one aspect of myself and present this as the meaningful whole, eclipsing or denying the other parts of self. But this is a destructive and fragmenting way to live. My fullest concentration of energy is available to me only when I integrate all the parts of who I am, openly, allowing power from particular sources of my living to flow back and forth freely through all my different selves, without the restriction of externally imposed definition." (Lorde 1984, 120–21, as quoted in Caesar-Richardson 2012, 132)

Integrating our multiple definitions of the term "overcoming" may also give it greater impact, and acknowledging its perceived and real limitations may make it stronger when used in ways that acknowledge its complex meanings. Recognizing these multiple meanings further validates overcoming as an internal and individual process but also as an expressive action for communities. Indeed, the development of the song "We Shall Overcome" reflected a similar development, starting as "I Shall Overcome," but members of the Student Non-Violent Coordinating Committee changed the phrase to show that individuals were vulnerable, but stronger if they worked collectively, relying on each other (Adams 2013; Library of Congress n.d.).

Implications and Recommendations for Higher Education

Student development, including identity development, is a critical part of the college experience. At HBCUs, there is a deliberate effort to connect individual development to broader experiences and cultural beliefs of African Americans, with an emphasis on developing African American leaders. Using resources referenced in this paper, we offer the following recommendations to campuses, in supporting dialogue about overcoming and in helping students think critically about race and disability.

Encourage students with chronic health conditions, disabilities, and mental or emotional struggles to link to the disability community and disability studies.

Students can benefit from considering the label of "disability" and exploring what that means to the disability community. Groups like the National Black Disability Coalition (http://www.blackdisability.org/), National Black Deaf Advocates (http://www.nbda.org/) or our own HBCU Disability Consortium (http://www.blackdisabledandproud.org) can help students, faculty, and staff find a community.

Create mentoring opportunities on campus. Whenever possible, Student Affairs should assist Black and disabled students in identifying mentors who can help them find support, assist in navigating college, direct them to campus resources, and validate their experiences.

Consider how diversity is defined, discussed, and welcomed on campus. While most campuses have an institutional commitment to diversity, this may not always extend to students with disabilities. It also may not acknowledge that many students have intersecting identities between carefully delineated definitions of "diverse" populations. Students must have formal and informal opportunities to gather with peers (however they define their peer group). Campuses should also consider how complaints are addressed for students, and whether groups are equipped to listen to, document, and act on complaints appropriately.

Academics teaching cultural studies must consider the limitations of their syllabi. For disability studies instructors, there should be an effort to include works by African Americans with disabilities, without making them tokens for their entire community. For African American studies or critical race scholars, the same holds true: if no people with disabilities are represented in courses, then disability becomes invisible or an issue of white people. In both cases, language and discourse around race and disability are silenced, and opportunities to discuss terms like "overcoming" become non-existent. It is also important to note that activists in both communities may not have the power and privilege to be published in texts and journals typically used in college courses. Faculty should consider hiring activists or using non-traditional works (e.g., videos, blogs, songs, stories) to supplement academic materials (with compensation for activists who visit classrooms, trainings, and conferences).

Consider discussions about oppression to be an important part of student development. While campuses often greet first-year students or new faculty with diversity trainings, difficult dialogue about race, disability, and other social justice issues may be better viewed as a foundation for enhancing student development and leadership, as HBCUs view it. This is also a way to connect theory to practice, with pragmatic consequences for campuses and students.

When students talk about "overcoming" and "being strong," ask what they mean. At both HBCUs and PWIs, we hope faculty and staff will pause when they hear students talk about "overcoming," "being strong," "fighting through it," or other terms similar to these. It is worth asking, "What exactly are you overcoming/being strong about/fighting?" Instead of presuming their rationales are good or bad, asking for individual interpretations may also foster constructive dialogue and student growth. We hope it would provide an opportunity to identify barriers and challenges on campus, and to begin identifying ways to address those without further self-sacrifice of students.

Utilize universal design and include Black students in the "universe" of users. Universal design (UD) is used in architecture, pedagogy, and computing. UD assumes there will be a variety users or learners, including people with disabilities (Burgstahler and Cory 2008; Meyer, Rose, and Gordon 2014; McGuire and Scott 2006; Rose, Harbour, Johnston, Daley, and Abarbanell 2006). UD is gaining traction as a tool for increasingly diverse campuses, but several authors have noted that faculty and staff may not be including people of color in their "universes" of potential users. They may also need training in multicultural or culturally relevant practices in order to be truly inclusive. (For more information, see, e.g., Higbee and Barajas 2007; Holbrook, Moore, and Zoss 2010).

Conclusion

In this chapter, we have discussed the term "overcoming" in disability studies, African American culture, and HBCUs. Rather than rejecting the term outright or risk using it in ableist ways, we have considered how "overcoming" may be framed, defined, and utilized to name oppressions and encompass a rich and empowering tradition in African American culture. When a disability services professional, professor, or student affairs administrator finds a student with a disability struggling to "overcome," this chapter provides tools to politicize students in understanding the history of the word and defining "overcoming" in ways that encourage critical resistance to racism and ableism. We have provided examples of African American students with disabilities who found ways to overcome ableism and racism during college, and discussed strategies for faculty, staff and researchers to support campus change; begin discussions of race and disability; and therefore ideally eliminate barriers students may need to overcome. We have provided a few recommendations for applying what we have learned about overcoming to improve the campus climate for African American students with disabilities, to infuse dialogue and change into campus culture and the broader curriculum, and to minimize the ableism and racism that college students need to overcome.

We ask that researchers in disability studies and African American studies continue their work exploring race and disability and the experiences of African American people with disabilities in and out of the academy. It is important to remember that students are not the only members of higher education who have disabilities—while little is known about students, even less is known about African American faculty, staff, and campus visitors (including disabled parents of current and prospective students).

We appreciate the many ways that HBCUs emphasize maintaining connections to activism and community; these may be replicable with other campuses and groups committed to social justice. We encourage HBCUs to remember that people with disabilities have been a part of the diaspora, the Civil Rights Movements, and HBCUs since the beginning, and we ask them to become more inclusive of disability in their teaching, outreach, and research.

We have provided our answers to the question "What do you mean by 'overcoming'?" and hope we have encouraged others to answer the same question for themselves and their campus communities.

References

Adams, Noah. 2013, August 28. "The Inspiring Force of 'We Shall Overcome.'" *NPR*. http://www.npr.org/2013/08/28/216482943/the-inspiring-force-of-we-shall-overcome

Adams, Rachel. 2001. *Freaks and the American Cultural Imagination*. Chicago: University of Chicago Press.

Annamma, Subini A., David Connor, and Beth Ferri. 2012. "Dis/ability Critical Race Studies (DisCrit): Theorizing at the Intersections of Race and Dis/ability." *Race, Ethnicity and Education.* 16 (1): 1–31. doi:10.1080/13613324.2012.730511

Arroyo, Andrew T., and Marybeth Gasman. 2014. "An HBCU-Based Educational Approach for Black College Student Success: Toward a Framework with Implications for All Institutions." *American Journal of Education* 12 (1): 57–85. doi:10.1086/678112

Asch, Adrienne. 2001. "Disability, Bioethics, and Human Rights." In *Handbook of Disability Studies*, eds. Gary L. Albrecht, Katherine D. Seelman, and Michael Bury, 297–326. Thousand Oaks, CA: Sage.

Banks, Joy. 2014. "Barriers and Supports to Postsecondary Transition: Case Studies of African American Students with Disabilities." *Remedial and Special Education* 35: 28–39. doi:10.1177/0741932513512209

Banks, Joy, and Michael S. Hughes. 2013. "Double Consciousness: Postsecondary Experiences of African American Males with Disabilities." *The Journal of Negro Education* 82 (4): 368–81. doi:10.7709/jnegroeducation.82.4.0368

Baynton, Douglas. 2001. "Disability and the Justification of Inequality in American History." In *The New Disability History: American Perspectives*, edited by Paul K. Longmore and Lauri Umansky, 33–57. New York: New York University Press.

Bell, Christopher. 2006. "Introducing White Disability Studies: A Modest Proposal." In *The Disability Studies Reader* (2nd ed.), ed. Lennard J. Davis, 275–82. New York: Taylor & Francis Group.

Bell, Christopher. 2007. "'We Do Not Talk About Such Things Here': My Life So Far as an HIV+ Academic." In *Disabled Faculty and Staff in a Disabling Society*, ed. Mary Lee Vance, 217–23. Huntersville, NC: Association on Higher Education And Disability.

Bell, Christopher. 2011. "Introduction: Doing Representational Detective Work." In *Blackness and Disability: Critical Examinations and Cultural Interventions*, ed. Christopher M. Bell. Münster, Germany: LIT Verlag.

Ben-Moshe, Liat, Chris Chapman, and Allison C. Carey. 2014. *Disability Incarcerated: Imprisonment and Disability in the United States and Canada*. New York: Palgrave Macmillan.

Burgstahler, Sheryl E., and Rebecca C. Cory, eds.. 2008. *Universal Design in Higher Education: From Principles to Practice*. Cambridge, MA: Harvard Education Press.

Caesar-Richardson, Nadia. 2012. *Strength that Silences: Learning from the Experiences of Black Female College Students with Mental Health Concerns at a Predominantly White Institution*. PhD diss., University of Alabama.

Cantey, Nia, Robert Bland, LaKerri Mack, and Danielle Joy-Davis. 2013. "Historically Black Colleges and Universities: Sustaining a Culture of Excellence in the Twenty-First Century." *Journal of African American Studies* 17: 142–53. doi:10.1007/s12111–011–9191–0

Centers for Disease Control and Prevention (CDC). 2013. "U.S. Public Health Service Syphilis Study at Tuskegee." *Center for Disease Control and Prevention*. http://www.cdc.gov/tuskegee/index.html

Cokley, Rebecca. 2015, July 6. "Police Violence against People with Disabilities." *Black Star News*. http://www.blackstarnews.com/us-politics/justice/police-violence-against-people-with-disabilities.html

Connor, David J. 2008. *Urban Narratives: Portraits in Progress. Life at the Intersections of Learning Disability, Race, & Social Class*. New York: Peter Lang.

Davis, Angela Thomas. 2006. "Disability Support Services at Historically Black Colleges and Universities." Ed.D. diss., Alabama State University.

Devlieger, Patrick, Frank Rusch, and David Pfeiffer, eds. 2003. "Rethinking Disability as Same and Different! Towards a Cultural Model of Disability." In *Rethinking Disability: The Emergence of New Definitions, Concepts, and Communities*, edited by Patrick Devlieger, Frank Rusch, and David Pfeiffer, 9–16. Philadelphia: Garant/Coronet Books.

Dolmage, Jay Timothy. 2014. *Disability Rhetoric*. Syracuse: Syracuse University Press.

Ferri, Beth. 2010. "A Dialogue We're Yet to Have: Race and Disability Studies." In *The Myth of the Normal Curve*, ed. Curt Dudley-Marley and Alex Gurn, 139–50. New York: Peter Lang.

Gabel, Susan, and Susan Peters. 2004. "Presage of a Paradigm Shift? Beyond the Social Model of Disability Toward Resistance Theories of Disability." *Disability & Society* 19 (6): 585–600. doi:10.1080/0968759042000252515

Harry, Beth, and Janette Klinger. 2006. *Why are So Many Minority Students in Special Education? Understanding Race and Disability in Schools.* New York: Teachers College Press.

Haughton, Jr., Claiborne D. 1993. "Expanding the Circle of Inclusion for African Americans with Disabilities: A National Opportunity." *Black Collegian* 23 (4): 63–68.

Heideman, Elizabeth. 2014, September 8. "Police Brutality's Hidden Victims: The Disabled." *The Daily Beast.* http://www.thedailybeast.com/articles/2014/09/08/police-are-failing-america-s-disabled.html

Higbee, Jeanne L., and Heidi Lasley Barajas. 2007. "Building Effective Places for Multicultural Learning." *About Campus* (July-August): 16–22.

Holbrook, Teri, Christi Moore, and Michelle Zoss. 2010. "Equitable Intent: Reflections on Universal Design in Education as an Ethic of Care." *Reflective Practice: International and Multidisciplinary Perspectives* 11 (5): 682–92. doi:10.1080/14623943.2010.516985

Hughey, Matthew W., and Marcia Hernandez. 2012. "Black, Greek, and Read All Over: Newspaper Coverage of African-American Fraternities and Sororities, 1980–2009." *Ethnic and Racial Studies* 36 (2): 298–319. doi:10.1080/01419870.2012.676195

James, Jennifer C., and Cynthia Wu. 2006. "Editors' Introduction: Race, Ethnicity, Disability, and Literature: Intersections and Interventions." *MELUS* 31 (3): 3–13. doi:10.1093/melus/31.3.3

Jeserich, Mitch, and Leroy Moore. 2013, September 19. "Audio Interview Leroy Moore on Letters and Politics on KPFA 94.1FM about Police Brutality against People with Disabilities." *POOR Magazine.* http://www.poormagazine.org/node/4908

Jewell, Joseph O. 2002. "To Set an Example: The Tradition of Diversity at Historically Black Colleges and Universities." *Urban Education* 37 (7): 7–21. doi:10.1177/0042085902371002

Jones, Ricky L. 2000. "The Historical Significance of Sacrificial Ritual: Understanding Violence in the Modern Black Fraternity Pledge Process." *Western Journal of Black Studies* 24 (2): 112–24.

Jones, Vita L. 2010. "Resiliency Instructional Tactics: African American Students with Learning Disabilities." *Intervention in School and Clinic* 46 (4): 235–39. doi:10.1177/1053451210389032

Kynard, Carmen, and Robert Eddy. 2009. "Toward a New Critical Framework: Color-Conscious Political Morality and Pedagogy at Historically Black and Historically White Colleges and Universities." *College Composition and Communication* 61 (1): W24–W44.

Lang, Paddy. 2003. *Understanding Deaf Culture: In Search of Deafhood.* Bristol: Multilingual Matters.

Library of Congress. No Date. "We Shall Overcome. Historical Period: Postwar

United States, 1945–1968." *Library of Congress.* http://www.loc.gov/teachers/lyrical/songs/overcome.html

Linton, Simi. 1998. *Claiming Disability: Knowledge and Identity.* New York: New York University Press.

Losen, Daniel J., and Gary Orfield, eds. 2002. *Racial Inequity in Special Education.* Cambridge, MA: Harvard Education Press.

McCaskill, Carolyn, Ceil Lucas, Robert Bayley, and Joseph Christopher Hill. 2011. *The Hidden Treasure of Black ASL: Its History and Structure.* Washington, DC: Gallaudet University Press.

Meyer, Ann, David H. Rose, and David Gordon. 2014. *Universal Design for Learning: Theory and Practice.* Wakefield, MA: CAST Professional Publishing.

McGuire, Joan M., and Sally S. Scott. 2006. "Universal Design for Instruction: Extending the Universal Design Paradigm to College Instruction." *Journal of Postsecondary Education and Disability* 19 (2): 124–34.

Mollow, Anna. 2006. "When 'Black' Women Start Going on Prozac: Race, Gender, and Mental Illness in Mari Nana-Ama Danquah's 'Willow Weep for Me.'" *MELUS* 31 (3): 67–99. doi:10.1093/melus/31.3.67

Moore, Antonio. 2015, February 17. "The Black Male Incarceration Problem Is Real and It Is Catastrophic." *The Huffington Post.* http://www.huffingtonpost.com/antonio-moore/black-mass-incarceration-statistics_b_6682564.html

Moore, Alicia L, and La Vonne I. Neal. 2006. "Resilience: Overcoming the Crippling Obstacles of Slavery." *Black History Bulletin* 69 (2): 2–3.

National Association for the Advancement of Colored People (NAACP). 2015. "Health Care Fact Sheet." *National Association for the Advancement of Colored People (NAACP).* http://www.naacp.org/pages/health-care-fact-sheet

National Center for Education Statistics (NCES). No Date. "Fast Facts: Historically Black Colleges and Universities." *National Center for Education Statistics, Institute of Education Sciences, U.S. Department of Education.* http://nces.ed.gov/fastfacts/display.asp?id=667

Nichols, Joyce Coleman, and Carol B. Tanksley. 2004. "Revelations of African-American Women with Terminal Degrees: Overcoming Obstacles to Success." *The Negro Educational Review* 55 (4): 175–85.

Obama, Barack. 2014, September 19. "Presidential Proclamation—National Historically Black Colleges and Universities Week, 2014." *Office of the Press Secretary, The White House.* https://www.whitehouse.gov/the-press-office/2014/09/19/presidential-proclamation-national-historically-black-colleges-and-unive

Owens, Janine. 2015. "Exploring the Critiques of the Social Model of Disability: The Transformative Possibility of Arendt's Notion of Power." *Sociology of Health & Illness* 37 (3): 385–403. doi:10.1111/1467-9566.12199

Petersen, Amy J. 2009. "'Ain't Nobody Gonna Get Me Down:' An Examination of the Educational Experiences of Four African American Women Labeled with Disabilities." *Equity & Excellence in Education* 42 (2): 428–42. doi:10.1080/10665680903245284

Pickens, Therí A. 2014. *New Body Politics: Narrating Arab and Black Identities in the Contemporary United States.* New York: Routledge.

Price, Margaret. 2011. *Mad at School: Rhetorics of Mental Disability and Academic Life.* Ann Arbor: University of Michigan Press.

Rose, David H., Wendy S. Harbour, Catherine S. Johnston, Samantha G. Daley, and Linda Abarbanell. 2006. "Universal Design for Learning in Postsecondary Education: Reflections on Principles and their Applications." *Journal of Postsecondary Education and Disability* 19 (2): 135–51.

Rosen, Shari. 2015, February 26. "Black History Speakers Discuss Racial Biases, Overcoming Barriers." *Soundoff!* http://www.ftmeadesoundoff.com/news/12577/black-history-speakers-discuss-racial-biases-overcoming-barriers/

Ruffins, Paul. 2008. "Creating an atmosphere of acceptance." *Diverse Issues in Higher Education* 25 (9): 14–16.

Samuels, Ellen. 2014. *Fantasies of Identification: Disability, Gender, Race.* New York: New York University Press.

Shakespeare, Thomas and Nicholas Watson. (2002). "The Social Model of Disability: An Outdated Ideology?" *Research in Social Science and Disability* 2: 9–28. doi:10.1016/s1479–3547(01)80018-x

Shapiro, Joseph P. 1993. *No Pity: People with Disabilities Forging a New Civil Rights Movement.* New York: Random House.

Shaw, Talbert O. 2006. "Character Education: The *Raison dÊtre* of Historically Black Colleges and Universities." In *How Black Colleges Empower Black Students: Lessons for Higher Education*, edited by Frank W. Hale, Jr., 89–100. Sterling, VA: Stylus Publishing.

Siebers, Tobin. 2008. *Disability Theory.* Ann Arbor: University of Michigan Press.

Skiba, Russell J., Lori Poloni-Staudinger, Sarah Gallini, Ada B. Simmons, and Renae Feggins-Azziz. 2006. "Disparate Access: The Disproportionality of African American Students with Disabilities across Educational Environments," *Exceptional Children* 72: 411–24. doi:10.1177/001440290507300301 01

Skloot, Rebecca. 2011. *The Immortal Life of Henrietta Lacks.* New York: Broadway Books.

Spiritual Workshop. No Date. "We Shall Overcome." *NegroSpirituals.com.* http://www.negrospirituals.com/songs/we_shall_overcome.htm

Taylor, Ashley. 2015. "The Discourse of Pathology: Reproducing the Able Mind through Bodies of Color." *Hypatia* 30 (1): 181–98. doi:10.1111/hypa.12123

Taylor, Steven J. 2011. "Disability Studies in Higher Education." *New Directions for Higher Education* 154: 93–98. doi:10.1002/he.438

Tettenborn, Éva. 2006. "Melancholia as Resistance in Contemporary African American Literature." *MELUS* 31 (3): 101–21. doi:10.1093/melus/31.3.101

Treatment Advocacy Center. 2014, November. "How Many Individuals with Serious Mental Illness Are in Jails and Prisons?" *Backgrounder, Treatment Advocacy Center.* http://www.treatmentadvocacycenter.org/problem/consequences-of-non-treatment/2580

Tushnet, Mark V. 1994. *Making Civil Rights Law: Thurgood Marshall and the Supreme Court*. New York: Oxford University Press.

Valente, Joseph Michael, Benjamin Bahan, and H-Dirkson Bauman. 2011. "Sensory Politics and the Cochlear Implant Debate." In *Cochlear Implants: Evolving Perspectives*, ed. Raylene Paludneiciene and Irene W. Leigh, 245–48. Washington, DC: Gallaudet University Press.

Wallace, Sherri L., Sharon E. Moore, Linda L. Wilson, and Brenda G. Hart. 2012. "African American Women in the Academy: Quelling the Myth of Presumed Incompetence." In *Presumed Incompetent: The Intersections of Race and Class for Women in Academia*, ed. Gabriella Gutiérrez y Muhs, Yolanda Flores Niemann, Carmen G. González, and Angela P. Harris, 421–38. Logan, UT: Utah State University Press.

Watts, Ivan Eugene, and Nirmala Erevelles. 2004. "These Deadly Times: Reconceptualizing School Violence by Using Critical Race Theory and Disability Studies." *American Educational Research Journal* 41 (2): 271–99. doi:10.3102/00028312041002271

Williamson, Carolyn E. 2007. *Black Deaf Students: A Model for Educational Success*. Washington, DC: Gallaudet University Press.

Wu, Cynthia. 2012. *Chang and Eng Reconnected: The Original Siamese Twins in American Culture*. Philadelphia: Temple University Press.

Risking Experience

Disability, Precarity, and Disclosure

KATE KAUL

Sitting at dinner around a large, busy table of conference participants, I turned to listen to a colleague who seemed to be telling me something to do with my paper. One of the people attending the session had tweeted something I'd said in my presentation, he told me. He was trying to show me the comment but I was halted by a sudden, sick feeling, as I replayed in my head the material from my paper presentation. I had added material without writing it down; I had not distributed drafts. What had I said? Who would read it? What, what, *what* had I been thinking? The small session I had participated in had never been private, but it had felt private. Without that illusion, it might have been impossible for me to speak.

The comment, it turned out, was about disclosing disability without disclosing impairment—and it didn't disclose (although I had in my paper) that this was personal; that I often disclose one without disclosing the other. To say that here, of course, is just to perform that careful refusal one more time. Disclosure is risky. Writing about disability and disclosure in the university as a part-time, contract instructor, I am aware that while my work is always already precarious, there are ways to make it more precarious, and that this may be one of them. Disclosure has risks and benefits; and we can never know in advance quite what a disclosure will cost, or what it will make possible.

My own experience of vertigo, of teetering between the private and the public, reminds me of Rosemarie Garland-Thomson's (2009) framing of invisible disability as always poised to erupt, to leap, into visibility. Weighing the risks and possibilities of disclosure involves more than a sudden sense of precariousness; as vertigo, it includes the fear that one won't just fall into vis-ibility, but jump. I have jumped. More than a year ago, I made an official dis-closure that I hoped would be a formality—surely people already knew—in order to begin an accommodation process. A year later, I moved my disability firmly into the realm of the visible, bringing a mobility scooter to campus. Seeking accommodations and recognition has been a long process, and it has involved a lot of meetings, a lot of people, a union, and the settlement of a grievance which is, of course, confidential. I had hoped for an ending to an episode of my accommodation process, which would make it easier to write about. A tenure-track position! A straightforward accommodation process! Not needing accommodations! But I am still falling, waiting for solid ground.

This essay takes up a few examples of the incoherence of living and work-ing with disability as a contract worker in a setting that frames both disability and contract work as extraordinary, each an unfortunate, if recurring, surprise. I want to consider the kinds of disruption involved in coherence, knowledge, and identity that seem to be asked of people at this nexus of disability and contract work, in the conflicting demands to disclose and to cover in the university and in academic life more broadly.

This writing is risky work. In the context of invisible and visible disability, in the uneasy moves between them, disclosing not just disability identity but impairment brings new risks, new possibilities. What if it is not practical, or even possible, for some of us to disclose disability or impairment? What kind of knowledge can we make out of not-knowing, or not-telling? How can we respond, as a field and a community, to the precarity that disability and dis-closure add, for some of us, to precarious work? Are we willing, in and as dis-ability studies, to risk recognizing accounts and analyses that occupy, rather than overcome, this tense margin between disclosure and non-disclosure? And what is the alternative? I'm interested in exploring how some of these risk factors translate into representation—what kinds of stories do we get to read, even within disability studies; are even compelling, important, accounts necessarily the stories that weren't too risky to tell? What does this leave us with as the shared discourse of our experiences in the academy?

This has been a difficult essay to write, a new direction in my work and, at the same time, something I am always thinking about. The Disability Dis-closure in/and Higher Education Conference gave me permission to think about disclosure as a problematic, rather than an immediate, ongoing, prob-lem. But without the resolution that would mark an ending, or at least an episode, it has been difficult to stop thinking about it long enough to write.

In part, this requires thinking through the ways in which disability counts, and is counted, in the academy, as well as the impact of this counting. We count, first, when we are recognized, important, noticed; and, second, when we show up as a statistic, a record, a factor, a number—as data. Altogether, counting points both to the research, the data which is not yet available, and to the tensions and vulnerabilities that make it so difficult to obtain; and this lack is tangible through my discussion.

I was at a workshop once where Garland-Thomson asked a question (2009). She introduced her question for the presenting feminist legal theorist by saying, "I work in literary criticism, and so I deal in conjecture." Then, something about a skirt. I work in critical theory, and so I would never call my conjecture "conjecture." But the kind of speculation that I do is not based in practical research. Instead of research, I have only experience. But I would hesitate to call this personal experience. My experience is not only private but public, not only individual but social. I'm using "experience" broadly, as not just what happens to us but as also how we make sense, meaning, self, out of what happens to us. I've argued elsewhere for the importance of this collective work of experience (Kaul 2016). Here, I want to focus on the work we are doing—we in the "here" of disability studies—on disclosure.

The word "disclosure" is a nexus in recent conversations about disability and, especially, invisible disability. These conversations include a wealth of new work, some of it problematizing this idea of invisibility. Garland-Thomson has herself suggested that invisible disability is just disability waiting to erupt into the visible (2009). This suggests that disability may disclose itself whether we choose to disclose it or not. I don't disagree with this entirely—I resisted it until I realised that I was walking through a library, trying to adjust my gait so that my ankle-foot orthotic (AFO) would stop squeaking in my shoe and the heads of the people I passed would stop turning towards me. My concern is with this idea of disclosure. It suggests that if we wanted to, if we felt safe, if it was in our best interests, if the costs were not too high, we could all disclose.

Disclosure suggests an underlying truth one has access to: an uncovering, with non-disclosure a covering of that truth. "Covering" in Yoshino's (2006) discussion of his painful journey towards his acceptance of his homosexuality--suggests one covers something one knows about. Yoshino translates Erving Goffman's "covering" from the context of disability to the context of sexuality but has little to say about this connection in *Covering: The Hidden Assault on Our Civil Rights*. What do we disclose when we disclose disability? In other places, I have taken a little more time to map out the ways that disability is always hyper-exemplary; rhetorically and discursively spectacular, it is always an example of something else (Kaul 2013). In the conceptual loop of disability itself, it is invisibility that is outside itself, not hyper but ultra-exemplary, beyond exemplary, incomprehensible—or suspect, always waiting to erupt unpredictably, *uncountably*, into the visible. One effect of this is, I think, that there *are* no good examples of disability. If even disability-as-wheelchair, in Fritsch's (2013) careful articulation, is a simplification, the full complexity of disability makes for bad examples.

Titchkosky (2011) has an interesting discussion of this problem of counting in her book, *The Question of Access: Disability, Space, Meaning*, in which she offers the example of the accessible classroom. In Titchkosky's example, her academic department secures "more than half a million dollars in grant money . . . in order to build an accessible, state-of-the-art classroom" (31). But this is in the context of the neoliberal university, which counts students, the time and space they will use, as "BIUs," "Basic Income Units" (31). The classroom is fully funded, with disability not an exception, an afterthought, or even a cofactor, but the original, basic, principle on which the grant was secured. But this does not stop disability from emerging as a funding issue, as an exceptional drain on resources. As "the university person responsible for space management" says:

> Who, exactly who, is to be included in this accessible classroom? And who is the adjoining special washroom for? You can't accommodate everybody. You've got to draw the line somewhere. Really, think about it, worst-case scenario, is your classroom for forty people going to fit forty people in wheelchairs? Your plan needs to include many more details about who, who exactly, is this space for. (AIF Accessible Classroom, Meeting Notes, November, 2007) (qtd. in Titchkosky 2011, 31)

No one lives their university life as BUI—no one is fully countable. But with disability defined as "exceptionally variable and in need of measurement" (32)—persistently, even definitively, uncountable—counting disabled people in advance, making space for them, accounting for them, simply *cannot* make sense. The accessible classroom threatens administrators with disabled people; it suggests they may show up, but it doesn't say how many of them, or when. It doesn't make them any easier to count. In the paradox that Titchkosky (2011) expresses as the gap between "they never show up" and "what are you doing here," even disability-as-wheelchair cannot contain forty disabled people, cannot make forty wheelchair users add up to forty.

I have a different example: an example of the inaccessible classroom. The first meeting of my new course, Women and Disabilities, was in a classroom that, clearly, wasn't going to work. I went to the course administrator and asked for a room change.

"It's not accessible," I say. "It only fits twenty-five people and I have forty enrolled. We can't get into it." "It's not accessible?" she asks.

I realize I need to put it differently but when fifteen of *some* people can't get into a room it's an access issue; when fifteen of *everybody* can't get into a room, it's a space allocation error.

"We need to move to a larger room," I say. "And I need it still to be accessible."

"Do you have a student who needs it to be accessible?"

"It's a disability studies class," I hedge/politicize. "So probably. Obviously, I can't ask."

"*Obviously*," stresses the administrator. "But . . ."

"But . . . ?"

"Well . . ."

"Really . . . ?"

We pause together in our ellipses. What will she need for her conversation with space allocation? I feign righteous ignorance for a while, and then I cave and answer her unspoken question:

"I didn't see anyone with a wheelchair or mobility stuff. Of course that doesn't mean no one needs an accessible space. And there are still a few students who haven't shown up yet. And it's a disability studies class. So chances are . . ."

"I would need a student to disclose," she says.

"I couldn't ask," I say.

"*Of course*," she agrees. "But . . ."

"But . . . ?"

"Well . . ."

We pause again. It's a long one. The administrator doesn't seem to be enjoying this; perhaps, like me, she's not sure where I'm headed.

"Ok," I say. "I need an accessible classroom. I need it for me. I need it because I have a disability that makes it hard for me to go up and down stairs. And I need to be able to reach the AV equipment." This may have seemed irrelevant but in another new disability studies course that year, for another new department, I had been surprised to find the AV console was welded to the wall, halfway up a flight of steep concrete steps. It hadn't occurred to me that I couldn't operate an AV console positioned at shoulder height, with my feet on different steps, until I gave it a try.

There's another pause. I'm confused; I thought I had given the administrator what she needed. But she tells me, "I'm going to need a thing."

"A thing?"

"A . . . thing."

"What kind of thing?"

"A letter from a doctor?"

An image flashes through my mind of the kind of letter my family doctor—a good sport in so many ways—might write that would set out the reasons why the disability studies course in the summer session of a mostly-newly built university should be held in a room the students and the instructor can be expected to get into. It's long and angry and it looks a bit like a paper I once wrote. I pat it down for now.

"I can get one," I concede. "But I also have this thing." I hoist my foot up on to the arm of the chair I've been standing next to, peel up the leg of my—cropped—trousers (it is, after all, the summer term), and point out the plastic brace. I can't believe she hasn't seen it before. She sees it now.

"Oh, of course," she says. "If they ask . . ."

"I'll get the thing," I finish.

But they don't.

At home, my girlfriend laughs: "Good thing you wore your splints today!"

I know that lots of us have these examples. But what's interesting to me is this: what are they examples *of*? This is not a story about an evil administrator; this administrator got me a new room, got me another room when the second room had tiny, broken seats, and generally made my life much easier than it might have been. Instead, this is a story about an institutionality—not a single institution, or university, but a way of organizing the academy, the world—which demands that disability be framed as something that an unfortunate individual—in particular, an unfortunate student—brings to the classroom. For example, there is no simple mechanism by which I can just let space allocation know in advance that I need an accessible room, whether I'm teaching disability studies or writing. In this framing of disability as something unfortunate students bring to the university, disability is by necessity a surprise and so it surprises people—*Really? What on earth did you do?* Of *course*—we will try to move things around for you in October. As a contract instructor, I have no routine input into room allocation or scheduling; I have to appear as a disruption and emergency. In fact, it's only as a disabled person—as a surprise—that I have any input at all. My disability experience and my contract experience have moved on from this point—my disability is visible, I have made an official disclosure and pursued accommodations, and I have more seniority in a unionized workplace. But I would be hard-pressed to find a simple mechanism in any of it.

I didn't just cave in my own story, above; I caved in so many ways—I reinforced the idea that disability is visible, even that invisible disability is just waiting to be made visible, and that an unfortunate individual (because those AFOs are very uncomfortable, especially the right one) brings disability to a classroom that was fine until she turned up. I also, of course, claimed disability; I asserted my authenticity, my right to teach from my experience. I weighed costs and benefits, although I weighed them in a situation in which my choices were narrowly constrained.

But showing someone a brace, an AFO, is not really disclosing, is it? In some ways, it's misdirection. It's a claim to identity without offering any information, any specifics. It does say: this invisible disability I'm claiming is physical—not a learning disability, not a psychiatric disability. My claim might be false, or—sneakier—partial; I might claim a physical disability and not mention depression, anxiety, other things that might be hard, or costly, to count. I imagine this reassures the university, if only to some extent, and I'm sorry to be participating in this hierarchy of reassuring and less reassuring disabilities myself. But I'm not separate from this university in which I have studied and taught for many years now, even if it's never quite gotten to know me.

If I was going to disclose my disability, really disclose, wouldn't I have to go further than saying that I'm not unsurprising but—surprise—disabled, go further than saying that my disability is physical; wouldn't I have to say what it is? Sometimes I go so far as to clarify that it's not temporary, or that it's not MS. But disclosing disability identity is a copout in a situation whereby "disability," the person asking means "impairment." As for what it is? Karen Kelsky, of *The Professor Is In* (2015), advises that even representing oneself as an adjunct can be disastrous for an academic career. I've probably said enough for now.

When I first started drafting this essay, I had not disclosed my disability in any consistent, official way at work, but I had disclosed it repeatedly—sometimes, I felt, relentlessly—in individual encounters, in conversations with academic staff, in the private and semi-private moments of committee and departmental work and events, in my teaching. These disclosures seemed to have little ongoing impact on my work life; for example, a disclosure in September usually got me an accessible room to teach in by October, but it had no impact on the following September. When rooms were already accessible, I didn't need to change them, so I didn't need, or risk, even informal disclosure.

One of the things I have learned over the last few years is that the accessible classroom that Titchkosky (2011) describes is not just a space. It is a matter of timing, of priority (and hierarchy), of communication, of legibility, recognition, imagination. A room is a time-slot, a space, a set of technological devices: lights, seats, a writing surface, a door, a floor, a media system, amplification. In an accessible room, by which I mean, one where I can use all the things that I need in order to teach, I may not have to disclose my disability to my students. If I had the early input into room allocation that many tenured and tenure-track instructors do (with room allocation, of course, only possible following teaching assignments), I would choose one of the rooms that are accessible, or mostly accessible, to me. Since I don't (or at least, don't yet) have this input and since other people do, it's not unusual for me to have to teach a tutorial in a room that has a computer system I can't use, for example. In this situation, I have the option of lying to my students and telling them the media system is not working, or the other option of telling them that I cannot operate the media system and—in either case—that we are waiting for a room change by the administration. In either case, I cannot show a film or video clip, I cannot use the doc-cam to replace writing on the board, and I cannot access the course web management site to illustrate my discussions of assignments and the syllabus with students. The first time a colleague covers a class for me may expose me as either a technophobe or a disabled instructor, as someone who wouldn't, or couldn't, use the technology in the classroom which does seem, after all, to be working. Whether we disclose or not, it's hard to imagine that restrictions like these will not be reflected in our student course evaluations. Those evaluations, and their life in hiring and promotion, represent one more under-researched area in which we cannot control or even anticipate quite how disability counts and is counted.

In suggesting that academic institutions conceptualize disability as a student problem, I don't mean to compare the resources available to students and to instructors. For one thing, I am part of a union which, while not at its strongest, is stronger than many. I have access to funds, grants, benefits, and provisions, which includes provisions related to disability—and I am glad to have this. My work on this article, for example, was supported by internal research funding for union members. Disabled students deal with a different set of obstacles and resources. Disabled student-workers, usually teaching assistants, occupy an especially uneasy position. My point is that instructors with disabilities don't make sense to the university because its conception of disability doesn't make sense—and that this failure to make sense—this un-countability—demonstrates the sadly unsurprising disaster of disability policy.

If this fails to make sense, it is part of a broader, more calculated, failure. Here, we can move beyond conjecture to, at least, the "data fragments" available (Bauder 2006, 229). The "casualization" of academic labor is intensifying, and this casualization is not just bad for casual workers themselves (or for their students), it supports what is left of the tenure system. Bauder (2006) describes the function of what Karl Marx called the "reserve army" of labor in the specific situation of the twenty-first century academy:

> The workers in the secondary segment of the labour market absorb the shock of fluctuations in the general demand for labour. In other words, the availability of a pool of "flexible" workers, who can easily be hired and fired, permits the relative stability of the primary segment, in which workers will keep their jobs when demand of labour temporarily declines. From this perspective, it could be argued that the stability of tenured faculty positions is functionally dependent on the existence of a sufficient number of flexible sessional and adjunct faculty. Without this flexible academic labour force, the stability of a segment of tenured professors would be threatened. (231)

In this case, though, Bauder argues, "segmentation becomes a strategy of reducing wages and labour standards in the entire academic labour market" (231).

Ivancheva (2015) maps out the demands of this generation of contract academic workers: one is internationalization, the necessity that a worker relocate (often with their family) from one region, country, or even continent, to another or settle for inferior working conditions (42). But it is not unusual now to relocate, not only for tenure-track jobs and the "celebrated 'internationalization'" Ivancheva describes, but even for short-term teaching contracts—for precarious work. This is a challenge to anyone whose impairment is exacerbated by travel or whose disability demands structures of care (accessible housing, accessible local transit, extra childcare, attendant care, insurance or government support benefits, specialized medical care) that do not travel easily. Immigration status restricts mobility, and immigration presents particular problems to many disabled workers. Moving from job to job, or cobbling together courses at different universities, can mean disclosing repeatedly in different environments. It can mean knowing that a disclosure in one setting may carry over into another setting that may be less protected. At the same time, disabled people are over-represented in casual academic work. Disabled people have served as a reserve labor pool since long before Russell (2002) articulated this in an intersectional analysis of race with disability in the U.S. labor market reserve. The relationship between disability and adjunct status is under-researched, but it is hardly casual.

I would love to have more data and less conjecture to offer here, but I hope I have been able to at least gesture toward the intense precarity of disabled contract instructors and the difficulties that disclosure presents, repeatedly, to many of us in this intersection. In disability studies itself, our conversation about disclosure has been concerned more directly with writing and research than with teaching. But I want to ask: what happens when we set our conversation about disclosure in disability studies into this broader context?

Michel Foucault frames his text "What is an Author?" with a quotation from Samuel Beckett: "What does it matter? What does it matter, who is speaking?" Imagine, for a moment, that it doesn't matter who is speaking. Imagine that you aren't looking for the thread that would lead you to an identification, a subject position, disclosure, a particular human—the particularity of being human. So many of us care who is writing and teaching disability studies. Should we?

We all live in a world that is structured by ability/disability—by what Garland-Thomson calls "the ability/disability system" (2002, 2). I agree with this and I agree, also, with Thomson's suggestion that many of us are "temporarily able bodied"; that people who are not disabled—TABs—may become disabled at any time. These suggestions are part of what I think of as a universalist approach to disability: it's happening to everyone; it can happen to anyone. This approach has been a way to present disability as both important and ordinary. It's happening to everyone; it can happen to anyone. This is true, but it's not true enough. Its truth obscures truths which are more important.

In a 2014 article for *Rhetoric Review*, Kerschbaum considers the demand that she bring her deafness into her academic writing, her varying response to this demand, and the sometimes unpredictable consequences of disclosure—of the disclosures through which she preempts, anticipates, responds to, or concedes to this demand. The four scenarios—examples—that frame

Kerschbaum's essay suggest more than a demand for disclosure but an insistence that deaf experience be centered as always important to the deaf scholar's work—because it is so important, so surprising, to the hearing person who is insisting. As Kerschbaum points out, disclosure may be met with "denial, resistance, or ignorance" (2014, 57).

Does it matter, when this demand is made, who is asking? Kerschbaum cites Lennard Davis, who writes, in *Enforcing Normalcy*, "that 'there is a powerful policing mechanism' that insists upon an answer to the question of a writer's disability status, which is not revealed in the written word unless it is explicitly identified (xvi–xvii)" (2014, 56). Kerschbaum's own scenarios suggest that the people who are asking her are not deaf, and that if the fourth involves someone she identifies as a "disability studies colleague," the other three likely don't; the demand to disclose often comes from nondisabled people or from colleagues working outside disability studies. In Davis' case, though, the force of the "policing mechanism" seems to come from disabled people or from *within* disability studies. What an awesome power "we" wield! Maybe the demand for disclosure undermines the ethos of nondisabled scholars working in disability studies but, if it does, it does so in the only area of knowledge production in which disability is not perceived—as Kerschbaum reminds us—as "disqualification" (69) but as a qualification.

In the classroom, the disabled instructor acts as a disruption of the epistemological negation of disabled people that positions us as not-knowers rather than knowers. Following Kumari Campbell (2009), we could imagine this disruption as characterizing only the epistemological force of the embodied disabled instructor in the disability studies classroom; that force is Kumari Campbell's immediate focus in the archly titled, "Having a Career in Disability Studies without even Becoming Disabled! The Strains of the Disabled Teaching Body." In the performance of a disabled teacher teaching disability studies, "The teacher's body rather than being a tolerated imperfection in the system instead is integral as, [citing Maria Angel 1994], '"the *site* and *sight* of authoritative display'" (2009, 3). Although the visibility of the disabled instructor, as a body in the classroom, is important to this analysis, the visibility of the instructor's disability is not as important as its disclosure. Thinking through theories of "experience," Kumari Campbell builds on Simi Linton's and Nancy Mairs' early suggestions that we pay attention to the phenomenological aspects of disabled people's lives that inform what Mairs calls "the disability gaze" (qtd. in Kumari Campbell 2009, 3). Kumari Campbell calls it "surprising" that we are still needing to make this argument, which

Linton and Mairs each articulated in 1998. I would be less optimistic, less disappointed, and say that it is surprising that we still need to make it within disability studies—or that I wish I were surprised.

If we move beyond teaching disability studies, or critical disability studies, to the writing that still qualifies people for that teaching, we find a broad conversation about disclosure, one that I can only sketch out here. Introducing her 2009 book, *Dangerous Discourses of Disability, Subjectivity and Sexuality,* Shildrick situates her project in, and as, "critical disability studies," arguing:

> One important difference that marks out critical disability theory from its predecessors is its willingness to step aside from the claim that disability studies not only is, but should be, territory occupied primarily, if not solely, by those who live with a disability. What has become clear is that as the ground for a form of oppression widely perpetuated in western societies, disability—like alternatives to heterosexuality, or racial differences—poses probing questions about the nature of those societies, both in terms of their overt organization and their social imaginaries. The responsibility for inquiry and analysis falls, then, not on disabled people alone but on all those who participate in the relevant structures. Just as the scholarship of recent years has identified racism as a problem of whiteness, so too ableism must be addressed by those who are identified with normative standards and those who are excessive to them. (15)

Shildrick here identifies the centering of disability experience, including the demand for disclosure, as unscholarly, uncritical—and she does so in a field-defining move if, as is increasingly the case, "uncritical" disability studies is read as *not* disability studies. In her influential 1998 "Disability Studies/Not Disability Studies," essay, Linton distinguishes the liberal-arts, humanities-based approaches to disability she names as "disability studies," from the "applied" fields' approaches to disability that she identifies as "not" (1998, 132–36). Linton moves from calling for representation of the phenomenological experience of people with various disabilities (140) to the importance of subjectivity in disability studies scholarship (142). Shildrick (2009) nudges the reader toward a newer distinction in which work that is concerned with situation and identity is not "critical disability studies," a term that otherwise seems still to apply to the work Linton would have called "disability studies" in 1998 (and might now) in distinguishing it from work that is steeped in the medical model. Shildrick's position actually inverts Linton's distinction, adding identity and experience to the detritus that critical disability studies needs to leave behind. I agree that disability is a world-structuring category in which all of us are implicated, and that all of us—not just disabled people—should be paying critical attention to it. My problem is this: the position that position doesn't matter is a valid one, but it's one we're overwhelmingly more likely to read, when the subject is disability, than the position that position does matter. Is this because it's more true, or because it's more palatable, or because the people who think it are more likely to write it and publish it? Should we allow it to define a field? Inquiry and analysis is not only a responsibility, or even an opportunity; sometimes, especially in the academy, it's a job.

Asking people to situate their work is not the same as asking them to stop doing it; Kumari Campbell (2009) is explicit in setting this out, suggesting in response to "the vexed question of a CDS [critical disability studies] academic's 'disability status'" a call to publicly acknowledge the ways one's own positionality intersects with disablement and the impact this may have on teaching and research" (7). And situating ourselves is something most of us might give more thought to, given other problems with representation in disability studies. In asking "What's so 'critical' about critical disability studies?" Helen Meekosha and Russell Shuttleworth (2009) map a critical disability studies genuinely informed by critical social theory and call for, in particular, "an explicit dialogue with human rights and emancipatory thinking from the diversity of cultures" (54). This global approach, they argue, "is crucial for CDS when the global majority of disabled people are excluded from the dominant disability discourse" (54).

Even in North America, the stakes are high around disclosure. It is hard to compare Davis' experience of "policing" in our field with the attempts by disabled adjuncts to cover and to pass, or with the struggles by disabled job applicants to decide when, whether, or how much to disclose as part of the same problem. A loss of authority, a failure to have one's full experience recognized, can be frustrating, but it does connect you to disability identity. For disabled academics, disclosure is sometimes a claim to authority and experience. Often, it is an attempt at access. It is hard to distinguish those two elements, but I know that—in my own experience—a claim to authority is a small compensation for the risks that disclosure exposes me to when I ask for accommodation, risks which I can no longer avoid if I want to write and teach. Fritsch's discussion of "access" reminds us that, etymologically, access is both entry and attack; it draws our attention to borders (2016, 28). One person's access is another person's threat, and that dynamic is something we might be aware of here.

Australian academic Newell suggests that, in bringing a complaint against his university under Australia's Disability Discrimination Act, he had a responsibility to fight, to tell his story, because he could: "As someone with a well-documented complaint, access to important resources, a supportive family and an adequate education, I felt that I had the best chance of many people with a disability in tackling the issue successfully" (Vance 2007, 119). Newell writes that in sharing his own story, he is trying "to show the importance of <u>doing</u> and <u>being</u> rather than mere talk"; we need to leave "the empty rhetoric about disability and reclaim the importance of rhetoric as powerful arguments and stories, which drive equal opportunity outcomes" (Vance 2007, 121, emphasis in the original). Telling and not-telling, disclosing and not disclosing, are part of this doing and being. But that is not to say that we should all disclose.

O'Toole's (2013) demand for disclosure is a demand that people situate themselves, an assertion that situation makes a difference. This situating, this disclosure, is part of the action through which disability studies can make change in the world. O'Toole articulates this demand as necessary, important, something "we" need to do as a field, as a movement. Here, O'Toole echoes Price's (2011) discussion of "kairotic spaces"—hallways, etc.—the liminal spaces of the academy, in which disclosures happen, or don't happen, which Kerschbaum also takes up (Kerschbaum 2014). O'Toole (2013) is frustrated that someone participating in a disability studies conference may disclose in a hallway, or at lunch, but not in their conference paper—and that many people bristle at the demand for disclosure. Asking all of us to respond to the question, "What is your relationship to disability?" O'Toole (2013) calls for "universal public disclosure" by disability studies scholars as a way to fight stigma, build community, and advance disability rights. O'Toole suggests that while disability information should be shared, "medical information is private," acknowledging that some impairments are highly stigmatized (2013, 7). Later, she writes that "The statement, 'I am disabled' is complete and does not necessitate an impairment discussion . . . With practice, accepting someone's answer such as 'I'm a nondisabled Disability Studies scholar' will become accepted" (11). I agree that O'Toole's open claiming of her identity as a queer disabled parent has made it possible for other people to approach her and to build community; certainly, I have benefitted from this personally. O'Toole acknowledges that disability experience is not static for anyone. But disability identity is not always straightforward either. The statement "I am disabled" has never been complete to me. How can I expect someone else to accept it?

In the same issue of *Disability Studies Quarterly* where O'Toole's essay appears, Rinaldi (2013) presents a different position, arguing that disclosure is too much to ask of too many of us in disability studies. And yet, noting that she is "caught up in a contradiction," Rinaldi centers her critique in a vivid, detailed, personal disclosure of her own disability experience. It is a discomfiting account and it accomplishes Rinaldi's purpose: "to illustrate that there are complications to coming out, that at least my coming out comes with baggage, and that not all moments of coming out lead to a community embrace." Rinaldi (2013) concludes that she remains "convinced that we have enough safe spaces, even and especially in our own field, for all of our stories" (11). Like O'Toole, Rinaldi grounds her position in her experience. As an academic whose disability is not usually visible, perhaps Rinaldi needs this authority to make the point that asking people to disclose is asking too much. But what about people for whom it really is too much to disclose—not just painful and personal, but too painful, too personal, too costly?

I don't have a clear position in this debate. I agree that disclosure builds community and fights stigma, but I think that it can be disastrous for individuals. Some people have complex relationships to disability and to impairment. The question, "what is your relationship to disability?" can be difficult to answer even privately, let alone publicly, for people without a clear diagnosis, for people whose disability experience has involved traumatic losses, or for people who expect their impairments to shorten their lives. My experience so far has been that a disability question does lead to an impairment question, and while this may improve, it can't change fast enough for many of us.

That said, I am not prepared to go as far as Kumari Campbell (2009) or O'Toole (2013) diplomatically do in valuing everyone's participation in disability studies equally. Vick (2014) writes, "for workers with episodic disabilities, it takes a lot of work to go to work" (8) and disability studies—whether we call it "critical" or not—is work, the work of research, writing, presenting, and teaching. Given current employment statistics, it is not unreasonable to assume that most (not all) working academics who do not disclose as disabled in their writing and teaching are, like most (not all) other working academics, not disabled.

Broadly speaking, it is harder—not easier—to get secure work in disability studies if you are disabled. There are exceptions—Rinaldi suggests that aspects of her own experience have been advantageous in the academy, for example (2013, 10)—and qualifiers; some disabilities, impairments, and related life circumstances have much less impact on academic opportunities than others. I am lucky to live in Canada, where I have good (but not perfect) healthcare, to have a partner with secure work, to be white and middle class, and to have a strong social network; these factors are part of my disability experience. But while disabled people are under-represented in academic work and concentrated in situations of precarity that do not support writing and research, I believe the following is important: We are overwhelmingly more likely to encounter the opinions of nondisabled academics, both in the classroom and in the discourse of academic disability studies—about disclosure, identity, and everything else—than we are of disabled academics. That discourse includes a very small percentage of the world's disabled and nondisabled population, as Meekosha and Shuttleworth (2009) remind us, and even within that percentage, it represents a limited set of experiences. While that is the case, we need to work to keep field-defining questions—our borders—open. We need to think about what we can do to support diverse perspectives in disability studies. We need to be willing to be surprised.

References

Bauder, Harald. 2006. "The Segmentation of Academic Labour: A Canadian Example." *ACME: An International E-Journal for Critical Geographies* 4 (2): 228–39. http://ojs.unbc.ca/index.php/acme/article/view/735

Fritsch, Kelly. 2013. "The Neoliberal Circulation of Affects: Happiness, Accessibility and the Capacitation of Disability as Wheelchair." *Health, Culture and Society* 5 (1): 135–49.

Fritsch, Kelly, Claire O'Connor, and A. K. Thompson, eds. 2016. *Keywords for Radicals: The Contested Vocabulary of Late-Capitalist Struggle*. Chico: AK Press.

Garland-Thomson, Rosemarie. 2002. "Integrating Disability, Transforming Feminist Theory." *NWSA Journal* 14 (3): 1–32.

Garland-Thomson, Rosemarie. 2009. Feminism and Legal Theory Workshop, "Feminist Disability Theories and the Law," 11–12 December 2009. Atlanta, GA: Emory University. Comments in discussion.

Ivancheva, Mariya P. 2015. "The Age of Precarity and the New Challenges to the Academic Profession." *Studia UBB. Europaea* LX (1): 39–47. https://www.academia.edu/11886905/The_age_of_precarity_and_the_new_challenges_to_the_academic_profession

Kaul, Kate. 2013. "Vulnerability, for Example: Disability Theory as Extraordinary Demand." *Canadian Journal of Women and the Law* 25 (1): 81–110.

Kaul, Kate. 2016. "Experience." In *Keywords for Radicals: The Contested Vocabulary of Late-Capitalist Struggle*, edited by Kelly Fritsch, Clare O'Connor, and A. K. Thompson. Chico: AK Press.

Kelsky, Karen. 2015. *The Professor Is In*. New York: Three Rivers Press. Kindle edition.

Kerschbaum, Stephanie. 2014. "On Rhetorical Agency and Disclosing Disability in Academic Writing." *Rhetoric Review* 33 (1): 55–71.

Kumari Campbell, Fiona A. 2009. "Having a Career in Disability Studies without even Becoming Disabled! The Strains of the Disabled Teaching Body." *International Journal of Inclusive Education* 13(7): 713–25.

Linton, Simi. 1998. "Disability Studies/Not Disability Studies" in *Claiming Disability: Knowledge and Identity*. New York: New York University Press.

Meekosha, Helen, and Russell Shuttleworth. 2009. "What's so 'Critical' about Critical Disability Studies?" *Australian Journal of Human Rights* 15(1): 47–79.

O'Toole, Corbett J. 2013. "Disclosing Our Relationships to Disabilities: An Invitation for Disability Studies Scholars." *Disability Studies Quarterly* 33:2.

Price, Margaret. 2011. *Mad at School: Rhetorics of Mental Disability and Academic Life*. Ann Arbor: University of Michigan Press.

Rinaldi, Jen. 2013. "Reflexivity in Research: Disability between the Lines." *Disability Studies Quarterly* 33 (2): 1–16.

Russell, Marta. 2002. "What Disability Civil Rights Cannot Do: Employment and Political Economy." *Disability & Society* 17 (2): 117–35.

Shildrick, Margrit. 2009. *Dangerous Discourses of Disability, Subjectivity, and Sexuality*. Houndsmills: Palgrave Macmillan.

Titchkosky, Tanya. 2011. *The Question of Access: Disability, Space, Meaning*. Toronto: University of Toronto Press.

Vick, Andrea. 2014. "Living and Working Precariously with an Episodic Disability: Barriers in the Canadian Context." *The Canadian Journal of Disability Studies* 3 (3): 1–28.

Yoshino, Kenji. 2006. *Covering: The Hidden Assault on Our Civil Rights*. New York: Random House.

III

Representation

Postmodern Madness on Campus

*Narrating and Navigating Mental
Difference and Disability*

BRADLEY LEWIS

––––––––

What is postmodernism? For that matter, what is madness? These simple questions are open to controversial responses and deep struggles over meaning. I do not plan to settle these questions, and indeed, it is because of the undecidability and ambiguity surrounding terms like "postmodernism" and "madness" that I find them helpful for considering contemporary mental difference on campus. Both of these terms invite humility with regards to language. We might even call them "anti-diagnostic" words in that they defy tight classification and categorization. They are open-ended, contested, and used in very different ways. Making sense of them is like trying to pin pudding to the wall. What does it mean to call someone "mad" or to identify with madness? What does it mean to say these are "postmodern" times? It can mean very different things in different contexts. Either term can have a positive or a negative valence, a source of hope or something to fear. Embracing the reality that there is much uncertainty surrounding this topic, I humbly use the signifier "postmodern" to investigate a swirl of contemporary forces on college campuses that are impacting student and faculty "madness."

Holding the two terms lightly, I will nonetheless start out with the fairly common usages of the terms "postmodern" and "madness." Postmodern is often used with a negative valence to signify intensified neoliberal forces driving society toward increasing commercialization, mediatization, globalization, deregulation, social cutbacks, competition, inequality, risk society, and environmental degradation. I will refer to this version of postmodernism as "neoliberal postmodernism." On the other hand, postmodern is also frequently used with a largely positive valence to signify emancipatory critical theory, which deconstructs dimensions of power and essentialism found at the heart of all representational practices, including the most seemingly neutral practices of science and medicine. I will refer to this version as "theoretical postmodernism."

Similarly, the term "madness" has two fairly common contradictory meanings. On the one hand, it conjures up frightening images of madmen and crazy people—the very emotionally loaded ideas that the term "mental illness" and the idea "it's a disease like other diseases" was supposed to sanitize. On the other hand, madness continues to be associated with creative genius and inspiration—a much more celebratory meaning that can be used to describe artists, poets, intellectuals, revolutionaries, and mystics who think and feel outside the limitations and constrictions of the norm. In this case, I will not mark this difference in language in order to keep the signifier "madness" open to a variety of meanings surrounding mental difference and disability.

Applying these loose meanings of postmodernism and madness to campus mental health, we can begin to articulate a contradictory story of challenge and opportunity. Postmodern madness brings awareness of the political challenges of neoliberalism and the emancipatory opportunities of critical theory to the different ways of making sense of and living with mental difference and disability on campus. To work through this story, I focus in the first section on some of the impact of postmodern neoliberalism on campus and in the second on the impact of postmodern theory. The third section brings these two together to consider ways to narrate and navigate the personal and scholarly dimensions of postmodern madness on campus.

Growing Up Postmodern: Campus Mental Health in Neoliberal Times

Understanding campus mental health in a time of postmodern neoliberalism requires a socio-cultural backstory that makes sense of both the increasing prevalence of mental health diagnoses and the consolidation of a biological model, or biomedicalization, of psychiatry as the main form of treatment (Clarke et al. 2010). We do not have to go far back in time to develop serviceable stories in these domains because much of today's trends regarding campus mental health can be traced to increasing neoliberal policies and cultural dynamics that emerged over the last few decades (Harvey 2005; Brown 2005). The year 1980 is a useful marker for a catalyst year. That year brings the election of Ronald Reagan, the rise of neoliberal policies, the publication of *Diagnostic and Statistical Manual of Mental Disorders*, third edition. (DSM-III), and the exponential growth of the pharmaceutical industry (Lewis 2011). These events came together to have a major impact on the prevalence and treatment of mental difference and suffering on campus.

Starting with increasing prevalence, epidemiologic studies of adult and childhood mental health tell a story that most of us already know—since the 1980s, the diagnosis and treatment of mental illness has been on the rise. Marcia Angell, the former editor in chief of *The New England Journal of Medicine*, recently reviewed the numbers: people who qualify for mental health disability increased nearly two and a half times between 1987 and 2007. The rise is even more dramatic in children—a thirty-five-fold increase in the same two decades—which makes mental illness the leading cause of disability in children. In addition, a survey of randomly selected adults, sponsored by the National Institute of Mental Health and conducted between 2001 and 2003, found that 46 percent met criteria for having had at least one mental illness within their lives and most met criteria for more than one diagnosis. Of a subgroup affected within the previous year, a third were being treated—up from a fifth in a similar survey ten years earlier (Angell 2011).

With regard to current biomedicalizing trends in mental health treatment on campus, from the 1950s until the 1980s, college counseling centers focused on the relatively benign issues of student development and adjustment to college. This meant college counseling centers were largely staffed by psychotherapists and relied on humanistic and psychodynamic therapeutic practices as their primary treatment paradigms. But moving into the late 1980s, college counseling centers found themselves dealing with what they understood as very different kinds of problems and a very different mental health climate. Counseling centers reported a sharp increase not only in service requests but also in what they called "severe psychological problems." They saw a rapid rise in the numbers of students with learning disabilities, self-injury concerns, eating disorders, substance abuse, bipolar disorder, depression, sexual assault, and sexual abuse problems. In addition, they saw a marked increase of students with previous mental health history and in the numbers of students who came to college already taking psychiatric medications (Kitzrow 2003, 168; Kadison 2004; Gallagher 2006).

College counseling centers responded to these shifts by transitioning their focus away from young adult developmental issues toward more medical models and psychiatric standards of care. Psychiatrists trained in medical models started to play an increasing role, not only in the administration of college programs but also in the assessment and treatment of students. As a result, more and more students today leave counseling centers with psychiatric diagnosis and medication as a key feature of their care (Gallagher 2006, 5). This shift toward medical model protocols shows up even in the names of these college centers as many drop the more humanistic/psychoanalytic signifiers of "college counseling center" and replace them with the more medical/scientific sounding signifiers of "college behavioral health."

Postmodern neoliberalism can be narrated as the catalyst for both the changes in prevalence and changes in treatment on college campuses. Neoliberalism contributes to prevalence by creating socio/cultural conditions of increased competition and decreased social support, both of which put increasing stress and distress on individuals. The distress among children is nicely summed up in the subtitle of a 2002 book, *Growing Up Postmodern: Neoliberalism and the War on the Young*. Strickland (2002), the book's editor and a humanities scholar, relates the notions of postmodernism, neoliberalism, and war on the young by noting that neoliberalism is "the hegemonic ideology of postmodern consumerism" (Strickland 2002, 2). Critics of neoliberalism, such as Strickland, argue that this globalist ideology promotes bottom line, free market economics that expands corporate rationality to the point that corporate profiteering is at war with other values—such as nutrition, healthcare, education, well-being, equality, compassion, childhood, environment, global climate, peace, risk reduction (environmental, financial, epidemic, nuclear), employment, labor conditions, social commons, news media, arts and culture, etc.

Economist Hewlettt and African American studies scholar West use their 1998 book, *The War against Parents: What We Can Do for America's Beleaguered Moms and Dads*, to articulate the equally aggressive and destabilizing role of neoliberalism on families and parents. As Hewlettt and West put it most succinctly, "market values destroy family values," a problem that continues through to the present and that has deeply impacted the childhood of today's college students (Hewlett and West 1998, 2). Hewlett and West make it clear that simply blaming the parents is not the answer. One has to pull back from the particulars of family life to see the social context. "Modern day mothers and fathers, like those before them, struggle to put children at the center of their lives. But major impediments and obstacles stand in their way, undermining their most valiant efforts" (2). For Hewlett and West, neoliberal values, at their heart, undermine the caring, nurturing, and cherishing values that are the central components of good parenting. This leaves children to be raised by corporate messaging and by their peers (who are also raised on corporate messaging). "Increasingly, these exposed, 'skin-less' children are being buffeted by a ruthless market and poisonous culture . . . their bodies and souls stunted and seared by the onslaught of neglect and greed" (Hewlett and West 1998, 1).

Giroux, a scholar of education and cultural studies, develops Strickland, Hewlett, and West's war theme by calling neoliberalism a "system of cruelty" comparable to the inequality and injustice of the nineteenth century's Gilded Age. The cruelty of neoliberalism has so established itself as to become a new common sense that reaches the soul of the citizen-subject: "It has become normalized, serving as a powerful pedagogical force that shapes our lives, memories, and daily experiences, while attempting to erase everything critical and emancipatory about history, justice, solidarity, freedom, and the meaning of democracy" (Giroux 2008, 2). These conditions, accompanied by the deadening neoliberal mantra "there is no alternative," create a culture of fatalism, resignation, and cynicism. "The ongoing attacks on children's rights, the endless commercialization of youth, the downsizing of children's services, and the increasing incarceration of young people suggest [that] adult society no longer cares about children" (Giroux 2008, 86).

The challenge of neoliberal childhood is worse in areas of the highest poverty, but it impacts other classes as well. Child psychiatrist Timimi (2010) articulates many of the specifics of childhood distress that cut across class: (1) demise of the extended family with an increase in separation and divorce, an increase in parental working hours, and a decrease of time parents spend with children; (2) family lifestyles have been uprooted by increased mobility and more time pursuing individual gratification; (3) children's lifestyles have been changed by a decrease in exercise and more indoor pursuits such as computers and TV; (4) commercialization/commodification of childhood with an increase in consumer goods targeted at children; (5) a shift in the education system to a teaching ideology that is rooted in continuous assessment and competition; (6) diets with increased sugar, saturated fats, salt, and chemical additives and decreased in certain essential fatty acids and fresh fruit and vegetables; and (7) exposure to a high anxiety narcissistic value system that has left many children in a psychological vacuum, preoccupied with status and survival and lacking a sense of emotional security and enduring sense of belonging (adapted from Timimi 2010, 692–95).

All of these critics of neoliberalism point to the challenges facing college students as they enter campus. The distress emerging from these challenges is an important dimension of the increasing prevalence of emotional suffering. And, as if this list were not enough, we can also add the impact of neoliberalism on college tuition and on the job market as neoliberal economies increasingly dominate and commercialize both college itself and any future employment the students may have.

The story of the dominant "biological psychiatry" treatment model that now prevails on campus can also be articulated as a neoliberal story. Once again, the story begins in 1980. This year was the year that the American Psychiatric Association turned away from psychoanalysis and psychotherapy through the publication of the *Diagnostic and Statistical Manual of Mental Disorders*, third edition. (DSM-III). The manual decisively and purposefully turned the field back to an earlier era of biological psychiatry. At the time, leading psychiatrist Andreason (1984) hailed the DSM-III as a revolutionary book that would create "a massive reorganization and modernization of psychiatric diagnosis" (155). True to her prediction, historian of psychiatry Shorter (1997) echoed the same themes years later when he argued that DSM-III signaled a "turning of the page on psychoanalysis" and "a redirection of the discipline toward a scientific course" (302).

The year 1980 also marks the moment when the pharmaceutical industry began riding the tides of neoliberalism to become a transnational colossus that competes with the financial industry as the most profitable industry on the globe. Angell (2005) explains that before 1980, the pharmaceutical industry "was a good business, but afterward it was a stupendous one" (3). Drug sales were fairly steady from 1960 to 1980, but during the next twenty years, sales tripled to more than $200 billion a year (2005, 3). The pharmaceutical industry remade itself starting in 1980 because, in one sweep, that year brought the election of Ronald Regan, a new business-friendly climate in Congress, and the passage of several pro-business legislations (such as the Bayh-Dole Act designed to speed technology transfers from tax-supported universities to the corporations). In the wake of these changes, the pharmaceutical industry unleashed a marketing blitz of staggering proportions.

The most well-known tools of this marketing blitz are *direct-to-consumer* (DTC) and *direct-to-provider* (DTP) advertising that now saturate the lay and professional media. The less well-known tools of the marketing blitz are *indirect-to-consumer* (ITC) and *indirect-to-provider* (ITP) promotions. These indirect methods follow the public relations tactic known as the "third man" technique—where promotion comes indirectly through a seemingly neutral "third man" and therefore sidesteps the usual scrutiny and skepticism people give to direct advertising (Rampton and Stauber 2002). For consumers, indirect promotion includes press and video news releases, product placement techniques, and setting up various patient- and disease-specific advocacy groups (which allow products to be promoted without it seeming like it comes from the corporations directly). For providers, indirect promotion includes an avalanche of continuing medical education materials, medical opinion leaders, and medical practice and treatment guidelines. Indeed, even the science of medicine itself has in many ways become a marketing arm of the pharmaceutical companies (Sismondo 2007; Matheson 2008; Applbaum 2009; Lewis 2012; Smith 2005; Dumit, 2012).

This transition of the pharmaceutical industry into a corporate colossus, at the same time that psychiatry moved into its second biological era, is not a coincidence. All of medicine was targeted, but psychiatry in particular provided an ideal site for manipulation. The vast bulk of the increased pharmaceutical sales after 1980 were life-style drugs and me-too drugs devoted to chronic conditions. This meant that psychiatry was the perfect focus for big pharma. Psychiatry, in other words, provided pharmaceutical public relations experts with a corporate "marketer's dream" (Angell 2005, 88). This marketing plan was so successful that psychiatrists put their patients on multiple drugs for multiple conditions and drug company profits soared. The global market for pharmaceuticals was $900 billion in 2010, and, after treatment for cancer, psychiatric medications were the second-best selling class of drugs that year—coming to a total of $50 billion (Healy 2012, 10).

For the industry to become this kind of colossus (especially when many of big pharma's psychiatric products do not seem to work that well), it has had to create a cultural climate of opinion and desire surrounding the product. Jan Leshley, the former CEO of Squibb pharmaceuticals, explains: "Suddenly information technology was so essential that we realized we are an information company more than we are a pill company. Because it's the software—all the research, networking, marketing—that's important in a pill. . . . It's not the pill that costs so much it's the software'" (quoted in Crister 2005, 61). In Leschley's analogy, the modern colossal drug company does not sell its products, the pills, as much as it sells the information that surrounds their pills. Today's neoliberal pharmaceutical industry has become an information industry, an industry of cultural change, not a pill industry. The lengths to which it will go have become so out of control that Peter Gotzsche, the cofounder of the Cochrane Center dedicated to evidence-based uses of pharmaceuticals, recently compared pharma's business practices to organized crime (Gotzsche 2013).

Putting the increasing prevalence of college mental health issues together with the biomedicalization of psychiatry and rising psycho-pharmaceutical treatments, students come to college extremely vulnerable to a form of neoliberal disaster capitalism. When college students come to campus, they are dealing with all of the stresses of neoliberalism—including the impact of neoliberalism on college itself—plus the stress of leaving home, often for the first time, losing the support system in which they were raised, having to build a new support network, and having to cope with new risks, new temptations, and a higher work load than they have ever faced before. As these students falter, have exacerbations of previous troubles, or attempt to move beyond normative expectations, the worldview of the campus behavioral health center—to whom they turn for help—abstracts out all of these many issues to focus exclusively on questions of diagnosis, biological variables, and pharmacologic treatments. Neoliberalism, in other words, creates a climate of distress that leaves college students highly vulnerable to difficulties and normative pressures. At the same time, neoliberalism creates a treatment system that exploits and profits from this same distress. The profits from this exploitation of distress are so high that there is very little incentive to make meaningful changes.

Postmodern Theory and the Birth of Mad Studies

On the other side of campus, 1980 marks a period of equally dramatic changes in the humanities. There had been a consensus by the end of WWII that humanities research rested on neutral distinctions between fact and value, theory and observation, and knowledge and power. Value neutrality and theory neutrality were hallmark principles of humanities scholars who, like their scientific colleagues, maintained an austere posture of objectivity. Humanities scholars Kreiswirth and Cheetam (1990) point out that by 1990, the "theory wars of the 1970s and 1980s" changed all that. The rise of theory, usually referred to as "postmodern theory" or more technically "poststructural theory," opened up emancipatory possibilities by deconstructing previously common sense distinctions between fact and value, theory and observation, and knowledge and power (Drolet 2003, Lewis 2006). Speaking for the humanities at that time, Krieswirth and Cheetam (1990) observed, "not only may we be 'theory-mad beyond redemption'—to borrow a phrase of Poe's—but we may even wonder how desirable such redemption might be, or indeed, how it might be possible to envision it without what we now call theory" (1).

A comparison of psychiatry and the humanities reveals a curious contradictory trend on two sides of U.S. campuses. Over the last forty years, psychiatry rallied itself with great fervor to champion scientific and objective knowledge. Meanwhile, over that same period, the humanities went in the exact opposite direction to deconstruct essentialist notions of truth and objectivity. The theory-madness that Kreiswirth and Cheetham talk about has lost much of its passion and excitement in the humanities since the 1990s, but it has hardly gone away. Indeed, it has now become the working common sense of much of contemporary scholarship. In this working common sense, theory has begun to influence areas of campus beyond the arts and humanities, including psychology and psychiatry.

In the world of mental health, in other words, one could say that for a significant number of activists, artists, scholars, and clinicians, the emancipatory possibilities of theory-mad humanities has migrated to become "mad theory"—or what many are now calling "mad studies" (LeFrancois, Menzies, and Reaume 2013; LeFrancois and Diamond 2014; Lewis 2009; Ostrander and Henderson 2011). From a mad studies perspective, biological psychiatry has lost legitimacy as the single truth of psychiatric conditions, and three core pillars of biological psychiatry's idealization of science are reconfigured:

1. from a quest for Objective Truth to a *crisis in representation,*
2. from Faith in Method to an *incredulity toward metanarratives, and*
3. from a Telos of Progress and Emancipation to a *telos of struggle and compromise.*

The reconfiguration by mad studies of these three pillars of dominant health models opens up to much more democratic possibilities for narrating and navigating mental suffering, disability, and difference (Lewis 2006, Lewis 2011). Before we can get to this more open structure of possibility, however, we must work through these pillars one at time.

Crisis in Representation

The quest for Objective Truth means that when biological psychiatrists create disease categories and causal explanations for mental difference, they aim to understand the universal truth, or the way the world "really is." Psychiatrists, in other words, do not give us possible ways to make meaning, they give us the Truth of our differences and our suffering. This Truth is stamped on our identity, and we either accept it or we are considered "in denial." Biological psychiatrists counter this description by claiming that they are more humble than this and the categories and explanations they use are mere hypotheses. But these so-called humble hypotheses will only change if the science changes, and biological psychiatry claims to be the "most scientific." As a result, biological psychiatry believes it is right until biological psychiatry itself decides to change its mind.

Incredulity toward Metanarratives

From a mad studies perspective, all knowledge about mental difference, including biological psychiatry, is necessarily formulated through the constraints of a nontransparent language. This *crisis of representation* does not mean language is "bad." Language is valuable for making meaning and is essential to the process of inquiry and intelligibility, but language does become problematic when it loses self-reflexivity, monopolizes other forms of knowledge making, and reinforces deeply problematic power dynamics. Biological psychiatry too often falls into all of these traps. It resists critical reflection, it fails to take seriously other approaches beyond its own, and it has become a handmaiden to neoliberal corporate profits (big pharma) and neoliberal ideologies (social problems are individual problems).

Faith in Method means that biological psychiatry has become a metanarrative that can no longer be debated or challenged. As a metanarrative faith, biological psychiatrists trust their knowledge and dismiss other knowledge possibilities. Knowledge that comes from nonscientific sources such as patients, families, clinical experience, case studies, humanities, social theory, creative arts, religion, or political activists are at best seen as conjectures that have not been "tested." At worst, these other perspectives are dismissed outright as myth, superstition, or idle speculation.

Mad studies, on the other hand, has lost faith in metanarrative and has become *incredulous of metanarratives*. This does not mean that metanarratives, like science in biological psychiatry, are worthless, only that they are not objects of faith. For mad studies, biological science is only one way to make sense of madness and mental difference. As such, biological science may be helpful, but there are other possibilities and hybrid combinations of possibilities. This multiplicity of possibilities for making meaning opens out to new kinds of questions. The scientific question, "what is the diagnosis?" for example, opens us up to much more human questions: "how shall we make meaning in this situation?" and "who should decide?" These questions can only be answered through a process of judgment that considers a complex interweaving of multiple aspects of knowledge. This includes scientific evidence but also includes the useful, aesthetic, ethical, and political consequences of knowledge. Without science as a final court of appeal, different people, or even the same people at different times, will make different judgments by weighing these criteria differently. Thus, for mad studies, there must be room and appreciation for a diversity of "legitimate" knowledge structures that are decided by people using differing values and differing preferred consequences of knowledge.

Telos of Struggle and Compromise

Finally, mad studies moves biological psychiatry from a telos of progress and emancipation to a *telos of struggle and compromise.* Riding on a faith in scientific method, biological psychiatry sees itself as making progress toward the Truth of mental difference and simultaneously that increased Truth will necessarily yield increased freedom and emancipation. But, alas, like so many other modernist projects, while biological psychiatry has brought some advantages, it has also brought many disadvantages. In the language of medicine, the positive effects have come with many side effects, many complications.

From a mad studies perspective, the ambivalent outcome of biological psychiatry is not surprising. Knowledge, and the particular ways of life organized by knowledge, always involves trade-offs. There cannot be progress without loss, emancipation without constraints. Anti-utopian in this sense, mad studies replaces the telos of progress with the telos of struggle and compromise. Humans struggle and compromise with the world—they always make trade-offs between gains and losses of alternative worldviews. And humans struggle and compromise with each other—they always negotiate competing worldviews that are constantly forced on the less powerful by the more powerful.

Theoretical work in mad studies, in sum, deconstructs normative science as the only "truth" of mental difference. Simultaneously, it opens to a diversity of approaches on campus and beyond for constructing additional ways of meaning-making and being with diverse mental states. This deconstructive work is invaluable for avoiding the traps of dominant models, but, at the same time, the deconstructive work has been more developed than the constructive work. The challenge of the next section is to further develop the constructive possibilities of navigating mental difference on campus.

Narrating and Navigating Mental Difference

After this consideration of postmodern madness on campus, both neoliberal and theoretical, we are left with the question of how to construct new and alternative approaches to mental suffering, diverse mental states, and mental disability. One of the first things to see is that this constructive work must be in at least two registers—both the scholarly and the personal dynamics of madness. The *scholarly* because mental difference involves a dense intertwining of social, cultural, political, economic, philosophical, representational, historical, artistic, religious, spiritual, psychological, biological, environmental, and interpretive issues. The *personal* because the challenge of mental difference can cause immense suffering and even be fatal for the individuals involved. Each register—the scholarly and the personal—is critical, but neither alone will suffice.

The Scholarly: Mad Studies

Starting with the scholarly, the proper response to the conceptual complexity of madness is the creation of interdisciplinary learning communities similar to programs devoted to gender and sexuality, race, and disability, among others. Mad studies programs, like other area studies programs and very much in coordination with these programs (particularly disability studies), can be a scholarly hub that generates courses, conferences, invited speakers, publications, artistic productions, certificates, degrees, and community. A key focus of this scholarship is to better understand the suffering, exploitation, and oppression caused by the contemporary power dynamics surrounding mental difference. As we have discussed, exploitation takes the form of neoliberal disaster capitalism at the hands of corporate-medical systems of care. Oppression takes the form of systematic and institutionalized stereotyping, discrimination, and social violence similar to ableism, racism, sexism, and homophobia. For mental difference, this discriminatory process, or *sanism*, runs much deeper than the more well known "stigma" to create a social climate of denigration, exclusion, and spoiled identity (Perlin 1992, Poole et al. 2012, Lewis 2013). Sanism, like other forms of institutionalized discrimination, hurts everyone. It causes a great deal of the isolation, segregation, and suffering of mental difference. Moreover it keeps the so-called "normal" people trapped in emotional and cognitive conformity—trying to achieve an often unliveably narrow band of experience and expression. And even when people do succeed, they are always haunted by a fear of falling into the spoiled categories of mental difference.

To address this exploitation and oppression, mad studies should be seen as an engaged scholarship designed not only to understand but to reduce the suffering of mental difference. The goal of mad studies programs is to work toward larger social change and also to take madness out of the closet and dance with it in the here and now. In other words, one does not have to wait until society changes to construct prefigurative social worlds where commercial exploitation is understood and actively avoided, where the impact of sanism across campus is countered, where the scholarly complexity of madness is actively pursued, and where one can meet and develop friends and colleagues involved in these issues and world views. This micro social world can be built on campus now while efforts are made to engage the larger social context.

Mad studies programs as engaged scholarship will need to have a robust relationship with activists on and off campus. As with other area studies programs, the effectiveness of mad studies will be greatest when there is a connection between scholarship and activism. In addition, mad studies programs would ideally cultivate connections with areas of campus working on the transformative and generative aspects of art (such as art therapy and community arts), spirituality (such as religious studies, pastoral counseling, and mindfulness programs), and political change (such as political science, cultural studies, and other area studies—particularly disability studies). Interestingly, this also means an engaged relationship with the more normative approaches to mental difference, such as biology, neuroscience, psychology, psychiatry, social work, and so on. The goal is to form relationships with researchers, artists, and scholars in these parts of campus that can do critical inquiry, ask different questions, and open up biological and psychological variables beyond the reductive and the deterministic to include the cultural and the political (Davis and Morris 2007, Malabou 2008, Slaby 2015).

The Personal: Creating Community, Clinical Services, New Narratives

The next register of concern on postmodern campuses is the personal aspects of mental difference and disability. Even while the campus is opening up, in a scholarly sense, to a much more robust understanding of the complexity of mental difference, there are people working through mental difference in their own lives now. Of course, from a mad studies perspective, separation of the personal and the scholarly should be seen as only a heuristic. Indeed, mad studies programs in and of themselves can have a deep impact on the personal register of madness because the very community of mad studies changes the cultural and subcultural context of people's mental life. Just as with other area studies, creating a community of friends and colleagues around an area of oppression means that one is no longer alone with the oppression. The experience of community can be lifesaving and the friendships developed can be the "best medicine" for the suffering of social difference (Icarus Project 2013). Imagine, for example, the experience of having questions about one's sexuality on campus in the 1950s, where there would potentially be no one to talk with except a clinician (who would immediately pathologize you), and the experience of having questions about sexuality on campus today, where one can often find events, talks, classes, degrees, and people with like-minded interests and concerns. One can work through similar thought experiments with regard to all the area studies programs, particularly disability studies since the personal experience of disability is also medicalized for most people before the emergence of disability studies programs.

In addition, the clinical services available through student health and campus referral systems will ideally participate and be aware of the mad studies program. This participation will impact the relationship between clinicians and service user in their appreciation of diversity and openness to a range of narratives surrounding mental difference, whether they are biological, psychoanalytic, cognitive, behavioral, family, existential, political activism, spiritual, recovery, or biopsychosocial, just to name a few. If we step back from the particulars, we can use a mad studies perspective to see that all these models work through root metaphors that structure our understanding and perception by foregrounding and backgrounding different variables. Biological models foreground biological variables, psychoanalytic models foreground mental conflicts, family models foreground family dysfunction, spiritual models foreground higher consciousness and compassion, artistic models foreground aesthetic creation, political models foreground social oppression and transformation, etc. Some of these are formal clinical models that have systematically developed a particular metaphor through a research and treatment community. These formal models then seep out of the clinic and become tools for storytelling about mental differences and troubles. Other models of mental difference have not been given significant formal development but remain viable options for meaning-making nonetheless.

This mad studies perspective on how mental models are used for meaning-making is already developing in clinical work under the banner of "narrative," "narrative psychotherapy," and "narrative psychiatry" (White and Epston 1990, Crossley 2000, Angus and McLeod 2004, White 2007, Lewis 2011, Hamkins 2013). The implication of narrative for mental health work is that there are many ways to tell the story of mental difference and suffering—not just one right way and many other wrong ways. All the models of mental difference work as potential tools for storytelling about mental troubles. No matter which model or combination of models one uses, the process of healing involves an initial set of problems that the person is unable to resolve. Through clinical dialogues, client and clinician use one or more models to bring additional perspectives to the client's problems, allowing clients to understand them in new ways. The perspectives vary greatly depending on the models used. The metaphors of broken brains, unconscious conflicts, cognitive distortions, family dysfunctions, artistic creativity, social transformation, and spiritual seekers differ greatly. But, from the vantage point of narrative theory, all of these perspectives, when used for storytelling, allow the possibility of reworking the initial story into a new one. Having a new story allows new degrees of flexibility for understanding past and present troubles and provides new strategies for moving into the future.

Mad studies programs can stimulate the embrace of these more narrative perspectives on campus so that when students go to the clinics they can meet clinicians that understand narrative diversity. These clinicians will also have a familiarity and openness to celebratory and generative models of recovery as much as the more common pathological models. Generative narratives see mental difference and suffering as a positive sign of sensitivity and yearning—the very narrative catalysts that can be turned into a life of art, spirituality, and political activism (Lewis 2012). To be sensitive and to be yearning is usually negative from a pathological frame ("stop being so sensitive," "quit being so idealistic," "did you take your medicine?"), but it is often positive in the context of art, spirituality, and activism. After all, we want our artists, our spiritual seekers, and our activists to help take us beyond the normative world to a place that is more beautiful, more compassionate, more sustainable, and more just.

This openness to alternative stories does not mean the end of normative stories or of biological models, psychiatric diagnoses, or medications. A narrative turn means that all the models are potentially valuable if used self-reflexively in dialogue with clients and in the service of recovery. Ultimately, it is the client's choice which model or combination of models best fits their goals and desires. The task of clinicians is to help narrate and navigate the process and the options. This kind of narrative self-reflexivity helps clinicians remember that their allegiance is to their clients, not to clinical models. Recovery and flourishing is the goal, not loyalty to models.

One of the most fascinating implications of a mad studies perspective for campus life is that one does not have to have a "single story" (Adichie 2009) for one's mental difference. Postmodern madness creates the possibility for tactical and strategic paradox and contradiction. From a mad studies perspective, it is very possible to tell a story about oneself using psychiatric diagnostic metaphors and plots for the purposes of gaining disability benefits and resources, while at the same time seeing these same diagnostic metaphors and plots as incomplete, inadequate, or even harmful. In other words, with a mad studies perspective, we do not have to have a mono-story of our mental difference. We can have a multiplicity of stories for making meaning of our differences and troubles. There is more than one way to relate to this multiplicity. It is possible to live that multiplicity simultaneously, it is also possible to have a preferred story (while using the others as backups for certain situations), and it is also possible to feel that there is only one story that is "the truth."

However we decide to live this multiplicity, since we are in a neoliberal time where social benefits are restricted to limited to hegemonic biomedical stories, there is no reason, from a mad studies perspective, that some people cannot take advantage of these benefits while at the same time being able to put the story of those benefits into a larger narrative frame they do not prefer. For example, because of my sensitivity to the suffering, impermanence, and injustice at the heart of the human condition, I can be clinically depressed on Monday (when I am negotiating the insurance company) and I can be a Buddhist philosopher or a poet or a political activist on Thursday and Sunday (when I am with my Sangha or at my poetry reading group or with my colleagues in mad studies). This kind of double and multiple coding is particularly important on campus as the support systems of clinics, therapists, disability offices, deans, bursars, etc. all think in terms of a dominant biological frame for mental disability. Mad studies allows individual students and faculty to navigate this dominant frame for strategic purposes while at the same time it works to help individuals and the university open and expand this frame.

Conclusion

Postmodern times are contradictory times of challenge and opportunity for living with and relating to mental difference. On the one hand, these are hard times. Postmodern times are times of aggressive neoliberal practices that are creating challenges of increased distress, hardship, and difficulty holding or desiring the "normative" position. As people inevitably fall out, opt out, or are pushed out of neoliberal norms, neoliberalism has remarkably situated itself to profit from the pharmaceutical interventions used to treat the difference and distress it helped create. On the other hand, these are times of opportunity and interpretive flexibility. Postmodern theoretical tools provide the critical and conceptual apparatus necessary to deconstruct the essentialism and power dynamics contained in normative psychiatric practices. These tools are increasingly available through the development of mad studies scholarship. As campuses begin to take seriously both the scholarly and the personal dimensions of madness for their students and faculty, they can start to open mad studies programs in coordination with other area studies programs where the many challenges of mental difference can be given the interdisciplinary attention they deserve.

References

Adichie, Chimamanda. 2009. *The Danger of a Single Story*. TEDGlobal. https://www.ted.com/talks/chimamanda_adichie_the_danger_of_a_single_story?language=en

Andreason, N. 1984. *The Broken Brain: The Biological Revolution in Psychiatry*. New York: Harper and Row.

Angell, M. 2005. *The Truth about Drug Companies: How They Deceive Us and What to Do about It*. New York: Random House.

Angell, M. 2011. "The Illusions of Psychiatry." *New York Review of Books*, July 14.

Angus, L. and J. McLeod. 2004. "Toward an Integrative Framework for Understanding the Role of Narrative in Psychotherapy Process. In L. Angus and J. McLeod, eds., *Handbook of Narrative and Psychotherapy: Practice, Theory and Research*. Thousand Oaks, CA: Sage Publications.

Applbaum, K. 2009. "Getting to Yes: Corporate Power and the Creation of a Psychopharmaceutical Blockbuster. *Culture, Medicine, and Psychiatry* 33 (2):185–215.

Brown, W. 2005. "Neoliberalism and the End of Democracy. In W. Brown, *Edgework: Critical Essays on Knowledge and Politics*. Princeton: Princeton University Press. 37–59.

Clarke, A., L. Mamo, J. Fosket, J. Fishman, and J. Shim. 2010. *Biomedicalization: Technoscience, Health, and Illness in the U.S.* Durham, NC: Duke University Press.

Crister, G. 2005. *Generation Rx: How Prescription Drugs Are Altering American's Lives, Minds and Bodies*. New York: Houghton Mifflin.

Crossley, M. 2000. *Introducing Narrative Psychology: Self, Trauma, and the Construction of Meaning*. Buckingham: Open University Press.

Davis, L. and D. Morris. 2007. "Biocultures Manifesto." *New Literary History* 38: 411–18.

Drolet, M., ed. 2003. *The Postmodernism Reader: Foundational Texts*. New York: Routledge.

Dumit, J. 2012. *Drugs for Life: How the Pharmaceutical Industry Defines Our Health*. Durham, NC: Duke University Press.

Gallagher, R. P. 2006. *National Survey of Counseling Center Directors*. Alexandria, VA. International Associations of Counseling Services, Inc.

Gøtzsche, P. C. 2013. *Deadly Medicines and Organized Crime: How Big Pharma Has Corrupted Healthcare*. London: Radcliffe.

Giroux, H. 2008. *Against the Terror of Neoliberalism: Politics beyond the Age of Greed*. Boulder: Paradigm Press.

Hamkins, S. 2013. *The Art of Narrative Psychiatry: Stories of Strength and Meaning*. Oxford: Oxford University Press.

Harvey, D. 2005. *A Brief History of Neoliberalism*. Oxford: Oxford University Press.

Hewlett, S.A., and C. West. 1998. *The war against Parents: What We Can Do for America's Beleaguered Moms and Dads*. New York: Houghton Mifflin Company.

Healy, D. 2012. *Pharmageddon*. Berkeley, CA: University of California Press.

Icarus Project. 2013. *Friends Make the Best Medicine: A Guide to Creating Community Mental Health Support Networks*. The Icarus Project.

Kadison, R. 2004. *College of the Overwhelmed: The Campus Mental Health Crisis and What to Do about It*. San Francisco: Josey-Bass.

Kitzrow, M. A. 2003. "The Mental Health Needs of Today's College Students: Challenges and Recommendations. *NASPA Journal* 41, no. 1 (Fall): 167–81.

Kreiswirth, M., and M. Cheetham. 1990. *Theory between the Disciplines: Authority/Vision/Politics*. Ann Arbor: University of Michigan Press.

LeFrancois, B. A., R. J. Menzies, and G. Reaume. 2013. *Mad Matters: A Critical Reader in Canadian Mad Studies*. Toronto: Canadian Scholars' Press.

LeFrançois, B. A., and S. Diamond. 2014. *Psychiatry Disrupted: Theorizing Resistance and Crafting the (R)Evolution*. Montréal: McGill-Queen's University Press.

Lewis, B. 2006. *Moving beyond Prozac, DSM, and the New Psychiatry: The Birth of Postpsychiatry*. Ann Arbor: University of Michigan Press.

Lewis, B. 2009. "Madness Studies." *Literature & Medicine, 28*(1), 152–71.

Lewis, B. 2011. *Narrative Psychiatry: How Stories Can Shape Clinical Practice*. Baltimore: Johns Hopkins Press.

Lewis, B. 2012. "Recovery, Narrative Theory, and Generative Madness." In A. Rudnick, ed. *Recovery of People with Mental Illness: Philosophical and Related Perspectives*. Oxford: Oxford University Press.

Lewis, B. 2013. "A Mad Fight: Psychiatry and Disability Activism. In L. Davis, ed. *Disability Studies Reader*, 4th ed. New York: Routledge.

Malabou, C. 2008. *What Should We Do with Our Brain?* New York: Fordham University Press.

Matheson, A. 2008. "Corporate Science and the Husbandry of Scientific and Medical Knowledge by the Pharmaceutical Industry." *BioSocieties* 3:3 55–82.

Ostrander, N. and B. Henderson, eds. "Special Issue: Disability and Madness." *Disability Studies Quarterly* 33 (1). http://dsq-sds.org/issue/view/100

Perlin, M. L. 1992. "On 'sanism.'" *Southern Methodist University Law Review* 46: 373–407.

Poole, J. M., T. Jivraj, A. Arslanian, K. Bellows, S. Chiasson, H. Hakimy, J. Pasini, and J. Reid. 2012. "Sanism, 'Mental Health', and Social Work/Education: A Review and Call to Action." *Intersectionalities: A Global Journal of Social Work Analysis, Research, Polity, and Practice* 1: 20–36.

Rampton, S. and J. Stauber. 2002. *Trust Us We're Experts: How Industry Manipulates Science and Gambles with Your Future*. New York: Tarcher.

Shorter, E. 1997. *A History of Psychiatry: From the Era of the Asylum to the Age of Prozac*. New York: John Wiley and Sons.

Sismondo, S. 2007. "Ghost Management: How Much of the Medical Literature Is Shaped behind the Scenes by the Pharmaceutical Industry?" *PLOS Medicine* 4 (9):1429–33.

Slaby, J. 2015. "Critical Neuroscience Meets Medical Humanities." *Medical Humanities* 41: 16–22.

Smith, R. 2005. "Medical Journals Are an Extension of the Marketing Arm of Pharmaceutical Companies." *PLoS Medicine* 2 (5): 364–66.

Strickland, R. 2002. *Growing Up Postmodern: Neoliberalism and the War on the Young*. Maryland: Rowman and Littlefield.

Timimi, S. 2010. "The McDonaldization of Childhood: Children's Mental Health in Neo-liberal Market Cultures." *Transcultural Psychiatry* 47 (5): 686–706.

White, M. and D. Epston. 1990. *Narrative Means to Therapeutic Ends*. New York: W. W. Norton.

White, M. 2007. *Maps of Narrative Practice*. New York: W.W. Norton.

Doing Disability with Others

REBECCA SANCHEZ

As this volume attests, in recent years, the rhetoric of disclosure has become the dominant way of framing conversations about disability in the academy. Job seekers debate the best time to disclose a disability to potential employers. Faculty develop strategies for disclosing their own disabilities to students on the first day of class, as well as for creating environments in which students feel comfortable disclosing their own (see Knight, this volume). Researchers question whether including disclosures of personal experiences with disability will strengthen their scholarship. For many people, thinking of such communicative exchanges specifically as disclosures has evoked a productive sense of openness, a sense that disability is an identity that can be proudly claimed rather than something that must be hidden. This language has mapped particularly well onto one of the most frequent formats for raising disability as a topic in universities: the accommodation request.

Despite these benefits, however, I will argue that framing disclosure as a singular communicative exchange carries with it a great deal of problematic ideological baggage that is counterproductive to the very goals of many disclosures. Put briefly, it reinforces preconceptions about disability as static, and it mischaracterizes the complex ways that most exchanges of information about disability unfold. After unpacking some of this baggage, I will explore alternatives to this paradigm through a consideration of three artifacts—wheelchair lights, a "DeafBlind and Badass" button, and a "Piss on Pity" t-shirt—that move away from the emphasis on a singular, formal moment of revelation inherent in the idea of disclosure and toward an articulation of more flexible ways of doing disability in public space.

Disclosure and Its Pitfalls

Today's disability disclosures take place within a broader cultural moment that valorizes both identification and information sharing. The proliferation of social media and personal technology has exponentially increased the frequency with which individuals are either required or strongly encouraged to provide details regarding their age, gender, ethnicity, relationships, and ability status. One way to understand the pressure to make globally public information that previous generations would have understood as private (or as public only to a select group of people) is in relation to what Samuels (2014) describes as the "crisis of identification" that emerged in the mid-nineteenth century over increasing social mobility. This mobility challenged established societal hierarchies and made individuals more difficult to classify and govern. In response to such boundary blurring, Samuels argues that "a range of fantastical solutions began to circulate . . . eventually becoming solidified into our twenty-first-century discourses about bodies and identities. These *fantasies of identification* seek to definitively identify bodies, to place them in categories delineated by race, gender, or ability status" (2).

Although Samuels is primarily concerned with the biological means through which these identities are validated, her account historicizes identification and serves as a reminder of the complex and, at times, contradictory ways that identity functions. While the investment in identity politics in our own historical moment has emphasized the powerful and self-affirming effects of the kinds of identifications associated with disclosures ("I am X"), identity categorization can also operate as a means of control, dividing populations so as to render them legible and effacing the complexities of individuals' understandings of themselves and their relationships to other subjects and to society.

The tension between these effects of identification is present in many accounts of the experiences surrounding acts of disclosure. In "On Rhetorical Agency," for example, Kerschbaum interrogates both the "deeply agentive" role disclosures can play and her own ambivalence over the microaggressions through which disabled faculty are pushed to explicitly discuss their physical, sensory, intellectual, and psychiatric differences in their scholarship (2014, 69). The pressure to disclose, to render one's body legible to the gaze of administrators, colleagues, and readers in particular ways, serves as a powerful reminder of the structurally conservative ways in which identification can function. Without losing sight of its productive functions, it is necessary to remain attentive to the extent to which these pressures are symptomatic of the framing of identity embedded in the idea of disclosure itself.

To disclose is to "reveal new or secret information" (*OED Online* 2015). When we talk about disclosing an identity, then, that identity is positioned as a secret, something hidden and associated with concealment and shame. Like the logic of the closet, disclosure operates to create a binary division between those who have already revealed the "secret" of their disability and those who have not. In so doing, it produces a closet, a space of nondisclosure into which those who cannot or do not wish to discuss their disabilities, or who do so in ways that are not legible under this paradigm, are forced. While disclosure places the emphasis on a different point in the process of revelation ("the closet" focuses on spaces occupied by individuals who, it is presumed, feel pressure to conceal their identities, whereas "disclosure" emphasizes the communicative acts through which individuals exit these spaces), both function to produce unhelpful divisions within minority populations that reinforce erroneous preconceptions about the meanings of those identities.

In "My Body, My Closet," Samuels (2013) draws attention to a number of complications that arise from engaging the rhetoric of the closet to describe the act of sharing information about a nonvisible disability, critiques that might also be applied to the structurally similar framework of disclosure. One of the problems Samuels identifies has to do with temporality. As she explains, "coming out [is not] a static or singular event . . . an over-the-rainbow shift that divides one's life before and after the event" (319). Unlike the disclosure of one's salary, exchanges of information about disability do not take place in instants of revelation but unfold over crip time, described by disability activist and artist Petra Kuppers as "lemonade time: tea, coffee, drip / time . . . time for us breathing" (2008) that exists outside of "productive, forward-leaning, exciting time" (Kuppers 2014, 29).

The fetishization of a single moment of disclosure perpetuates fantasies of identification that hold that identities constitute the kind of information that can be revealed in a single word or sentence, on a single form, through a blood test. Such fantasies are dangerous. They emphasize reductive labels that leave no space for bodies (and our understanding of bodies) to change over time. And they efface the role of context and conversational partners in determinations about the presentation of disability, the particularities of the power differentials across which we are always communicating in academic settings, and the complex calculations of probabilities of increased or decreased personal safety (physical, emotional, financial) that shape people's decisions about when, where, and how to discuss disability. By attempting to produce disability as a stable truth, something that can be revealed in a single exchange, disclosure simultaneously causes us to overly invest in utterances we recognize as such and to fail to register forms of communication that we don't. These implications haunt the language of disclosure itself, regardless of the intentions of the individual disclosing.

By means of illustration, let us consider the information conveyed in a statement readily legible as a disclosure: "I am blind." "I am blind" clearly constitutes a revelation of information. What is less apparent is precisely what information it conveys (and, by extension, what information it doesn't). The assertion informs conversational partners of the fact that "blind" is a label the speaker claims for herself. It might be reasonably extrapolated that it is also the term she prefers others use to describe her. While the speaker may intend to embed additional information in the statement, however, it is not self-evident that she does so. The disclosure does not, for example, specify the level or quality of the speaker's vision, whether she has always been blind or if her vision has deteriorated (or is continuing to deteriorate), the accommodations she might prefer, whether she considers blindness a part of her identity or a biological fact (or both, or neither). It is also silent on the matter of what she wants her conversational partner to do with this information.

When we assume the statement "I am blind" contains deep insight into its speaker, we increase the chances for misunderstanding, even in situations in which the speaker does mean for it to carry this weight. For such statements to be useful, they must be seen to constitute the beginning of a communicative exchange rather than the end. But once a secret (or a label, or a diagnosis) is revealed, the disclosure is over. Emphasizing (by naming) the revelatory instant, in many ways the least informative component of a communicative exchange about disability, distracts us from the much more significant subsequent communication. Through this emphasis, by failing to call attention to the times and spaces in which extended conversations about disability occur, disclosure makes such spaces difficult to conceptualize. In a troublingly self-perpetuating cycle, they therefore become less likely to be created.

In addition to predisposing us to overly invest in identificatory statements, the ideology of disclosure also establishes a line between revealed knowledge and hidden secrets, between speech acts and silence. This division predisposes us to overlook information about disability that is shared in situations that do not seem like disclosures. One example of the consequences of this can be observed in the preface to Helen Keller's 1908 essay "The World I Live In," in which Keller explains her frequent use of the genre of autobiography. While the essay itself presents Keller's understanding of deafblindness in terms that are legible under a paradigm of disclosure (she specifically references her disability and the insights it has given her into sensory perception), the preface rails against a publishing world and reading public that demanded that her writing adhere to this formula:

> Every book is in a sense autobiographical. But while other self-recording creatures are permitted at least to seem to change the subject, apparently nobody cares what I think of the tariff, the conservation of our natural resources, or the conflicts which revolve about the name of Dreyfus. If I offer to reform the educational system of the world, my editorial friends say, "That is interesting. But will you please tell us what idea you had of goodness and beauty when you were six years old?" . . . The Editors are so kind that they are no doubt right in thinking that nothing I have to say about the affairs of the universe would be interesting. But until they give me opportunity to write about matters that are not-me, the world must go on uninstructed and unreformed, and I can only do my best with the one small subject upon which I am allowed to discourse. (Keller 2009, xi)

Looking for literal references to her disabilities, Keller's editors were incapable of considering what her writing about the Dreyfus affair or the tariff could have contributed not only to readers' thinking about those topics but also to their understanding of disability. In addition to capturing Keller's frustrated sarcasm at the limitations others' perceptions of her imposed on her writing practices, the passage significantly highlights the silencing that can ironically (and often invisibly) occur when we approach disability in the binary terms associated with disclosure.

Were Keller's editors to have taken seriously her assertion that "Every book is in a sense autobiographical," a potentially very different image of deafblindness could have emerged between the lines, in the gaps and silences surrounding words that did not explicitly pertain to disability. Like a disabled academic choosing not to begin an essay by explaining his or her personal relationship to disability, Keller's writing about "matters that are not-me" would have performed a different kind of disability politics by forcing readers to confront the fact that the interests of disabled people are not always or only linked to their own embodied experiences and that, even more significantly, the connections between these interests and their states of embodiment emerge in unexpected and unpredictable ways.

Developing tools for understanding such insight, working toward a more flexible vocabulary that accounts for the range of ways in which individuals express meaning, therefore, necessitates learning how to better interpret the kinds of information about disability shared beyond explicit assertions of identity. As Foucault explains in *The History of Sexuality* in relation to sexually marginalized identities,

> Silence itself—the things one declines to say, or is forbidden to name, the discretion that is required between different speakers—is less the absolute limit of discourse, the other side from which it is separated by a strict boundary, than an element that functions alongside the things said, with them and in relation to them within over-all strategies. . . . We must try to determine the different ways of not saying such things. . . . There is not one but many silences, and they are an integral part of the strategies that underlie and permeate discourses. (1990, 27)

While it is certainly the case that some silences result from silencing, and that work in disability studies needs to continue attempting to ameliorate the complex factors that prevent individuals from discussing disability when they want to, to assume that all silence, empty space, or communication that does not fit into the box of disclosure results from such silencing is to ignore vital insights about disability and to ensure that only perspectives that are legible under our current paradigms enter the discourse.

Academics experience a great deal of pressure to disclose information surrounding their disabilities, not only to institutions in order to receive accommodation and to avoid the insinuation that they are "hiding" impairments but also socially, out of a sense that to "fail" to disclose is to indicate that they are not comfortable with their identities, that they are at a more nascent stage of personal development than those who speak openly with colleagues and students about their bodies. Rather than helping us to move beyond the limited and limiting ideas about disability that contribute to these pressures, the binary logic of disclosure serves to perpetuate them.

Designing Encounters: Disability as a Verb

In addition to the rhetoric of disclosure, then, we need to think more broadly about the "different ways of not saying" (Foucault 1990, 27) and of saying differently, the diverse forms in which people speak, sign, draw, point, and are silent about disability, and to develop more effective toolkits for interpreting intentional and productive silence. One way to begin doing so is to replace disclosure's emphasis on labels (on something that one is) with the idea suggested in the title of this essay, of disability as something that one does. Developed out of models of "racial formations" and of "doing gender," Brown, Hamner, Foley, and Woodring explain, "doing disability" employs

> an interactionist perspective showing how constructions of identity are *made and remade* through interactions with individuals and with institutions. Disability is not viewed as an individual attribute, but as a process variable that emerges in specific sociohistorical contexts. Thus, understandings of disability are not static or necessarily holistic, but dependent on the social interactions and contexts in which disability is understood. (Brown et al. 2009, 4)

By recognizing the ways individuals slide between modes of identification associated with various models (medical, social, political, cultural), "doing disability" takes the focus away from the individual body without eliding the importance of embodied difference. The activities that constitute "doing" disability combine attention to diverse physical, sensory, intellectual, and neurological states of being with the political, social, and cultural factors that shape the ways disability is discussed and performed in various contexts. The extended temporality of the verb "to do" also enables a space for playfulness and humor in discussions of disability that is missing from the bureaucratic frame of disclosure, with all of its legal connotations. In what follows, I will examine three examples of artifacts used as parts of strategies for doing disability in and through interactions with others in order to excavate components that could be productively incorporated into academic conversations. The first are decorative wheelchair lights.

In a 2012 TED Talk entitled "We Are All Designers," journalist John Hockenberry describes the way that adding flashing colored lights to his wheelchair changed his experience of navigating public space and the kinds of communicative exchanges he was able to engage in surrounding his paraplegia. For many years, he explains, his presence ignited a kind of panic in those around him. Strangers would rush to pull children out of his way while awkwardly avoiding eye contact lest they be perceived to be staring at him. Despite attempting various strategies to alter these interactions (making "no eye contact . . . dress[ing] up really, really sharply . . . mak[ing] eye contact with everyone") none were successful (Hockenberry 2012).

This narrative provides another example of the unexpected consequences of disclosure's ideological baggage, specifically of the ways that disclosure's positioning of disability as a secret (something that has to be revealed) may limit opportunities for those with visible disabilities to engage in conversations about their experiences. Disclosure's bifurcation of time into a "before" and "after" of revelation separates nonvisible disabilities that need to be disclosed and visible disabilities that are supposedly already apparent in ways that ignore the crucial difference between sharing information about one's body and being interpolated into a particular identity based on the (mis)perceptions of others. Believing that the visual evidence of disability (Hockenberry's wheelchair) constituted a disclosure, and that what was being disclosed was a narrative that fit within their preconceived notions of disability as tragedy, onlookers reacted to him according to a limited number of scripts. Trapped by their preconceptions about what conversations about disability needed to look like, they were unable to recognize the information Hockenberry was attempting to communicate through his various nonverbal strategies: dressing up to dispel the perception that all disabled people are economically disadvantaged, making eye contact to demonstrate that he was not ashamed or hiding.

For Hockenberry, the solution to this impasse ultimately came not through developing new strategies for narrating his body or experiences, but by expressing an attitude toward disability through the flashing wheels that disrupted people's assumptions, particularly the idea that the "truth" revealed by a wheelchair is a fundamental difference between the wheelchair user and those around him. By creating a situation in which Hockenberry did not need to awkwardly (and counterproductively) declare his similarity with onlookers ("I am like you. Please acknowledge that."), but in which others could recognize that for themselves, the wheels opened a space for more productive interactions to take place. "To be recognized," as Garland-Thomson has explained, "is to become familiar, no longer strange, to be seen and accorded the status of fellow human. The trajectory of recognition is this: I recognize you by seeing your similarity and your difference to me, and then I make your strangeness familiar" (2009, 158). The flashing wheels encourage such recognition by helping onlookers to identify points of similarity with Hockenberry: an interest in design or technology, a sense of whimsy, a taste for colorful accessories. These shared qualities did not erase Hockenberry's difference. They made the chair more, not less, visible. But they altered the ways in which that difference was understood. "Instead of blank stares and awkwardness," Hockenberry describes, "now it is pointing and smiling! People going, 'Awesome wheels, dude! Those are awesome! I mean, I want some of those wheels!' Little kids say, 'Can I have a ride?'" (Hockenberry 2012).

When we think in terms of disclosure, we are waiting for the revelation of a medical diagnosis, or a story of injury; we are predisposed to expect a situation in which the scripted response is either pity or the fulfillment of a need. What the wheels communicate instead, what makes the chair with the flashing wheels different from the chair without them is, as Hockenberry explains, "intent . . . I'm no longer a victim. I chose to change the situation . . . It conveys authorship" (Hockenberry, 2012). This authorship is specifically not expressed through a disclosure. The lights themselves are silent. Indeed, they operate to reduce the frequency with which Hockenberry is called upon to describe his accident and injuries. But that silence operates in Foucault's sense, as an "integral part of strategies that . . . permeate discourse" (1990, 27) by expressing agency. In so doing, the lights, as well as the other artifacts I will discuss, reveal something critical about disability design.

As Pullin has noted, design for disability has traditionally aimed to "be discreet and uncontroversial, unseen or at least not remarked on" (2009, 113). The lights do just the opposite, drawing attention to both Hockenberry and his chair. They also run counter to the principle of utility, the "imperative to produce something immediately useful," that similarly dominates disability design and has led to the vast majority of items for disabled people being produced with a strict sense of functionality rather than an interest in critical design more broadly understood as that which helps us to actively interrogate our surroundings (Pullin 2009, 113). In one sense, Hockenberry's wheels serve no purpose; he specifically notes that they are not there for safety. Like hearing aid jewelry, colorful canes, or tattoos for prosthetics, the lights are purely aesthetic. But despite, or perhaps because of, the fact that they are not designed to be useful, the lights end up performing vital work by enabling people to perceive disability and its accouterments in aesthetic terms, as something that can be desired ("I want some of those wheels!") rather than only needed or feared. Unlike the very goal-oriented ways in which disability disclosure is framed in academic settings (recognizable disabilities are revealed in the hopes of receiving specific accommodations), the sense of disability as aesthetic, desirable, and critically engaged rubs against the grain of commonly held assumptions, necessitating the creation of new vocabularies and forms of interaction that are not bound to limited understandings of bodily difference.

The second artifact I consider here, a 2.25-inch purple button with the words "DeafBlind and Badass" written across it in a bold black font, similarly undermines popular perceptions about what and how disability signifies. Riffing on the "Deaf and Low Vision" or "deaf and blind" slogans worn by some DeafBlind individuals as a form of disclosure that (it is hoped) will increase the personal safety of the wearer; the button makes visible an otherwise potentially nonvisible disability. It therefore serves as a reminder of the disability that always surrounds us even when we are unaware of it. Its revelation of a specific disability also makes it useful in the sense Pullin describes; it "solv[es] problems" by highlighting disability's presence (Pullin 2009, xv). "Badass" might also be understood as pragmatic in as much as it counteracts the sense of vulnerability that deafblindness may connote. Although they take different approaches to doing so, both terms, then, attempt to increase personal safety. These pragmatic elements are crucial to the work that the button does, but it also operates in excess of both the slogans from which it derives and the ideology of disclosure. This combination of pragmatics with elements of critical design offers insight into how such factors might similarly be balanced in academic environments, where the desire to design social encounters in new and creative ways around disability must always be negotiated in relation to the current pragmatic necessity of making sure that one's self-presentation fits into the boxes that will enable one to receive accommodation.

Like Hockenberry's lights, the "DeafBlind and Badass" button reveals authorship, not only of the artifact itself but of the individual's experience of disability. Both the color and the profanity convey information about the wearer's personal preferences that may provide others with a way of recognizing similarity that undercuts the fear or pity potentially evoked by the idea of deafblindness. Insisting that the identity of the individual not be subsumed by disability, the button capitalizes both "DeafBlind" and "Badass" and gives the terms equal space, indicating that the latter is just as important as the former in understanding the wearer. In addition to emphasizing the importance of playfulness in both design and disability, these strategies function to produce recognition in the terms that Garland-Thomson (2009) advocates.

The fact that the button presents this information in language that must be read, an activity that necessitates looking at, rather than away from, the wearer also increases the chances that the wearer will be acknowledged as an individual rather than interpolated as a symbol of perceived tragedy. The choice of "DeafBlind" rather than "deaf and blind" or "deaf and low vision" is also, to borrow Depoy and Gilson's definition of design, "purposive and intentional" (2013, 487). Whereas "deaf and blind" calls attention to the existence of specific disabilities, "DeafBlind" asserts an identity, capitalizing both and running them together to create something new: a DeafBlind way of being that is more than a medical descriptor or than either of the two labels separately.

For the button's owner, the mixture of messages it conveys serves to productively frame encounters with strangers. As she explains,

> Having the button on my backpack enables me to fast-forward past the first few awkward conversational moves. It makes people aware of my disability without me having to figure out the best time to interrupt them to tell them I can't hear. It sometimes deflects questions about why I'm not moving or responding in predictable ways. And it sets a certain tone. "DeafBlind and Badass" doesn't leave much space for sympathy. It provides information, but it also confuses people. How is this girl moving around independently if she can't see or hear? I find that confusion useful. It means that people are less likely to approach me with the assumption that they already know all about deafblindness because they read a book on Helen Keller in first grade. (Anonymous 2015)

The disconnect between people's assumptions about the meaning of deafblindness and the ways it is presented in both the button and its wearer's behavior destabilizes the script for how disability is engaged. Rather than offering a bite-sized "truth" about the disability of the wearer, the button creates confusion that can open up spaces for questions to be asked and deeper understandings of disability to emerge over more extended time, understandings that involve both attention to pragmatic physical needs (for those around the wearer to move out of her way or to adjust how they communicate with her) and a sense of play. By functioning as a kind of prosthetic disclosure, that is, the button enables conversations about disability to "fast-forward" past the revelatory instant and focus instead on the next steps in the process of information sharing.

The social model has trained us to think about the relationship between disability and the environment primarily in a singular direction: inaccessible built and social environments are disabling and need to be adapted so as to maximize the number of people who can move through them safely and comfortably. The responsibility for this adaptation is usually assumed to be that of primarily nondisabled government officials, architects, and contractors. One of the other things the button highlights is the role disabled people play in restructuring these spaces by designing social encounters using various conversational techniques and material artifacts to move beyond unproductive exchanges and to maximize the chances for more meaningful communication to take place.

The third, and final, example I will consider is a "Piss on Pity" t-shirt. Coined by disability activist and musician Alan Holdsworth in 1992 as a means of protesting the infantilization of telethons, the slogan encapsulates a rejection of paternalism that has been central to the disability rights movement. As Hahn explains with reference to his own shirt, "the movement is to treat disability as a source of dignity and pride. And as something positive. And to reject the sympathy, the paternalism, and the pity with which the non-disabled world has traditionally approached this issue" (1995).

As Hahn's comments indicate, in addition to restricting the possibilities within individual encounters, sympathy is also structurally problematic for the advancement of disability rights. When disability is perceived primarily through the lens of personal tragedy and the disabled understood as subjects to whom the most ethical response is pity, public policies and laws designed to enable the disabled are positioned as acts of charity rather than the responsibility of governments, universities, and communities in recognition of disabled peoples' civil rights. Like the symbolic baggage placed on wheelchairs or presumptions about the meaning of deafblindness, pity functions as a means of separating people, dividing those who feel pity from those they pity in ways that run counter to strategies of recognition. By rejecting both this distancing and its implications, and drawing a direct connection between individual interactions and larger structures of power, "Piss on Pity" poses a challenge to ideologies that are at once global and intimate.

An important component of this challenge is the preservation of the possibility of silence surrounding the body of the wearer. The shirt neither names disability in general, nor provides specific information about its owner. Instead, it discloses an attitude toward social relationality designed to destabilize viewers' understandings of their own investment in questions of diverse embodiment. Rather than focusing on individual authorship, as does the button, the shirt moves the conversation away from identity, which relies structurally on a division between individuals ("I am X," "I am not X"). While not precluding a discussion of personal identification with disability, the work of the slogan does not require it. This reframing helps produce a space for conversations about disability that emphasize the political components of

disablement and the shared stakes of everyone, regardless of how they identify, in undermining problematic forms of relationality like pity.

To achieve this reframing, the shirt highlights both social and embodied
elements of disability. As Serlin notes, it combines "the image of pissing as a
natural biological function with the image of pissing as an aggressive act of
individual and group disobedience" (2010, 185). Silence about the body of the
wearer, that is, does not translate into silence about bodies generally; the reference to pissing evokes both physicality and physical need. Significantly, this
is a need that is shared by all people. Just like the reference to pity, an emotion
with which everyone has personal experience, this framing invites interlocutors to take ownership of their personal responsibility in either perpetuating
or ameliorating disabling discourse. As opposed to a disclosure, which can
potentially create a line between speaker and viewer (most people to whom
one discloses will not share one's particular identity), "Piss on Pity" works to
develop coalition. Though its approach is more politically focused than that
of the other two artifacts, then, the balance of the slogan's aggressiveness—
not demurely asking for recognition but demanding it—and silence works
similarly to challenge assumptions about the kinds of communicative exchanges that can occur around disability and to foster new kinds of interactions in those spaces.

Conclusion

There is a different kind of pragmatics to this approach to communication
about disability; unlike disclosure, which emphasizes presenting disability
in ways that are legible under current paradigms (thereby reinforcing those
paradigms), these artifacts present modes of engaging disability that could
ultimately lead to the development of more effective and meaningful institutional thinking about accommodation. What kinds of conversations about
human diversity might be possible, for example, if universities were archi-
tecturally and socially designed in ways that encouraged all members of the
community to recognize their investment in questions of diverse embodiment, if conversations about disability were not assumed to be the responsibility of those with disabilities to initiate, often through personal disclosures? What relationships could emerge if we stopped viewing the bodies of
disabled faculty as texts through which their students and colleagues might
be educated about disability? What kinds of critical thinking would develop
in environments where disability was perceived not merely as something to

be accommodated but as something to be genuinely desired, an occasion for humor and playfulness rather than a topic that evoked fear and trepidation?

If part of the goal of communication about disability must of necessity take place within the confines of current attitudes and policy structures, we must also work to design these exchanges so that they can serve as components of strategies for calling into being the kinds of crip futures we want. Language operates not only as a means of describing our existing reality but as a way of making possible something other, what Muñoz describes as the "not-yet-conscious" (2009, 3). Despite the many benefits associated with disclosure, thoughtfully detailed throughout this collection, the word itself creates divisions between a before and after of disability's revelation, between those who have and those who have not disclosed, that are not only inaccurate descriptions of the way most communication about disability takes place but that reinforce problematic assumptions about disability (and disabled people). While the fact that many people now feel comfortable disclosing disability within employment and educational environments represents a major step forward and should not be taken for granted, we also need to remain conscious of the problematic conceptual baggage that the language of disclosure carries with it and continue, through both our language and our silences, pushing on the ways conversations about disability are framed. The emphasis on design and agency, on productive confusion, and on the shared responsibility for initiating conversation about physical, sensory, and intellectual difference invoked by the artifacts discussed above represent just a few of the ways this work might proceed.

References

Anonymous. 2015. In discussion with the author, March 10, 2015.

Brown, Keith, Doris Hamner, Susan Foley, and Jonathan Woodring. 2009. "Doing Disability: Disability Formations in the Search for Work." *Sociological Inquiry* 79.1: 3–24.

Depoy, Elizabeth, and Stephen Gilson. 2013. "Disability, Design, and Branding: Rethinking Disability within the 21st Century." In *The Disability Studies Reader*, 4th ed., edited by Lennard J. Davis, 485–93. New York: Routledge.

"disclosure, n." 2015. OED Online. Oxford University Press. http://www.oed.com/view/Entry/53779?redirectedFrom=disclosure (accessed March 20, 2015).

Foucault, Michel. 1990. *The History of Sexuality*, vol. I. Translated by Robert Hurley. New York: Random House.

Garland-Thomson, Rosemarie. 2009. *Staring: How We Look*. Oxford: Oxford University Press.

Hahn, Harlan. 1995. Interview in *Vital Signs: Crip Culture Talks Back.* DVD. Directed by David Mitchell and Sharon Snyder. New York: Fanlight Productions.

Hockenberry, John. 2012. "We Are All Designers." Presentation at TED. Long Beach, CA, March 2012.

Keller, Helen. 2009. *The World I Live In & Optimism: A Collection of Essays* (1908). Mineola, NY: Dover Publications Inc.

Kerschbaum, Stephanie. 2014. "On Rhetorical Agency and Disclosing Disability in Academic Writing." *Rhetoric Review* 33.1: 55–71.

Knight, Amber. This volume.

Kuppers, Petra. 2008. "Crip Time." *Disability Studies Quarterly* 28.2. www.dsq-sds. org

Kuppers, Petra. 2014. "Crip Time." *Tikkun* 29.4: 29–31.

Muñoz, José Esteban. 2009. *Cruising Utopia: The Then and There of Queer Futurity.* New York: New York University Press.

Pullin, Graham. 2009. *Design Meets Disability.* Cambridge, MA: MIT Press.

Samuels, Ellen. 2014. *Fantasies of Identification: Disability, Gender, Race.* New York: New York University Press.

Samuels, Ellen. 2013. "My Body, My Closet: Invisible Disability and the Limits of Coming Out." In *The Disability Studies Reader,* 4th ed., edited by Lennard J. Davis, 316–32. New York: Routledge.

Serlin, David. 2010. "Pissing without Pity: Disability, Gender, and the Public Toilet." In *Toilet: Public Restrooms and the Politics of Sharing,* edited by Harvey Molotch and Laura Noren, 167–85. New York: New York University Press.

Science Fiction, Affect, and Crip Self-Invention

—Or, How Philip K. Dick Made Me Disabled

JOSH LUKIN

Social movements have long struggled with people who don't feel the way they're supposed to feel. Late in 2014, a guest speaker in my "Dissent in America" class was telling the students about the history of ADAPT, about his own activism, and about current legislative battles in the disability movement. About halfway through his presentation, he decided to introduce the social model of disability by asking the students, "Finish this sentence: 'Disability is . . .'" Perhaps he expected an opportunity to rebut such clichés such as "tragic" or "an occasion for inspiring heroism." I had given the students some instruction on disability history and activism in the previous week, so the speaker, to his delight, received answers such as "environmental" and "diversity" and "a basis for oppression." One young woman, however, went off-script, saying "disability is anxiety." The speaker had no idea what to do with that one and quickly moved on to other topics—among them, ironically, how activists should listen and learn what their constituency wants.

Significantly, the noncompliant student was the only member of the class who had disclosed a disability to her classmates: early in our discussions of disability and stigma, she'd mentioned that on more than one occasion, upon learning about her chronic condition and the treatment it required, someone had said to her admiringly, "Whoa. If I were you, I'd kill myself." So the experience of disability, along with the idea that disabled people's lives are terrifyingly undervalued, were not unfamiliar to her. Nonetheless, even after a thorough study of the 504 sit-ins and the anti-telethon movement and the fight for the ADA, she wouldn't get with the program and express a positive attitude. After the course was over, I realized how much the sentiment she'd expressed overlapped with my own. Once one realizes that one's disability is not a moral failing, one is supposed, judging by the syllabi, books, and blog posts I have encountered, to embrace the social model of disability, become a proud activist, and write a memoir. I do have an unpublished draft of a memoir (*Urgency: Growing Up with Crohn's Disease*), and I have been credited with activism in my teaching and scholarship. But the social model part and the pride part don't work well for me, and I know from a number of students and from conversations in the disability community that I am not unique in that. So I want to consider why that might be, and how theoretical and science-fictional models offer alternative ways of being disabled—ways that are not really new discoveries on my part but that are already immanent in crip culture.

Discussions of disabled people's varied responses to the social model—its power and its limitations—are necessary. One exemplary account that I use regularly in the classroom is Egan's (2012) "I'm Not a 'Person with a Disability': I'm a Disabled Person," written for the webzine *XOjane*. Egan begins with the thesis that she is "disabled by a society that places social, attitudinal and architectural barriers in [her] way" and goes on to illustrate how disability is a social problem and not an individual problem. Understanding disability as a social problem leads Egan to argue for the universal and therapeutic nature of the social model, and she suggests that those who would disagree with her "haven't noticed the social model's distinction between 'impairment' (the things you can't do because of your body/brain) and 'disability' (the social barriers disabling you on the grounds that you have an illness or impairment)." Egan alternates between discussing the external injustices she was able to recognize thanks to the social model and recounting the revolution it inspired in her self-image:

> When I was a child I would wonder "why me?" on a daily basis. I would wonder why my spirit had been put into this body that hurt so much of the time. I hated my body when I was not allowed on school trips or when I was left in the classroom on my own while my classmates were doing something more fun. . . . Once I learned about the social model, I realized that my body wasn't the problem at all.

That awareness of the social model ended Egan's self-hatred is a great argument for its dissemination: if she found it to be so revolutionary, doubtless many others do.[1] But conversion narratives, as we know, have a way of becoming prescriptions—one is tempted, when saved, to evangelize—and there's a hint of that tendency in her claim that her opponents just don't understand what the social model is all about.

Criticisms of the social model have proliferated over the past twenty years.[2] Price (2014), for example, has pointed out that there are aspects of madness and pain that it doesn't cover, and Tremain (2001) has explained that the disability/impairment binary doesn't hold water. Recently, the rhetorician Hassler (2015) articulated several thoughtful criticisms of the binary between disability and impairment. She has suggested, for instance, that it reifies impairment both as something fixed—rather than a process that itself varies contextually—and as somehow *distinct from* the social, as if there is a realm into which the social doesn't reach. Further, she argues, it phrases the disabled experience in deficit terms because impairment in this context comes to mean "I cannot do this thing that my society values." And it often makes that claim en route to adding, "But we're not here to consider what the somatic and psychic barriers mean: we're here to consider the sociopolitical barriers we can fight. Soldier On. Rah."

The stigma against disability can easily shift to a negative valuation of impairment, which is dealt with by abandoning considerations of the experience of, and the materiality of, the body. Finally, the doings of our bodies and psyches may present intractable difficulties that don't always fit into an understanding of disability as something that societies impose on the impaired, or even as the interaction of an anomalous bodymind with an inhospitable environment. As Hassler says, "Falling is *hard*. Executive function struggles are *hard*. Society is what declares disability Bad, but often not what makes it hard" (2015). Oliver (2004), originator of the social model, dismissed theoretical criticisms of it by saying that the social model was not a theory but a hammer—a tool for social change. I agree with Oliver that it has been used to good effect in that way, but we need screwdrivers and pliers and little IKEA Allen wrenches in our tool belts, too.

While the social model has received some significant critique, a less frequently criticized imperative in disability self-narration is that of pride. For many years, it has seemed completely natural to base group solidarity on pride—to go from the realization that one's cultural identity does not have to be a source of shame to feeling pride and thence to an enthusiastic sense of communion in an activist project. That ideal trajectory is one aspect of Clare's great cripqueer memoir, *Exile & Pride* (2009). Clare begins with a critique of the social model, opining that "Oliver's model of disability makes theoretical and political sense but misses important emotional realities" (8). He describes a difficult project of transforming the anger and self-hatred that he suffers as a queer disabled person and a survivor of long-term sexual abuse, reclaiming his body, and—in raw, corporeal imagery—expelling the past: "I can feel slivers of shame, silence, and isolation still imbedded deep in my body. I hate these fragments" (110). And his answer to all of these struggles, repeatedly articulated in the first-person plural, is "pride": "Without pride, individual and collective resistance to oppression becomes nearly impossible" (107). "Pride works in direct opposition to internalized oppression" (109).

I want to emphasize again that I hope to avoid reproducing the problems I am criticizing. I don't want to tell anyone, "Your narrative makes no theoretical sense so you should give it up," nor do I want to claim that anyone's feelings are bad for progress. Tireless activists such as Clare find that their model of transformation and resistance to shame works to sustain them; objections to, for example, invoking internalization and expulsion on the grounds that we don't have a presocial self into which harmful things come from the outside may be academic.[3] And there is nothing irrational in saying you're proud of having survived in the face of social forces trying to destroy you. But once he turns to prescribing affect, I get rattled on a deep level. I once found myself rereading the passages on pride in Clare and muttering in some distress, "don'ttellmewhattofeel don'ttellmewhattofeel don'ttellmewhattofeel." Not everyone follows the shame-pride-praxis trajectory.[4] Clare's chronicle and historical narratives of proud disability heroes are invaluable in that they celebrate the *possibility* of pride as a response to ableist oppression, uttering bold and indispensable cries of defiance against the world that expects us to be complicit in our obliteration. But once that's been articulated, can there be space for other possibilities? Can't we at least—as Halperin (2009) has suggested in a gay pride context—get a shame break now and then?[5] What about access for the pride-impaired?

And just what is this "shame" feeling that we're supposed to transcend? In the 1970s, Lewis argued that "In order for shame to occur, there must be a relationship between the self and the other in which the self cares about the other's valuation . . . Fascination with the other and sensitivity to the other's treatment of the self renders the self more vulnerable to shame" (1987, 107). More recently, Sedgwick (2003)—and to some extent Nussbaum (2005)—have offered an account of shame's origins that focuses on the infantile experience of unfulfilled needs or processes. In Sedgwick's case, this unfulfilled need is specifically identified as something like a recognition wound. The proto-affect of shame becomes not the result of a transgression but the feeling that accompanies thwarted recognition, originally in the form of the care-giver failing to give the expected attention to the infant. Sedgwick, invoking Sylvan Tomkins and more recent researchers on affect, specifically invokes "the moment when the adult face refuses to play its part in the continuation of mutual gaze; when . . . it fails to be recognizable to, or recognizing of, the infant" and asserts that shame becomes a more general "reaction to the loss of feedback from others, indicating social isolation" (36). She cites Michael Basch's claim that "shame-humiliation throughout life can be thought of as an inability to effectively arouse the other person's positive reactions to one's communications" (qtd. in Sedgwick 2003, 37). I feel a great sense of affirmation reading this account: it resonates deeply with my sense of shame and with that of friends who were also hospitalized from an early age or for other reasons denied the expected recognition of supportive adult faces at lengthy intervals from infancy on. But does it encompass other experiences that we identify as shameful?

Is Sedgwick's account, for example, robust enough to address feelings of undeservingness? Disappointment in oneself? Failure to adhere to communal standards? The question of an individual's deserts is of some urgency; a common form of shame leaves one continually asking oneself, "What business do you have thinking you can do this or should receive that or belong in the space reserved for your betters?"[6] Clare articulates such feelings most often in the context of class shame, at one point movingly remarking, "I span the distance, able to sit in a posh Boston hotel with well-dressed New York butch and Boston femme dykes and not feel *shame*, only *embarrassment*" (42). Such experiences suggest that shame becomes not only about the *experience* of a recognition-wound, but the *anticipation* or the *dread* of one. A similar extension can explain the question of failure to live up to norms: by a straightforward psychological process, the recognizing caregiver becomes abstracted into the community or society or authority.

Considering the effect of shame on members of oppressed groups, Gould points out that the "sense of not being acknowledged, or even seen, [the] experience of social nonrecognition by an audience that is at least to some degree a desired audience, is common for members of socially marginalized and subordinated groups who are part of society but also exiled from it owing to their perceived difference" (2009, 222). Sedgwick goes further and takes a more provocative approach: she considers the question of shame and subordinated groups not only to raise the issue of nonrecognition but to question whether pride movements—which she defines quite broadly—are successful at disavowing shame. Sedgwick's claim is so striking that the editors of the

Gay Shame anthology single it out for attention, styling it a "radical conclusion" that allows for nonessentialist views of identity and modes of queer resistance. As she writes,

> strategies aimed directly at getting rid of individual or group shame, or undoing it . . . may "work" . . . but they can't work in the way they say they work . . . The forms taken by shame are not distinct "toxic" parts of a group or individual identity that can be excised; they are instead integral to and residual in the processes by which identity itself is formed. They are available for the work of metamorphosis, reframing, refiguration, *trans*figuration, affective and symbolic loading and deformation. (62)

This is a useful formulation but not, at least at the time of the 2003 Gay Shame Conference that the anthology documents, a novel insight. Even someone whose model of the self is as vulnerable to queer critique as Clare (2009) talks at length about *transforming* his shame and about accepting deformation[7] and indeed, memoirs like his, no less than the Henry James prefaces Sedgwick likes to cite, *are* literary performances and transformations of shame.

What do such performances do for readers, then? I have spoken of these theoretical concepts, in part, as consciousness-raising tools. I encounter them and I say, "Oboy, this names a thing I recognize: I am in a world where others experience it." Indeed, it was only my discovery of Adamson and Clark's (1998) *Scenes of Shame* anthology that prompted me to call my pain "shame." And I may only have begun thinking of *living* with the shame of disability when I heard Ellen Samuels speak on a panel at the Disability Disclosure Conference (Dalke, Gould, Lindgren, Mullaney and Samuels 2013). My experience of *literature* feels different: I'm on the other side of the gaze here. Although I will in the remainder of this essay speak of having recognized familiar experiences in literature, I actually tend to feel that the text has recognized *me* rather than the reverse.[8] And in being so recognized, I get, paradoxically, assured that responding, or having responded, with shame (or indeed with other intense affects) to past or ongoing experiences may not in fact be shameful. To illustrate this paradox, I want to consider two science fiction (SF) writers by whose work I have felt verified[9]: Philip K. Dick and Vandana Singh.[10]

Philip Kindred Dick's work is antithetical to that of Robert Heinlein and other chroniclers of science-fictional superheroes. A novel such as his *The Man in the High Castle* (1962), for example, follows the adventures of four ordinary people living under a fascist government, each of whom surprises him- or herself with a small-scale existential triumph against the inexorable forces of oppression; although a popular success, it was unintelligible to some of the readers accustomed to heroes transforming planet-wide civilizations. Dick's interest in vitiated heroes and timid schleps likely has its roots in his own history of shame, poverty, and abjection, which began in his childhood. In the wake of her divorce, young Phil's mother sought expert psychiatric advice and was told that it was her duty as a single parent to eschew displays of affection. She did not excel at displays of validation either: Dick remembered having heard, at the age of twelve, the news on the radio on December 7, 1941, and called home to tell his mother, "Mom, we're at war with Germany, Italy, and Japan!" Dorothy Kindred replied to her overimaginative son, "No, I don't think so, Philip" (Sutin 1989, 35).

Disability is ubiquitous in Dick's work. The embittered thalidomide child in *Dr. Bloodmoney* (1963), the benign intellectually disabled recluse in *Do Androids Dream of Electric Sheep?* (1966), the legless pilgrim of *Deus Irae* (1964), the autistic prophet in *Martian Time-Slip* (1962), the deaf, wheelchair-dependent film composer of *VALIS* (1978) . . . and everywhere, madness. The setting of *Clans of the Alphane Moon* (1964) is a world formerly used as a mental asylum, abandoned by its administrators, where the population has developed a functional society of tribes who identify by psychiatric diagnosis: the paranoids, the manics, the obsessive-compulsives, *et alia*. When a failed comedy writer from Earth, his estranged wife, his nubile neighbor, and an unfathomably wise slime mold from Ganymede arrive on the moon, hijinks ensue. In *A Scanner Darkly* (1973), the madness is the result of recreational drug use, a crime promoted by the state in the service of a nominally higher goal. The perceptions of its victims as their minds deteriorate are alternately hilarious and terrifying. Both novels imagine a disability community that is rare in literature.

The great 1969 novel *Ubik* contains an image of physical disability that has stayed with me since I first encountered it twenty-odd years ago. Our protagonist, Joe Chip, and his coworkers have encountered a strange force that increases their entropy, causing them and the objects around them to age and disintegrate rapidly. Joe is in the lobby of a high-class Des Moines hotel in 1939—the characters are from the twenty-first century but have slipped backward in time as well—and Joe is wearing out. "'I just feel tired,' he said, and realized how really tired his body had become. He could not remember such fatigue. Never before in his life" (170). And a couple of pages later, "Joe said, 'I want to go upstairs. I want to lie down.'" (172).

This is not a situation I had seen in fiction before. When a protagonist wants to lie down, it's generally an old person who's ending a significant life or someone who's been through a dramatic conflict. Joe Chip is feeling exhausted, after having done nothing in particular, for reasons he can only speculate on, and he wants to lie down! His fatigue manifests itself in a desire not to have to deal with anyone, a drive that I understand better now than I did in my twenties: "But the longing within him had grown greater, the overpowering need to be alone . . . entirely unwitnessed, silent and supine. Stretched out, not needing to speak, not needing to move. Not required to cope with anyone or any problem . . . he wanted to be unknown and invisible, to live unseen" (174). After he has been climbing the steps to his hotel room for four pages, Joe begins to develop a strategy or craft of negotiating them, as cripples do: "He did not talk; he did not even see. Going by the hardness of the surface against which he rested, he crept snail-like from step to step, feeling a kind of skill develop in him, an ability to tell exactly how to exert himself, how to use this nearly bankrupt power" (177). *Ubik*, I propose, is about the phenomenon that Zola (1982) and others have styled crip time.[11]

The shame and madness in Dick's life and work come to a head in the 1970s, perhaps most explicitly in his semi-autobiographical novel *VALIS* (1978). This witty, gripping, tedious, compassionate, misogynistic, sprightly, turgid novel takes as its focus Dick's alter ego, one Horselover Fat, who, traumatized by a friend's suicide, "continued his insidious, long decline into misery and illness, the sort of chaos that astrophysicists say is the fate in store for the whole universe." The diegetic narrator—also named Phil—says "Fat was certain that God had healed him completely. That is not possible. There is a line in the *I Ching* reading, 'Always ill but never dies.' That fits my friend" (18). Again, I was more than familiar with the frustration that people feel with a chronically ill person whose disease is never resolved by cure or death. Even my gastroenterologist, when I was fifteen, once came to my hospital bed on rounds and said, "I wonder whether you're having such frequent pain because you spend time lying here *thinking* about pain. You should get up and around more." But I had never seen that impatience rendered in writing.

As Sontag (1978) and others have observed, the tendency to hold patients responsible for their own suffering is deeply ingrained in our culture. This insistence is a powerful shame-generator for sick and disabled people: there's always someone around to start us wondering whether, if we'd tried a little harder or approached things a little differently, we would have been able to overcome the obstacles we faced. So it is exhilarating to see Dick in *VALIS* repeatedly condemn victim-blaming and other attempts on the part of the healthy to impose a reassuring narrative on the lives of the sick. Here is a passage in which Phil grows impatient with one of his friends' response to illness:

> Being a Catholic, David always traced everything wrong back to man's free will. This used to annoy even me. I once asked him if Sherri's getting cancer consisted of an instance of free will, knowing as I did that David . . . would make the mistake of claiming that Sherri has subconsciously wanted to get cancer and so had shut down her immune system. (28)

Sherri is not a sympathetic character; nonetheless, Dick, or at least the fictional Phil, refuses to blame her. This is a radical position in the Seventies, and not just in California: "Happy people don't get cancer" was a more widespread conviction everywhere than it is now. Phil maintains his antivoluntarist attitude when faced with his fellow Christians' attempts to make sense of pain. Ruminating over how suffering is supposed to have empowered Parsifal (there's lots of Wagner in Dick), Phil says, "Please show me how Gloria's suffering and Sherri's suffering contributed anything good to Fat, to anyone, to anything. It's a lie. It's an evil lie. Suffering is to be abolished. . . . What we really need is a doctor, not a spear" (133–34).

As in most of Dick, when the medical establishment appears, it's in the context of mental disability; and not all of the doctors in that field are better than spears. But Horselover Fat, in a psychiatric ward, has the good fortune to encounter a brilliant physician. This man, one Leon Stone, listens as Fat spins his elaborate theories of reality based on the pre-Socratics and Lao Tzu and the Dead Sea Scrolls and can match him citation for citation. At Fat's exit interview from the hospital, he asks Dr. Stone if his Gnostic discoveries are accurate.

> "You would know," Stone said, and then he said something that no one had ever said to Fat before. "You're the authority" . . . Stone had saved him: he was a master psychiatrist . . . I've always told people that for each person there is a sentence—a series of words—which has the power to destroy him. When Fat told me about Leon Stone, I realized . . . that another sentence exists, another series of words, which will heal the person. (65, 67)

The situation here fits Sedgwick's model perfectly: it offers a completed circuit of recognition from the caregiver. And the fact that it is recognition in a context where the subject has every reason to expect *in*validation—a shaming response—makes it a characteristic Phildickian moment. From his literary novels of the fifties on, there are a number of Dick books in which someone encounters the suffering protagonist, recognizes his condition and—to his astonishment—doesn't blame him.

Thanks perhaps to the pressures of the mid-century SF market, only a few of Dick's science fiction novels follow their own logic to leave us with the slimmest of hopes at the end. Many others proceed along the lines of a bleak Modernist or naturalist novel in which nobody has much agency and then force an optimistic ending via some science fictional trope or other, whether it's a religious encounter or a reassuring robot. What I'd like to see is a story taking the opposite tack, one in which being a benevolent alien or knowing how to enter parallel worlds doesn't make you any less fucked up. And it'd be nice if such a story contained the kind of affirming intersubjective recognition that is so moving in Dick, and if that recognition did not have to come from The Father, whether in secular or theological guise. There is a great scene in *VALIS* wherein Fat, convinced he has remembered a former life wherein he hung out with Jesus and His disciples, says "I saw him—sort of—and I want to see him again. That love, that warmth, that delight on his part that it's me, seeing me, being glad it's me: *recognizing* me. . . . He *recognized* me!" (130). Possibly, for validation to work, we have to feel that the person recognizing us has more freedom or power or *jouissance* than ourselves: that sense would correspond to the "[f]ascination with the other" that Helen Block Lewis (1987) argues is necessary for shame. But in several Dick novels, *VALIS* among them, the desire for recognition seems synonymous with yearning for an absent Dad's respect—a desire that not everyone will be able to identify with.

Fortunately, fiction that eschews some of these problems with the Dick canon is being written in our time, in Framingham, Massachusetts, by a physics professor named Vandana Singh. Singh began publishing science fiction at close to forty and so far her oeuvre includes two novellas, two children's books, one collection, and a few uncollected stories and essays. Her work for adults tends toward witty but melancholy stories of exile and cultural conflict. Singh is an expert at depictions of people surviving loss or grief or debility. Her most acclaimed shorter story, "Infinities" (2008) concerns a Muslim mathematician in a state torn by sectarian violence, who has to come to the shameful realization that the interdimensional beings he alone can see are not, as he had once imagined, angels of the Lord but uncomprehending observers of our world, and that Allah has only given us each other to rely upon for love, guidance, and recognition. When disability is central to one of her stories, it often appears in relation to hyperability: *Of Love and Other Monsters* (2007), for example, features an alien who has lost his shape changing power. The heroine of *Distances* (2009) is her world's—or her solar system's—greatest mathematician, able to derive equations through a combination of intellectual, sensory, and aesthetic brilliance: the novella involves how she copes with the loss of those gifts.

Distances, which in 2009 won the Parallax award for best science fiction by a person of color, is an intercultural odyssey whose heroine, Anasuya, starts out with a distressingly ableist if not eugenicist aesthetic. Living in a desert land that is in every way at odds with the aquatic realm she comes from, Anasuya passes harsh judgments upon her coworkers in the temple of mathematics. Of its Master, who is rumored to be an interspecies hybrid, she thinks, "She knew she should feel sorry for him, but he disturbed her too much, even for that. What kind of thing was he, not human, not [bird], not worm, but a bit of each? At least she knew what she was . . ." (13). And of the temple's intellectually disabled doorkeeper, Amas, "He was a broken geometry: he contained voids. He was a stone rattling in a gourd. She thought, if I had been born like Amas, I would have wanted my mothers to throw me to the sharks of the deep sea" (47).

Anasuya's own judgmental tendency is in part borne of guilt for having left her native realm—one expects that such a temperament will be most judgmental of itself, and sure enough, when her mathematical vision begins to fade, "She thought, if I don't get it back, I want to die" (111). Her confidence that she knew what she was is destroyed, "because she was turning into something else" (123). The word "shame" does not appear in the story, but the feeling that prompts Anasuya to flee her spouses—she is in a relationship with four other people—and her workplace, to go into hiding, to starve herself, and to believe upon returning to her house that she can do nothing whatsoever for her partners is clear enough. Anasuya's condition here is a powerful variation on the Sedgwickian model in which shame arises from recognition denied: her artistic and mathematical achievements are getting worldwide recognition, but the recognizing gaze doesn't validate her, as she is no longer the person who created them.

By the end of *Distances*, Anasuya is only beginning to consider how she will fulfill her duties to her native realm and live with her partners as a disabled woman. There's a heartbreaking exchange with one of her lovers in which she tries to recite by rote the mathematical truths she can no longer perceive intuitively. But, like Dick, Singh has shown us people surviving the anguish of disablement, persisting through their losses rather than having them resolved by cure or death. And both have imagined nonstandard and nonpunitive responses to disability, projecting positive relationships between disabled and nondisabled people, based in mutual recognition. The science fiction writer and literary critic Delany likes to explain that

> science fiction is far more concerned [than literary fiction] with the organization (and reorganization) of the object, that is, the world, or the institutions through which we perceive it. . . . How is the subject excited, impinged on, contoured, and constituted by the object? How might beings with a different social organization, environment, brain structure, and body perceive things? How might humans perceive things after becoming acclimated to an alien environment? (2012, 178)

Hence, works of science fiction have long been in conversation about interactions of anomalous bodyminds with their environments: in a sense, much science fiction starts out taking the social model for granted and then goes on to problematize its implications.[12]

A literature that delineates "why it's hard" to be disabled, that confronts the inevitability of shame, and that dwells on the problems of nonrecognition without any assurance that those injustices will be vanquished might be vulnerable to accusations of complicity with ableism. But to value such literature is not tantamount to letting down the drawbridge and inviting Peter Singer and Rand Paul into the crip fortress. For all the pain these characters endure, there is nothing in Anasuya's or Fat's experience to support such ableist claims as "Those people can't enjoy life" or "They're a burden on society." Without any disability movement allegiances but simply by virtue of their commitment to literature, Dick and Singh (and Nisi Shawl, and Lois McMaster Bujold, among other science fiction writers) eschew eugenic clichés and present brave, aesthetically sensitive, and witty disabled protagonists whose presence in the world is as valuable as anyone's. Read or taught in a disability studies context, science-fictional tales of shame and anguish over changing abilities offer nuanced perspectives that question whether we can always redefine disability as a Good Thing or understand it via epiphanies gained through the social model.[13] These stories can give us permission to face our pain, and they can speak to what disabled students are experiencing now, not just what they might encounter after the movement has wrought extensive social and emotional transformations. As Love (2007) says of narratives in the gay shame archive, "they describe what it is like to bear a 'disqualified' identity, which at times can simply mean living with injury, not fixing it" (4).

My student's consciously rebellious "Disability is anxiety," along with many of the conversations at the 2013 Disability Disclosure in/and Higher Education Conference, demonstrate that accounts of pain, shame, loss, and intractable bodies can exist alongside fights for disability justice. Simi Linton, talking of the Society for Disability Studies in her great memoir *My Body Politic*, wisely observes that

> Personal sufferings aren't discounted by an organization bent on social and intellectual change, but we are adept at sorting the preventable suffering from the inevitable. . . . Our symptoms may at times be painful, scary, unpleasant, or difficult to manage, and that may never change no matter what policy is implemented or what scholarly paper is written. (2006, 138)

She quickly moves on from that caveat to argue that the most frustrating of our sufferings comes from remediable social oppression. But her disclaimer gestures toward an important fact: "the movement from abjection to glorious community" (2007, 28), as Love has called it, isn't a one-way journey. We never get to leave abjection for good, and we can even feel its impact in the *midst* of glorious community.[14] Space for shame, more or less free of the imperative to transcend or mobilize that shame, remains an inextricable part of disability culture.

References

Adamson, Joseph, and Hilary Clark, eds. 1998. *Scenes of Shame: Psychoanalysis, Shame, and Writing*. Albany: SUNY Press.

Baldwin, James. 1974. *If Beale Street Could Talk*. New York: Vintage, 2006.

Cameron, J. M. 1962. "Poetry and Dialectic." *The Night Battle and Other Essays*. Baltimore: Helicon. 119–49.

Chandler, Eliza. 2013. "Interactions of Disability Pride and Shame." In *The Female Face of Shame*, edited by Erica L. Johnson and Patricia Moran. Bloomington: Indiana University Press. 74–86.

Chandler, Eliza. "Sidewalk Stories: The Troubling Task of Identification." *Disability Studies Quarterly* 30 (2010). http://dsq-sds.org/article/view/1293/1329

Clare, Eli. 1991. *Exile & Pride: Disability, Queerness, & Liberation*. Cambridge, MA: South End Press, 2009.

Clare, Eli. "Metaphor." (blog post). *Eli Clare* (website). 11 July 2008. http://eliclare.com/disability/metaphor

Crow, Liz. 1996. "Including All of Our Lives: Renewing the Social Model of Disability." In *Encounters with Strangers: Feminism and Disability*, edited by Jenny Morris. London: Women's Press. 216–25.

Dalke, Anne, Kate Gould, Kristin Lindgren, Clare Mullaney, and Ellen Samuels. "Unbinding Time." Panel presented at the Disability Disclosure in/and Higher Education Conference, Newark, DE. 25 October 2013.

Delany, Samuel. "The Art of Fiction, No. 210." Interview with Rachel Kaadzi Ghansah. *Paris Review* 197 (Summer 2010). 24–55.

Delany, Samuel. 1977. *The Jewel-Hinged Jaw: Notes on the Language of Science Fiction*. Middletown, CT: Wesleyan University Press, 2009.

Delany, Samuel. 1984. *Starboard Wine: More Notes on the Language of Science Fiction*. Middletown, CT: Wesleyan University Press, 2012.

Dick, Philip K. 1977. *A Scanner Darkly*. New York: Doubleday.

Dick, Philip K. 1964. *Clans of the Alphane Moon*. New York: Ace Books.

Dick, Philip K. 1968. *Do Androids Dream of Electric Sheep?* New York: Doubleday.

Dick, Philip K. 1965. *Dr. Bloodmoney, or How We Got Along after the Bomb*. New York: Ace Books.

Dick, Philip K. 1962. *The Man in the High Castle*. New York: Vintage, 1992.

Dick, Philip K. 1964. *Martian Time-Slip*. New York: Ballantine.

Dick, Philip K. 1969. *Ubik*. New York: Vintage, 1991.

Dick, Philip K. 1981. *VALIS*. New York: Vintage, 1990.

Dick, Philip and Roger Zelazny. 1976. *Deus Irae*. New York: Doubleday.

Egan, Lisa. "I'm Not a 'Person with a Disability': I'm a Disabled Person." *XOjane*. 9 November 2012. http://www.xojane.com/issues/i-am-not-a-person-with-a-disability-i-am-a-disabled-person

Examined Life. Directed by Astra Taylor. Performed by Sunaura Taylor, Judith Butler, Cornel West, Martha Nussbaum. Toronto: Filmswelike, 2008. Film.

Finger, Anne. "Pity Is Always Shadowed by Contempt" (interview with Josh Lukin). *Wordgathering: A Journal of Disability Poetry and Literature* 7 (2013). http://www.wordgathering.com/past_issues/issue26/interviews/finger.html

Gotkin, Kevin. Personal conversation. 16 April 2015.

Gould, Deborah. "The Shame of Gay Pride in Early AIDS Activism." In Halperin/Traub. 221–55.

Halperin, David. "Why Gay Shame Now?" In Halperin/Traub. 41–48.

Halperin, David and Valerie Traub, eds. 2009. *Gay Shame*. Chicago: University of Chicago Press.

Hassler, Elizabeth. Facebook chat with the author. 8 April 2015.

Jones, Pattrice. 1999. "Personality Complex: Eli Clare Dives Deep into the Muddy Waters of Identity Politics." 1999. *texts by pattrice jones*. 18 July 2008.

Kafer, Alison. 2013. *Feminist Queer Crip*. New York: New York University Press.

Koyama, Emi. "The Uses of Negativity: Survival and Coping Strategies for Those of Us Who Are Exasperated by the Empty Promise of 'It' Getting 'Better.'" *Eminism* (blog). 26 October 2013. http://eminism.org/blog/entry/404

Kuppers, Petra. "Toward a Rhizomatic Model of Disability: Poetry, Performance, and Touch." *Journal of Literary & Cultural Disability Studies* 3 (2009): 221–40.

Le Guin, Ursula. 1993. Introduction to *The Norton Book of Science Fiction*, edited by Ursula Le Guin and Brian Attebery. New York: Norton. 3–34.

Lewis, Helen Block. 1987. "Shame and the Narcissistic Personality." In *The Many Faces of Shame*, edited by Donald Nathanson. New York: Guilford Press. 93–132.

Linton, Simi. 2006. *My Body Politic: A Memoir*. Ann Arbor: University of Michigan Press.

Love, Heather. 2007. *Feeling Backward: Loss and the Politics of Queer History*. Cambridge, MA: Harvard University Press.

Mollow, Anna. "When Black Women Start Going on Prozac: Race, Gender, and Mental Illness in Meri Nana-Ama Danquah's Willow Weep for Me." *Melus* (2006): 67–99.

Moore, C. L. "Heir Apparent." *Astounding Science Fiction*, February 1950.

Moore, C.L. "Promised Land." *Astounding Science Fiction*, July 1950.

Morris, Jenny. *Pride against Prejudice: A Personal Model of Disability*. London: Women's Press, 1991.

Negrón-Mutaner, Frances. "*Boricua* Gazing" (interview with Rita Gonzalez). Halperin/Traub. 88–102.

Nussbaum, Martha. 2005. *Hiding from Humanity: Disgust, Shame, and the Law*. Princeton: Princeton University Press.

Oliver, Michael. "The Social Model in Action: If I Had a Hammer." *Implementing the Social Model of Disability: Theory and Research* (2004): 18–31.

Price, Margaret. "The Bodymind Problem and the Possibilities of Pain." *Hypatia* 30 (2014): 268–84.

Price, Margaret. (PriceMargaret). "Ellen Samuels: Crip time is sometimes 'grief time,' notes that sometimes crip time can mean 'loss and its crushing undertow.'" 25 October 2013, 12:18 p.m. Tweet.

Price, Margaret. 2011. *Mad at School: Rhetorics of Mental Disability and Academic Life*. Ann Arbor: University of Michigan Press.

Sedgwick, Eve Kosofsky. 2003. *Touching Feeling: Affect, Pedagogy, Performativity*. Durham, NC: Duke University Press.

Shakespeare, Tom. 2013. "The Social Model of Disability." In *The Disability Studies Reader, 4th Edition*, edited by Lennard J. Davis. New York: Routledge. 214–21.

Siebers, Tobin. "Disability in Theory: From Social Constructionism to the New Realism of the Body." *American Literary History* 13 (2001): 737–54.

Singh, Vandana. 2009. *Distances*. Seattle: Aqueduct.

Singh, Vandana. 2008. "Infinities." In *The Woman Who Thought She Was a Planet and Other Stories*. Delhi: Zubaan. 55–88.

Singh, Vandana. 2007. *Of Love and Other Monsters*. Seattle: Aqueduct.

Sontag, Susan. 1978. *Illness as Metaphor*. New York: Farrar, Straus, Giroux.

Sturgeon, Theodore. 1949. "Prodigy." *Astounding Science Fiction*, April 1949.

Sturgeon, Theodore. 1953a. *More Than Human*. New York: Farrar Straus, 1953.

Sturgeon, Theodore. 1953b. "The Clinic." In *A Saucer of Loneliness: The Collected Stories of Theodore Sturgeon, Volume VII*. Berkeley: North Atlantic Books, 2000. 297–310.

Sutin, Lawrence. 1989. *Divine Invasions: A Life of Philip K. Dick*. New York: Harmony Books.

Tremain, Shelley. "On the Government of Disability." *Social Theory and Practice* 27 (2001): 617–36.

Zola, Irving Kenneth. 1982. *Missing Pieces: A Chronicle of Living with a Disability*. Philadelphia: Temple University Press.

Satire, Scholarship, and Sanity; or How to Make Mad Professors[1]

THERÍ A. PICKENS

The discourse of ability lurks as an undercurrent within the academy, sometimes creating a riptide between the turbulent waters of superior thinking and the threat of madness. As such, it lingers—ebbs and flows, if you will—with the constancy of the school year's rhythms. The rigors of tenure and promotion decisions often expose how contingent a professor's reputation and livelihood is upon their relationship to sanity. To be clear, some are allowed to tip-toe closer to madness than others based on the other combination of identities they occupy. Those that can safely embrace their "crazy" (without threatening their prospects or livelihood) do so with the implicit acknowledgement that this behavior is germane to their identity as a professor. "Nutty professors" or "absent-minded professors" become (or remain) socially permissible when they are tenured, straight, white, male, and/or able-bodied (Harris and Gonzales 2012). There are a few classic cultural examples of this archetype including the titular character of the film *The Absent-Minded Professor* (1961), Robin Williams' character in *Flubber* (1997), and Sheldon Cooper of *The Big Bang Theory*. Nonacademic examples include Sherlock Holmes and all his televisual kin: Gregory House (*House*), Adrian Monk (*Monk*), and Spencer Reid (*Criminal Minds*), among others. Their oddity, in other words, is a function of their genius. Others—usually people of color, queer, untenured, women, and/or disabled—fall into another category of "mad professor": specifically, their behavior and outlook is supposedly the result of their sojourn in the institution or germane to the identities understood to be the antithesis of professorial. There are fewer cultural representations of this archetype, but they include Eddie Murphy as Sherman Klump in *The Nutty Professor* (1996) and *The Nutty Professor II: The Klumps* (2000). In recent events, professors Saida Grundy and Steven Salaita faced significant public scorn mobilizing just this sort of rhetoric after they expressed antiracist views on Twitter.

In what follows, I wish to examine the representation of the so-called mad professor, specifically the kind whose craziness results from the constant assault of micro-aggressions and hostility within the college environment. Methodologically speaking, this essay sits at the nexus of literary and cultural analysis. I take for granted that representations of marginalized subjects often get called upon to correct misconceptions or champion positive or respectable images. If it were my aim to assist in that endeavor, Mat Johnson would be the wrong author to discuss here. Instead, I look to his work precisely because he mobilizes satire and irreverence as a central part of his oeuvre in order to level a critique of some sort at various institutions. Looking to representations (of all kinds) to explain or correct reveals an expectation that narrative does cultural work. To be fair, that expectation is not entirely misplaced. However, "focusing on whether or not a particular image is either good or bad does not necessarily address the complexity of representation. Rather it is important to examine the ideological work performed by images and story lines" (Alsultany 2012, 13). Thus, I analyze Johnson's *Pym* (2012) for what it reveals about the ideological stakes operating within one of the academy's most important evaluative and validating procedures: the tenure process.

Pym begins with a black male professor's tenure denial; his subsequent depression and confrontations are subtended by the idea that he has supposedly gone crazy. Johnson's succinct twenty-page depiction disrupts the facile causal relationship often presumed between be(com)ing a professor and the onset of insanity. I choose to analyze Johnson's brief portrayal for how it offers a counter-narrative to this causal relationship by foregrounding the complex constellation of relationships at the heart of being an academic of color. Thinking of the professoriate as a generative ground for madness creates a linear narrative that does not account for the multiple intersections of race, gender, and ability. Discourses about in/sanity also require a nonlinear narrative since madness usefully disrupts the adherence to Western rationality—the backbone of the academic enterprise. In unpacking Johnson's narrative, I argue that the facile scripts regarding madness, race, and gender fail to attend to the profound complexities present within the academy. An insufficient understanding of how these scripts function leaves racism, sexism, and ableism unchecked and, as a result, more insidiously influential.

As my use of terms like *mad* and *crazy* might suggest, I accept the linguistic and cultural slippage these more common words allow, in contrast to more academic terms such as *neuroatypical, cognitive impairment,* or *mental illness.* Certainly, none of these words are neutral (Price 2011, 1–25). I prefer *mad* and *crazy* because they highlight the large concern of this essay (that of representation) while allowing for the intentional vagueness and lexical baggage accrued to each term. In being offensive, they call attention to themselves in such a way as to highlight how they function as delegitimizing discursive terrain. In addition to their invocation of sanity, *mad* and *crazy* also carry with them charges of excess, obsession, impracticality, singularity, and excellence. When linked to the requirements and habits of the professoriate, the two words index a set of expectations regarding how professors ought to represent themselves to each other as well as the rest of the world. Alas, it needs to be said that those expectations change dramatically when the mad, nutty professor in question holds a marginalized identity or even several.

The Road to Tenure Denial

Within Johnson's *Pym,* Professor Chris Jaynes does not receive tenure because he has, according to the college president, neglected to fulfill the duties for which he was hired. The faculty votes favorably for him, but the president overturns their vote for two reasons. First, his research takes him to Edgar Allan Poe as a way to think through the operational impulses of whiteness in the American literary imagination. The president asserts that Chris's desire to steer himself into researching and teaching nineteenth-century white authors does not dutifully fulfill the obligations of an African American literature professor. Second, Chris refuses to serve on the Diversity Committee. The president claims that Chris's lack of wider professional acknowledgment (i.e., Fulbright, Rhodes) should have made him embrace his local role more (Johnson 2012, 14). *Pym* has a similar structure to the Poe novel it satirizes, *The Narrative of Arthur Gordon Pym of Nantucket* (2012). First, there is a preface written by Chris Jaynes affirming the veracity of the events to follow, naming Mat Johnson as another professor. The reader enters the text several months after the tenure decision has been made and just after Chris has cancelled the last week of his classes and holed himself up in a hotel room in Harlem with his cousin by his side. Upon his return to campus, Chris finds all his belongings taken from his office, so he goes to the president to lobby for his reinstatement as a faculty member, but only succeeds in losing his temper and emasculating the president by ripping off his bowtie. Chris then returns to his home to find that his priceless book collection has been unceremoniously dumped on his porch in the rain. So, he goes to his local bar, only to be beat up by Mosaic Johnson, a hip-hop theorist/literature professor hired to replace him. As he pummels Chris, Mosaic shouts "Poe. Doesn't. Matter" (21).

Johnson's text layers into itself, through its simultaneous participation in satire, memoir, and realist fiction, a stringent commentary on the presumption of authority for black professors. Chris Jaynes's so-called preface invites a reading akin to that of a memoir—contingent on real-life happenings but also participating in the flourish narrative creates. It does not mention Chris's identity as a professor, but rather, marshals its authority from the fictional Mat Johnson's identity as such. Since it is at Mat Johnson's urging that Chris reveals the narrative, Johnson's profession becomes the ideal way to give the narrative the veracity Chris worries it lacks. *Pym's* preface is nearly identical to Poe's (2012) original, a choice that marks the text as satire but does not alone undo the authority Mat-Johnson-as-professor holds. Certainly, those familiar with Poe's work may question the authority within the text because Poe's version uses similar tactics (i.e., insertion of the actual author as fictive character, use of preface as verification) to undermine its own authority. Readers familiar with Johnson's trademark sardonic wit and the troubling of power within his oeuvre might also be skeptical of Johnson's insertion of himself as an authority figure. In the preface, Johnson is identified as part of a group of "brothers" (raced and gendered language implying he and Chris are black men), and Chris writes that Johnson works at Bard College, "a historically white institution, in the town of Annandale, along the Hudson River" (4). The explanation appears straightforward enough, but when read alongside the satirical impulse of the text, it widens the gap between the stated presence of authority and its actual locus. The preface upsets the easy alignment between professors and authority by calling attention to the irrationality germane to satire. The figure of the black professor (here, Johnson, and later Chris Jaynes) does not assume the intellectual gravitas accrued to the profession. Instead, the link to irrationality—a precursor to madness to be sure—undermines any claim to expertise.

Given this preface and introduction to his character, Chris Jaynes's failed tenure case invites scrutiny not only about its merits but also the expectations for black literature professors. Successful tenure cases tend to demonstrate excellence in research and teaching. Service, either to the college/university or to the field, often functions to indicate commitment to the institution or, in more nebulous terms, fit.[2] Obviously, weighing the merits of Chris' case is not possible, but the components of his case require some attention. There is no explicit mention of his research, which could indicate a wide range of possibilities from excellence to nonexistence—though a faculty "yes" vote suggests that Chris had some research completed. Chris mentions his analyses and discoveries as an avenue toward "curing America's racial pathology" since Poe and other early American writers evince "the very fossil record of how this odd and illogical sickness formed" (8). Yet, Chris does not mention his research as reason for his denial. Read alongside the deauthorization in the preface, the inattention to Chris's research agenda suggests that his research does not matter. I am aware that I have just signified on Mosaic Johnson, a moment of intertextuality that should speak to the deep irony embedded with in the words. Poe does not matter for Chris Jaynes, but only because Chris was not assessed based on his analyses of Poe or anyone else. Interpreting this situation with the cynicism satire requires expands the scope of Chris's predicament, suggesting that no black professor's research actually matters. If one is not considered an expert, why then would one's research need to be read, digested, or used to shape policy?

At the center of Chris's denial seems to be his teaching. He offers the course, "Dancing with the Darkies: Whiteness in the Literary Mind," twice a year regardless of enrollment. His intention to teach America's racial pathology to students meets with low enrollment, not only because of the subject matter but also perhaps because the course is offered at eight o'clock in the morning. In terms of subject matter, Chris has not strayed far from African American literary practice. As Toni Morrison (1993) makes clear in *Playing in the Dark*, a consideration of "this black presence is central to any understanding of our national literature and should not be permitted to hover at the margins of the literary imagination" (5). Chris's course title invokes Morrison's monograph and participates in a set of reading strategies that engage whiteness and black presence specifically. It would appear that his emphasis on America's racial pathology alienates students. Chris's sarcastic defense that "the greatest ideas are often presented to empty chairs" (Johnson 2012, 8) suggests that he is a mad professor: obsessively insisting on his subject matter after students have decided it is not worthy of study and proceeding to talk to himself.

Interpreting Chris's behavior as mad dovetails with common scripts regarding putatively nutty professors, but it also shifts the locus of madness from the institution to Chris himself. Consider that Chris cannot be trusted as a reliable narrator. His defense of his own actions, then, becomes suggestive rather than conclusive. In other words, Chris's conversations with himself (if indeed they take place) result from the lack of support he receives from the institution. Regardless of whether we believe it is strategic to offer the course twice a year to low enrollment (it isn't), there appears to be no incentive for students to take his courses either within his own department or the larger institution. They do not appear to be required since filling required courses is never a problem even if they are taught at eight o'clock in the morning. Moreover, Chris's portion of the academic enterprise—teaching African American literature—rests solely on him, requiring that he shoulder the entirety of the African American literature curriculum. Unfortunately, this is not a portion of *Pym* that readers can dismiss as the *reductio ad absurdum* of satire, since it apes the reality of many an African American literature professor at small liberal arts colleges. Therein lies the slippage between the novel's satirical and realist impulses: the fictive college does not allow room for Chris's teaching to evolve, nor does it support the teaching of necessary, but uncomfortable, interpretive strategies for understanding race.

Chris's service record shares space with teaching at the crux of his tenure denial. In particular, his work on the "toothless" diversity committee (8) receives the brunt of Johnson's satirical pen. Chris refuses to sit on this committee because, as he explains to Mosaic Johnson, "the Diversity Committee has one primary purpose: so that the school can say it has a diversity committee" (18). Since this is the only service work required of Chris, it would appear that his refusal justifies his tenure denial, especially since service speaks to the nebulous concern of whether a professor fits in with the school environment. Mat Johnson holds up both the singularity of the request and its implications to ridicule. Chris's school can envision him serving only on this particular committee. Their crisis of imagination intimates that they believe diversity must be sequestered and remanded into a specific space for it to be useful to the administration. That is, to contain diversity is to own it, wield it, for their own purposes rather than allow diversity to precipitate the transformative power of difference. Moreover, the administration metes out consequences for Chris's refusal, further suggesting that the committee functions not as a space to reform the school but as a disciplining mechanism for its faculty (and perhaps staff and students).

Chris's supposed failure in this area puts pressure on the commonly accepted wisdom about diversity committees. He understands them not as indicators of progress but as roadblocks thereto. Chris's ideas are worth quoting at length:

> They need that for when students get upset about race issues or general ethnic stuff. It allows the faculty and administration to point to it

and go, "Everything's going to be okay, we have formed a committee." People find that very relaxing. It's sort of like, if you had a fire and instead of putting it out, you formed a fire committee. But none of the ideas that come out of all that committeeing will ever be implemented, see? Nothing the committee has suggested in thirty years has ever been funded. It's a gerbil wheel, meant to "Keep this nigger boy running." (18)

Though Chris declares his ideas in a rant, they cannot be easily shunted aside for the same reasons that concerns about his teaching cannot be dismissed as absurd. Again, his so-called failure highlights the destructive logics with which his college operates. Diversity only functions as a glossy fixture to which administrators can point if a problem arises. It mollifies. It pacifies. It does not effect change. Chris's evokes Ralph Ellison's *Invisible Man* ("Keep this nigger boy running"), gesturing toward the emptiness of the committee and its function to discipline him (and others) into their proper places. Mosaic Johnson, then, as the newest member of this committee only serves as the black punishing hand—literally, since he beats Chris up—which reminds Chris of obligations. Moments earlier in the text, Mosaic Johnson forms his hand into a black power fist, suggesting that black power ideology gets enfolded into the hegemony of the institution in the form of the diversity committee. Ellison ghosts the text again here for it is not within Mosaic's power to change the joke and slip the yoke. The diversity committee is the yoke and the joke is (on) him.

One more aspect of Chris's tenure denial troubles the facile correlation between his action and the final decision: the faculty voted "yes" for Chris's tenure and the president of the college overturned their decision. Chris locates the blame for his misfortune with the president himself, choosing to confront him and emasculate him by stripping him of his "itty-bitty microphallic [bow]tie," thereby taking away his "power source" (14). Chris's fixation misdirects the narrative since it assumes that the faculty and the president worked at cross-purposes. What Chris's critique of the diversity committee and the very quick hire of Mosaic Johnson suggests is that his firing was anticipated. The faculty, then, do not necessarily vote favorably out of a belief in Chris's skills, but from a milquetoast impetus to deal with conflict by avoidance, the same inclination that causes them to form a diversity committee. Chris Jaynes's hire (and Mosaic Johnson's, by extension) functions according to the same rationale as the diversity committee. They only exist to be a physical stopgap between the institution being racist and being called so.

They allow that one (or one's institution) does not have to do anything about racism if the bodies of black and brown people are present. The components of Chris's tenure denial are interpreted according to the logic that buttresses the institution's power and abets the ableist charge that Chris has gone crazy: instead of examining their willful disregard of his research, they charge him with straying from his expected intellectual enterprise. It is not that they did not provide the structural support necessary for his teaching; he did not teach the proper topics. His refusal to participate on the diversity committee reads not as a strategic use of his time but rather evidence of his acting out.

(And the Whole World Has to Answer Right Now Just to Tell You Once Again) Who's Mad

The discussion of why Chris does not fit in this college setting incorporates an entangled web of racial, gendered, and ability discourses. His focus on the president's bowtie and temporary embrace of Mosaic Johnson as a fellow brother (and the preceding embrace of Mat Johnson and others) pinpoints how Chris understands this experience as raced and gendered. The college's focus on the diversity committee further clarifies how much the tenure denial resulted from Chris's disruption of acceptable black male behavior in the college setting. Though Chris does not explicitly discuss it, his tenure denial hinges on the school's conception of him according to discourses of madness. Chris disrupts the kairotic spaces of the institution by skirting behavioral protocols. Price (2011) defines kairotic space as the "less formal, often unnoticed, areas in academe where knowledge is produced and power exchanged" (21). Tenure decisions and personnel meetings carry the mark of formality, but the committee meeting is not a formal space. The interactions between Chris and his colleagues—in the main office, in the hallway, et cetera—also factor into his tenure decision, particularly because they inform his colleagues' conception of him. As Price notes, kairotic spaces are not set up to accommodate multiple forms of being in the world. They do not disambiguate the extent to which fit determines tenure decisions or the strategies required to best create a successful tenure case. The result is that university pressures facilitate the use of madness as an invalidating accusation, rather than a consideration thereof as a subject position.

Without diagnosing Chris Jaynes as a mad professor, I index how madness lurks within the narrative about him. For instance, his unsuccessful tenure case hinges on his putative misuse of time. He spends the wrong kind of time on research, inappropriate time on teaching, and no time on service. In other words, Chris's tenure decision relies on a series of temporal upsets. That is, he does not adhere to the constraints placed upon his time by others. This is not merely a matter of how to strategically spend one's time but about the temporal mandate of blackness before the tenure clock. As Holland (2012) notes, the black body (and other non-normative bodies) occupies space as excessive and the white body (and other normative bodies) controls time in the Western imaginary (1–17). As a result, the Western institution of the college attempts to discipline blackness rather than create room for it. For this reason, Chris's refiguring of time—also informally referred to as "colored people's time" and/or "crip time"—becomes evidence of his lack of compliance with the institution. Since the institution and behaving according to its rules evinces sanity and genius, Chris's lack of conformity implies madness as a result. Here, Chris's inability to appropriately occupy the time set before him functions as *prima facie* evidence of his madness to those deciding his tenure decision. The temporal mandate about how to spend his time, the controlling of his temporal space, relies on a logic that dictates and disciplines Chris's behavior vis-à-vis tenure. When he does not comply, he becomes disruptive to the so-called intelligent and rational system.

The genre of satire also makes it possible to question the extent of madness within the narrative. Satire opens up a gap between a first person narrator and the narrative, facilitating a metatextual commentary. In *Pym*, the gap between Chris Jaynes's first person narration and the events of the novel (even when Chris creates his own commentary via footnotes) clarifies how much the tenure case relies implicitly on viewing him as crazy. To my mind, understanding this discourse becomes even more urgent because Chris is unaware of how it operates even though he is acutely aware of how it operates vis-à-vis blackness and masculinity. His unawareness makes madness-as-accusation more insidious because it surfaces as an enactment of privilege that others have in relation to him, a silent stealth process that jeopardizes his chances without his understanding. In this way, college pressures converge with social pressures requiring Chris to perform a certain kind of sanity in order to excel at his job.

Simultaneously, diegetic space between narrator and narration allows the text to question the way this narrative facilitates Chris's tenure denial. If reading the novel in straightforward terms, it would appear that the tenure denial causes Chris's depression. After he is denied, he "gets bourbon drunk and crie[s] a lot and roll[s] into a ball on [his] office floor" (7). He also retreats to Harlem "to be among [his] own race and party away the pain" (7). On the one hand, the narrative supports a causal relationship between the tenure decision and Chris's depression, a sequence of events that validates the emotional freight tenure carries. Yet, the narrative does not support a causal relationship between the academy and madness, since depression is not the only version of supposedly going crazy within the novel. The primary relationship between the two is accusative: madness gets mobilized against Chris while it undergirds his tenure denial. Since Chris does not explicitly acknowledge this discourse in the same way that he does race and gender, the silence in his narration allows the events in the novel to foreground the unfairness of how that discourse works. In this gap arises the insidiousness of the accusation, and the invalidity of the unquestioned affiliation of the academy with rationality.

Even if Chris's depression is interpreted as causal, the circumstances of that depression trouble a facile narrative that all Chris feels is sadness or grief about his job. In reading Cvetkovich (2012) reading Cornel West, racism and depression are not simply causally linked (115–53). Cvetkovich points out that depression clinically occurs for everyone, but the responses and triggers thereof require a more substantive engagement especially within the American context. She takes seriously the idea that "depression, in the Americas at least, could be traced to histories of colonialism, genocide, slavery, legal exclusion, and everyday segregation and isolation that haunt all of our lives" (115). West and Cvetkovich concur that structural racism for those who experience it permits a stasis of sadness. Tracing depression through history and linking it to the quotidian praxis of racism resonates with Chris's experience within the college without pathologizing him. His tears and escape to Harlem is the apogee of what he has been experiencing all along. Chris's reaction comments on the vulnerability of black bodies within the academic institution and indicts the system that perpetuates it.

To understand Chris's depression solely as an instantiation of madness or to dismiss it as mere grief participates in the same delegitimizing discursive action as the institution. Without having to utter the words *crazy* or *mad*, madness gets mobilized as a way to do violence to the bodies most vulnerable within the academy. We have to note that the institution's objections to Chris came in the form of rejecting his understanding and usage of time as well as dismissing his ability to fit (and exacerbating his misfitting).[3] Both of these ideas—time and fit—speak to an undercurrent of rationality. When he is accused of poorly using time or not fitting (while having a black male body), he is also understood as *de facto* crazy. After that institutional violence has occurred (in Chris's case, firing him), madness lingers discursively to justify itself by implicating the actions of the one to whom it was done. Johnson's depiction of Chris adds to what Cvetkovich terms an "archive of ordinary racism," where the black intellectual in the form of a novelist participates in "the only available strategy [of] 'speculation,'" when "there has been no public life around certain kinds of experience" (121–22). Johnson's satire speculates and prods such that depression can take on the multiple valences disavowed in other narratives.

Discharge and Denouement

Moving out of satire for a moment and into the critique it offers raises concerns about who gets to be mad. What bodies are allowed to safely occupy craziness as a legitimate subjectivity? Madness delegitimizes Chris's claim to the academic enterprise based on his raced and gendered body. That is, Chris cannot inhabit an acceptable form of madness because his body is not an acceptable professorial body. His black maleness takes away the option—that might be available to others—to perform madness without repercussion. To be clear, I do not suggest that faculty who experience cognitive difference or mental health concerns are safe. They are not. In fact, this fictional experience indexes the extent to which madness can only be performed by certain able bodies and be considered legitimate. Consequently, madness cannot be marshaled for gain when yoked to a body already associated with it (regardless of whether that link is constituted in ability, racial, or gendered terms). Neither can this critique of the institution simply label the institution mad, for that would invalidate the analysis by participating in the behavior it denounces. Instead, this reading censures the academy's relationship to social protocol as a violent, dehumanizing process that mobilizes madness as insult.

After his tenure fiasco, Chris Jaynes proves that he is a consummate scholar. He throws himself into a research project. Johnson's *Pym* continues on for another three hundred some odd pages, depicting Chris's travel to Antarctica, enslavement by giant snow monsters, a 200-year-old Arthur Gordon Pym, and global destruction. No topic and no character is safe from Johnson's pen. Yet, the first twenty pages, to my mind, represents that danger as it surfaces seriously in all spaces, even in the ivory tower. The pages that follow suggest that this danger is only the precursor to more pernicious events: in true satiric fashion, global destruction. In some ways, Chris's research—and where it takes him—relies on the idea of the nutty professor, obsessively seeking answers at all costs. Yet, it also reminds us that the school could not make room for Chris's kind of brilliance, nor the body to which it belonged. Instead, the faculty embarked on a disciplining enterprise to subdue Chris by muting his sound objections to structural inequality.

Sadly, the road to tenure requires intellectual production of a certain kind and reproduction as well: that of the norms of the institution. These twin processes create a fundamentally unsafe space for faculty who identify as mad and those against whom madness is mobilized as insult or disciplining practice. As I mentioned before, my stake in this argument is not to compel positive representation or correct stereotypes. Instead, I uncover how madness functions so that it does not remain as dangerous a presence because of its persistent silence. Yet, naming the discursive processes of madness should not coax people to invoke it only to dismiss it and avoid the consequences of identifying as, identifying with, or working alongside the putatively crazy. To do so would recapitulate the same effects of silence using the language of dismissal. The discouraging fact is this: Resistance to marginalized bodies and minds is both entrenched and systematic. It will not resolve itself, especially if those in power refuse or neglect to do the emotional and intellectual labor required to do so or if those in power revel in the protection that resistance provides.

References

Alsultany, Evelyn. 2012. *Arabs and Muslims in the Media: Race and Representations after 9/11*. New York, NY: New York University Press.

Cvetkovich, Ann. 2012. *Depression: A Public Feeling*. Durham, NC: Duke University Press.

Garland-Thomson, Rosemarie. 2011. "Misfits: A Feminist Materialist Disability Concept." *Hypatia*. 26.3: 591–609.

Harris, Angela P., and Carmen G. Gonzales. 2012. "Introduction," *Presumed Incompetent: The Intersection of Race and Class for Women in Academia*, edited by Gabriella Gutiérrez y Muhs ,Yolanda Flores Niemann, Carmen G. Gonzales, and Angela P. Harris. Boulder, CO: University Press of Colorado.

Holland, Sharon. 2012. *The Erotic Life of Racism*. Durham, NC: Duke University Press.

Johnson, Mat. 2012. *Pym*. New York, NY: Spiegel & Grau.

Morrison, Toni. 1993. *Playing in the Dark: Whiteness and the Literary Imagination*. New York, NY: Vintage.

Poe, Edgar Allan. 2012. *The Narrative of Arthur Gordon Pym of Nantucket*. New York, NY: Atria Books. Kindle.

Price, Margaret. 2011. *Mad at School: Rhetorics of Mental Disability and Academic Life*. Ann Arbor: University of Michigan Press.

Rockquemore, Kerry Ann, and Tracey Laszloffy. 2008. *The Black Academic's Guide to Winning Tenure without Losing Your Soul*. Boulder, CO: Lynne Reiner Publishers.

Diagnosing Disability, Disease, and Disorder Online

Disclosure, Dismay, and Student Research

AMY VIDALI

Many classroom assignments invite student disclosure, often in the form of personal essays, argumentative claims, or reading responses. Scholars have been justly critical of how such assignments might impact disabled students; in her piece on disability disclosure and personal essays, Wood (2001) argues that "personal essay writing, due to its tacit invitation to write about traumatic experience, is troublesome for students with disabilities" (38). Less conspicuously tied to disclosure, however, are research assignments, where students are asked to locate, summarize, synthesize, and sometimes critique the sources they have found. In this chapter, I focus on online health research, which raises complex issues of disclosure as students negotiate their identities in research spaces that are typically populated by negative representations of disability, disease, and disorder. I suggest that we must more thoughtfully evaluate the disclosures that research requires from teachers and students; examine the ways that research discloses certain ideas of disability, disease, and disorder to students; and develop approaches for more productively realizing the progressive goals of disability studies when teaching students to research disability topics and perspectives.

To explore these issues, I trace fourteen student responses to an assignment in my senior-level argumentation course, which asked students to research health symptoms online and formulate diagnoses in research narratives. I begin by examining the narratives of students who disclosed and analyzed symptoms they were experiencing, and I suggest that students claiming their own bodies—and disclosures—resulted in useful searches, though I question how I might replicate this success without requiring student disclosure. Next, I examine the narratives of students who researched symptoms their loved ones were experiencing, noting students' anxiety level and inattention to the ramifications of disclosing for others. Finally, I linger on narratives that jocularly diagnosed multiple sclerosis, AIDS, and chronic fatigue syndrome, which reified damaging views of disability, disease, and disorder.

Obviously, this was not how I hoped this assignment would play out, and this article also narrates my teaching failure, which is its own kind of disclosure. I find stories of teaching failure to be the reality television of academia, as I read them avidly and sometimes heckle, improbably imagining how much better I would perform in the same set of circumstances. However, rather than spectacle or side-note, I want to suggest that stories of pedagogical misconnection and failure be treated as tender disclosures that are invaluable in translating students' lack of learning into broader pedagogical gain. In this chapter, I disclose my own teaching failure to reflect on what went wrong and to understand the deeper issues my teaching experience reveals about disability disclosure in undergraduate learning and research.

In the final portion of this chapter, I broaden my scope to consider disability research in any undergraduate course. I offer four tenets of an embodied approach to undergraduate research, which include using critiques of disability simulation to rethink the risks of disability research, encouraging critical engagement with cyberchondria, disclosing the difficulties of disability studies research, and engaging in discussions of trigger warnings to encourage thoughtful, prepared research. Adding a final layer of disclosure, I conclude this piece by disclosing my own needs in online health research, as I grappled with an undiagnosed condition while writing this chapter.

In all, disability disclosure loops through this piece, and I use it as a touchpoint through which I can make arguments about other things (undergraduate research, teaching failure, cyberchondria). I mark disability disclosure as central and important, while I avoid presenting a more direct argument about what disability disclosure does or does not achieve, which many of the other chapters in this book already do so well.

"Googling a Diagnosis" and Student Response

My assignment, entitled "Googling a Diagnosis, or Twenty Minutes to Cancer," was the fourth and final unit in an upper-level undergraduate argumentation and logic course. As noted on the assignment sheet, the goal was to "demonstrate an understanding of the rhetorical choices you make online, which ultimately articulate an argument (or diagnosis)." The assignment asked students to select three symptoms, perform two online health searches based on those symptoms, and reach tentative diagnoses. In the first search, students were to use the rhetorical research strategies from class to perform their best online health search, which I refer to as the "best practices" search. The second part of the assignment asked students to employ the fallacious logic we had critiqued to construct what I call the "worst practices" search. At the time, I was aware that the worst practices search came with some risk, but I felt it was important for students to recognize both good and bad rhetorical choices in online health research. For each search, students wrote a reflective, chronological narrative detailing their online choices in the context of class concepts and readings. I directed them to spend twenty to thirty minutes on each search (plus writing time), and I intended the writing process to slow down less thoughtful searching/clicking.

Course readings and related class discussions focused on fallacious reasoning, online decision-making and search engines, and disease and disability representations.[1] Our class discussions sometimes took disability as topic but, more often, engaged disability through the lens of argument and audience, and my pedagogical approach emphasized class discussion, modeling, group work, and drafting. We discussed the stakes involved in researching your own symptoms, the symptoms of a loved one, or fairly random symptoms. The language on my assignment sheet reveals the complicated disclosure issues the assignment invited:

> This project will likely be more meaningful if you choose symptoms that you truly understand and that have meaning for you. You can choose symptoms for a diagnosis you have, though this may bias you toward picking that diagnosis. You do not need to disclose your relationship to the symptoms if you do not want to—you have the right to keep your health information private from your classmates in peer review, and/or me.

Contradicting my memory of class discussions, the assignment preferences symptoms students are or were experiencing, and my attempt to avoid requiring student disclosure reads somewhat like advice not to disclose. In retrospect, I can see that several students likely researched their own symptoms but did not claim them, and I believe that I needed to more deeply probe the ways that disclosure functioned in the assignment so that students could respond in ways that were most comfortable and productive for them.

I created an assignment focused on online health searches because, as I note on my assignment, such searches are "a common and high-stakes rhetorical internet exercise." The "Generations 2010" report, produced by the Pew Internet & American Life Project (Zickuhr 2010), notes that despite differences among age groups, "certain key internet activities are becoming more uniformly popular across all age groups," with "seeking health information" being the "third most popular online activity for all internet users 18 and older." A primary motivator for my assignment was to discourage cyberchondria, which is typically defined as "unfounded escalation of concerns about common symptomology, based on the review of search results and literature on the Web" (White and Horvitz 2009, 2). This was particularly important because the student population at my university is largely without health insurance and claimed that they often researched health issues online. In their study of cyberchondria, Starcevic and Berle (2013) note that improving "'health information literacy'" would "involve measures to educate Internet users [on] how to critically appraise online health information, interpret results of Internet searches and apply retrieved information to their own health problems or personal situations."[2] I sought to teach these skills, as most people researching health issues online fail to check the validity of a source (Muse et al. 2012, 190), and one study "found a significant, positive association between an individual's ability to understand, interpret and use the medical information online and the frequency with which an individual uses the Internet as a source of information on health issues" (Paré et al. 2009, 13). However, research on cyberchondria encourages users to fear what the internet is most famous for serving up in online health searches: significant disability, disease, and disorder. As I discuss further in the final section of this chapter, I needed to critique concepts of cyberchondria more directly.

Broadly, the narratives students produced for their best practices searches detailed their navigation to no-name websites that cropped up on the first page of Google, which they adopted or abandoned before moving to another site or search. I asked that all students begin with Google,[3] and though we had discussed the benefits of Google's advanced search at length, only one student started there. Nearly all the best practices narratives mention fallacies, as well as frustration with less-than-useful websites. In all, the best practices narratives describe mostly effective searches. In contrast, the worst practices searches were more intuitive, using a "I know a crappy website when I see it" logic. Many students wrote their worst practices narratives in over-the-top ways, positioning their diagnoses in these searches as highly unlikely or impossible, even though many students used similar strategies in both of their searches.

Fourteen of twenty-five students in the course consented to participate in the project. In table 3 below, I identify the symptoms students selected and the outcomes of each search, sorted by students' relation to their symptoms (self, loved one, or unknown).

Table 3. Participants, symptoms, and diagnoses

Diagnosed	Name	Chosen Symptoms	Best Practices Diagnosis	Worst Practices Diagnosis
self	Joshua	mid-back pain, nausea, moderate dizziness	ankylosing spondylitis	Aneurysm
self	J.J.	fluid buildup behind kneecap, rapid fluctuation of swelling, and chronic swelling	arthritic injury to knee cartilage	Gout
self	Lisa	overheating, insomnia, irritability	hyperthyroidism	chronic fatigue syndrome
self	Hope	lower back pain, sleeplessness, anxiety	muscle strain, plus pre-existing issues	cocaine addiction
loved one	Hannah	insomnia, loss of appetite, irritability	Adderall addiction/ withdrawal	Graves Disease
loved one	Cynthia	severe abdominal pain, nausea, loss of appetite	acute pancreatitis	acute pancreatitis
loved one	Nita	numb face, tingling arms, dizziness	contact a physician	MS
loved one	Risa	eye mucus, red swollen eyes, under two years	viral conjunctivitis	cataract disease
unknown	Ashton	coughing up blood, back pain, swollen eyes	tuberculosis	tuberculosis
unknown	Nick	headache, nausea, diarrhea	viral gastroenteritis (stomach flu)	giardia
unknown	Delilah	blurred vision, forgetfulness, slurred speech	low blood sugar (or MS)	MS
unknown	Rosa	imbalance, rash	Lyme disease	MS
unknown	Kendra	swollen glands in neck, difficulty swallowing, headache	pharyngitis (inflammation or infection of larynx)	AIDS
unknown	Kelsey	soreness in ear, nose bleed, difficulty hearing	Otitis media (allergy-related)	impacted ear wax & heart disease

Four students disclosed that they were researching their own symptoms, and these searches most clearly demonstrated fruitful online research. In three of the four cases, I was already aware of the student's condition based on prior discussions, and these students used the internet to research and confirm much of what they already knew, with their attention focused on website evaluation (rather than diagnosis). Both in the assignment and in discussions with me outside of class, Joshua discussed his symptoms of mid-back pain, nausea, and moderate dizziness. His best practices narrative thoughtfully considers ankylosing spondylitis with interest but little concern. Lisa also mentioned her symptoms to me outside of class, and in her narrative, she notes: "In other words, the information retrieved matched some of the rhetorical information I already knew about myself." Early in the course, I invited all students to discuss their learning needs, and Hope came to me to explain that she experiences severe anxiety, depression, and post-traumatic stress. She was particularly pleased with the information she found on anxiety, which she described as "correct." J. J. was the only student who did not disclose his symptoms to me prior to submitting his assignment, though he researched the comparatively less-stigmatized experience of having a knee injury. In all, these best practices narratives were focused on critically evaluating online health information and avoided shunning disability, disease, or disorder.

These narratives suggest that having disclosed, students could focus on the research task; they had little need to cautiously adopt certain identities, and this highlights how student disclosure can be freeing instead of primarily dangerous. The students were also invested, particularly Joshua, who did not yet have a diagnosis, and avoiding cyberchondria is easier when a diagnosis already exists, as it did in the other three cases. However, replicating this success is difficult, as I obviously cannot require all students to disclose, and it seems that engagement might be reduced, though disclosure issues less fuzzy, if students picked a specific diagnosis and then researched related symptoms to see if they landed on that diagnosis. Also, these four narratives sometimes "approved" online content in place of critically engaging it, and connecting disclosure and critical representation might be achieved by having students analyze how their symptoms and/or diagnosis are represented online.

Another four students selected symptoms that their loved ones were currently experiencing, and these students' research narratives expressed the most anxiety. These searches seem most likely to mirror typical online health searches, where diagnoses are unknown and the stakes are real, whether for yourself or a loved one.[4] Disclosure functions in complicated ways in these searches, as students typically shared little about themselves, yet provided much detail about their loved ones. In class, we spoke about possible anxieties created by researching symptoms for elderly family members, but each of the four students researched symptoms of loved ones who were their own age, plus one child. Hannah researched symptoms for a friend with "insomnia, loss of appetite, and irritability," and while she carefully detailed her search, she followed her intuition more than the research, noting: "I know that this person has a poor diet due to lack of money and I have witnessed on several occasions their drug abuse." She ends with a diagnosis of Adderall addiction, but no clear sense of how to move forward with her friend. Similarly, Cynthia performed a relentless search regarding her friend's GI issues, noting that "the doctor's assumptions were wrong" when her friend was prescribed an antibiotic. She ends with a convincing diagnosis of acute pancreatitis, though after coming to the same diagnosis in her worst practices search, she questions the usefulness of online health research. In researching symptoms for her young daughter, Risa expresses stress and relief noting, "Finally, I was breathing alright, my daughter would be fine, not blindness or cancer."

These three narratives mostly fail to recognize the ethical tensions involved in disclosing another's condition or symptoms, which reveals the need to emphasize how good intentions can lead to colonizing effects when teaching about disclosure. I cannot know if these students' asked their loved ones if they could write about them, but I assume not, as there is no trace of the voices of the disclosed in the narratives. Instead, each response assumes a solid understanding of the symptoms and an ability to speak for (not with) the loved one. My assignment is partly to blame here, but next time, I will ask students to consider what it means to disclose for another and seek permission, then detail this process in their narrative.

In contrast, the fourth student who researched a loved one details symptoms but hesitates to declare a diagnosis. Nita researched symptoms her boyfriend was experiencing, and she begins her best practices narrative by justifying her desire to search online before seeing a doctor: "For someone like me, who does not have medical insurance, I like to know what I am walking into (or how much money I will be leaving without) before visiting a professional." She also defended using blog-like forums to find information (also see Fox and Jones 2009), which I had critiqued in class. At the same time, she claims, "While I would never personally diagnose myself via the internet, I can certainly see myself becoming paranoid about the possible causes of my symptoms. So paranoid that I would schedule a costly doctors [*sic*] visit consumed with the idea that I have a terminal disease." Despite her tentative enthusiasm for online health research, she was the only student to reach a diagnosis of seeing a physician. She justified this with the claim, "Both [web] sites clearly stated that the information contained within the site is intended for educational purposes only and should not be used as a medical diagnosis." While this is a smart decision, the assignment and in-class modeling focused on arguing tentative diagnoses, which Nita steadfastly refused to do. Conversely, in her worst practices narrative, she diagnoses her boyfriend with MS in lock-step fashion. She claims, "While I am not a doctor and cannot be certain that multiple sclerosis is the cause of my boyfriend's symptoms, it did seem probable." Revealing the complications of disclosure, Nita can only disclose a possible diagnosis of MS within the context of doing "bad" online research, making the diagnosis irrelevant, despite her rigorous search. In all, Nita seems to fear disclosing too much, not so much to me, but to herself in claiming a feared diagnosis.

Two other students diagnosed themselves with MS in their worst practices narratives, and again, I recognize that I encouraged students to do unreasonable searches which would likely end in typically-feared diagnoses. Still, it's interesting to note how students embraced the opportunity to perform "ridiculous" searches and place distance between themselves and the significant disability, disease, and disorder disclosed in their searches. Delilah's search intentionally focused on MS symptoms, yet she discards MS as a valid diagnosis for nearly anyone. In her best practices search, Rosa diagnoses herself somewhat casually with Lyme disease,[5] and in contrast, in her worst practices search, she jokingly diagnoses herself with MS, noting, "It had dizziness, difficulty balancing, and itchiness under the list of symptoms, and 3 out of 21 total symptoms isn't a terrible proportion. MS was a very likely candidate." Joshua notes, "So I've been wiggin' on it all day: do I have cancer?" and another student diagnoses herself with AIDS with the quip, "All of my symptoms match up. I am a dead man walking." Finally, a student named Ashton researched symptoms of TB (after we read Sontag [1990]), and she keeps the diagnosis at arm's length: "I was dually impressed by the comforting effect of the site's thorough description, installing major ethos before I even clicked, to the point that I was feeling not only ok about having TB, but *excited* to delve further into what knowledge the site could impart me, regardless of the indication that I am in fact infected with tuberculosis." Students who selected symptoms they seemed to have not experienced tried on and tossed aside various disabled, diseased, and disordered identities. However, in one case, a student who jocularly engaged chronic fatigue syndrome in her worst practices narrative added this post-script: "Just to be sensitive to the topic of CFS, I want to say that although controversial, this is generally believed to be a real medical issue that many people suffered from and feel strongly that doctors need to keep trying to find the cause and the cure." She was the only student to defend the condition she mocked.

It is important to remember that this course did include disability studies content—I felt I had prepared students to avoid fearing disability, disease, and disorder in their research. I cannot fully account for what seems like the failure of the disability studies content to do the work I thought it would; however, stories of struggle and failure in teaching are common in disability studies because teachers who engage these topics often serve as students' first contact with non-normative disability perspectives. In the introduction to *Fictions of Affliction*, Holmes (2009) describes more diffuse resistance by an entire class, though she defends them as "thoughtful, interesting, smart people." She instead argues that her students ultimately could not challenge the "dominant cultural narratives" of disability, which "teach us that it is alien, terrifying, tragic; that it transforms your life in overwhelmingly negative ways; and that it is normal to feel horrified, relieved, and inspired, all from a safe distance, when we encounter disability" (ix). I was similarly unsuccessful in getting students to resist the "dominant cultural narratives" of disability, as students spoke/wrote for others or only jocularly engaged significant diagnoses. I believe much of this resistance had to do with my indirect engagement with disclosure in the class, as we did not spend much time thinking about what it really means to claim one's own, another's, or random symptoms. Instead, my engagement with disclosure simplistically boiled down to warning students not to disclose something they didn't want to share with me or the class. Instead, in the time between selecting symptoms and beginning their searches, I might have asked students to discuss and write about the disclosure entanglements of their approach, with more diverse options to skip peer review or be semi-anonymous, rather than adopt the falsely comforting disclosure categories of self, loved one, or other. Put another way, while I felt I needed to emphasize search strategies to teach online health research, I really needed to emphasize the politics of disclosure.

Embodied Student Research

I've indicated a number of things I might have done differently, but there are also broader pedagogical problems that arise whenever disability research is taught, many of which involve issues of disclosure. In this section, I offer four approaches to making disability research in undergraduate courses more critically engaging, which grow from my class experience and my anecdotal understanding that disability studies courses often focus on class and close readings (particularly in the humanities), perhaps because of somewhat justified fears of what disability research tends to disclose. First, I highlight the dangers of "ill-informed" disability research by repurposing critiques of disability-simulation exercises, which can have similarly negative effects. Next, I argue that teaching disability research means dispelling myths of cyberchondria, which falsely suggest that "bad health research" exists in individual bodies. Third, I suggest that as disability studies scholars and teachers, we more directly disclose the circuitous and sometimes frustrating nature of disability studies research. Finally, I examine how we can teach students about possible anxiety and trauma when researching disability, without exacerbating disability fears or demanding that teachers disclose their own traumas.

Critiques of disability simulation exercises suggest that they typically increase participants' fear of disability, and encouraging undergraduate research on disability without adequate preparation risks the same outcome. As noted by Burgstahler and Doe, in disability simulations, "participants learn how difficult it is to maneuver a wheelchair, how frustrating it is to be unable to hear or read, how frightening it is to be visually impaired, or how impossible it is to participate in activities without the use of their hands," without emphasis on the realities and joys of disabled life.[6] Likewise, when students research disability online, they are likely to encounter representations that confirm disability stereotypes, as my students did in play-acting diagnoses they quickly cast off. Burgstahler and Doe instead offer alternative "simulations" (also see Blaser 2003), which emphasize the need to "debrief thoroughly and reflectively acknowledge discomfort." Similarly, in the process of researching disability, students must be encouraged to react to what they're finding, with space to "debrief" and "acknowledge discomfort." Teaching about disability simulations can encourage such processing, as students can gain practice in disclosing their fears and concerns before mapping such disclosure strategies to their research.

Teaching students to research disability also means critically engaging with cyberchondria. I engaged discussions of cyberchondria in my course and sought to modulate student knowledge and behavior through increasing students' understandings and abilities. While I meant well, my assumption that my students' behavior was the problem problematically accords with discussions of cyberchondria scholarship, which are focused on the cyberchondriac. For example, Starcevic and Berle (2013) note that to "cure" cyberchondria, "the relevant factors that fuel cyberchondria . . . would need to be targeted," which "might include perfectionist tendencies, intolerance of uncertainty and ambivalence about what should be perceived as trustworthy."[7] From a disability studies perspective, this is textbook medical model, where the "problem" is located in the body rather than in the interaction of bodies and environments.

Instead, as Lewis (2006) notes in her study of cyberchondria, we must challenge "[t]he image of the lone 'cyberchondriac,' obsessively hunting for information about their own health," which "needs to be tempered . . . by the recognition that much health-related activity on the internet is occurring within the context of interpersonal and communal exchanges" (525).[8] The idea of cyberchondria as defined by personal and economic "excessiveness" (McElroy and Slevin 2014) fails to account for the ways we are taught to understand our bodies, especially online. In response, when teaching students to research disability, cyberchondria must be positioned as a socially and culturally ingrained fear-reaction to disability, disease, and disorder, which responds to societal fears and the over-representation of "severe" conditions on the web (Lopes and Ribiero 2011). We must create assignments where student researchers can disclose what they fear and what they found in doing disability research, especially if we are to claim online health research as purposeful, not pathological.[9]

Preparing students, particularly undergraduates, to research disability also means disclosing the pragmatic difficulties involved in performing such research. Most disability studies researchers are accustomed to wading through much information that is firmly "not disability studies" (Linton 1998), such as medical- and science-oriented articles that contain damaging perceptions of disability. In her study of library subject headings, Koford (2014) documents the difficulty of locating disability studies scholarship by studying the research habits of nine disability studies scholars, and she notes that disability studies, like women's studies or queer studies, is a "high scatter" field. Such fields tend to span several disciplines, be "traditionally devalued in society," and have inadequately or even offensively labeled headings that make relevant materials hard to find (389–90). Disability studies reclamation of the term "disability" can also be complicating, as a feminist scholar in Koford's study notes: "'Disability, you know, unless you search disability studies, which isn't always a word that people use, you're going to get lots of medical stuff, and that's really frustrating'" (397–98). While it is important to gather and critique such problematic representations and materials (and this is sometimes the goal of disability scholars or student researchers), it's also important to emphasize ways *through* these materials so that meaningful, progressive disability studies analyses and stories can (also) be located.

While this isn't news to most disability studies scholars, my sense is that we don't frequently or consistently disclose these research challenges to students; instead, we assume that our in-class discussions and readings will discourage students from engaging research that is "not disability studies" or we avoid research altogether. Instead, I suggest that we disclose how hard this research can be and outline the sorts of strategies needed to find disability studies research, which, combining my ideas with Koford's, include using the search term "disability studies" in quotes, building from existing bibliographies, incorporating Google Scholar, and modeling how to comb through long lists of search results. But more than this, we must have frank discussions about the "scary" representations of disability students are likely to find in their research, and probe the cultural assumptions and fears that create and shape such reactions. In revising my own curriculum, this would mean modeling the process of encountering significant disability, disease, and disorder in researching health symptoms, and questioning, though perhaps not entirely dispelling, the "panic" that can arise in such searches. I might model a search bound to turn up MS, then explicitly place medical sources alongside disability studies sources, such as Krummel's (2001) "Am I MS?" In doing this, we encourage students to identify the internet as agentive; it deftly clothes us in certain identities ("I am rationally searching about my health") and not others ("Oh no, that tragic person with MS does not seem like me"). We must re-think the internet as (only) a passive location one can disclose *to*, and instead imagine the internet as an agent that *discloses* certain identities to internet users, which must be critiqued through disability studies.

In teaching disability research to undergraduates, we must also engage the trauma that research on disability can, but not does always, invoke.[10] This is trickier than telling research stories or modeling search techniques, because engaging the trauma that is sometimes inherent in disability experience risks reaffirming students' worst fears about disability. At the same time, if we are to move beyond the carefully chaperoned spaces of class readings, discussions, and responses, then we must prepare students for the ways that research will disclose potentially traumatic embodied pasts, presents, and futures. As Kafer (2016) notes in "Un/Safe Disclosures: Scenes of Disability & Trauma," "attending to violence and trauma does not run counter to but is actually an essential part of a critical politics of disability," meaning that we can teach "anti-ableist politics" while accounting for the trauma disability may cause (6). In the undergraduate classroom, this may include students challenging their immortal views of themselves, facing the realities and complications of conditions they already have or are at risk for, and understanding the traumas they or their disabled loved ones have experienced or may experience.

There is methodological work on embodiment that can be helpful here. In a piece on embodied knowledge and qualitative health research, Ellingson (2006) contends that "the erasure of researchers' bodies from conventional accounts of research obscures the complexities of knowledge production and yields deceptively tidy accounts of research" (299). Similarly, students must be encouraged to consider themselves in the context of their research. In another piece on qualitative research, Dickson-Swift et al. (2009) consider the "emotional labor" of thirty public health researchers (67), and the authors emphasize how the researchers had "to be able to undertake a level of 'self-care' to ensure that they are not adversely affected by the work that they do" (74). While this research can problematically position disability as something that "wears down" abled others, so does it invite opportunities to consider the "emotional labor" inherent in rigorous disability studies research. It also introduces new ways to disclose, as these scholars clearly identify their own bodily states as central to their work, and the ways they position themselves can be modeled and critiqued. As a teacher, I can also identify my own trauma and why I don't want to disclose the details, to model the process of personally engaging but not necessarily sharing such productive moments.

A final idea is to engage the debate around trigger warnings to encourage students to identify how they might interact with disability in their research. As Price (2014) suggests in her brief comment in *The New Yorker*, "Trigger warnings serve to prevent panic attacks or flashbacks that impede one's ability to engage in discussion. . . . They are intended to enable everyone to remain present and alert enough to be challenged and discomfited." Similarly, after engaging a portion of the larger debate on trigger warnings, ("On Trigger Warnings" 2015; Friedersdorf 2014; Johnson 2014; Roff 2014; Shaw-Thornberg 2014; Zehner 2015, among others), my approach would emphasize how students can identify their triggers so they can be better researchers who are "challenged and discomfited." In class, this might mean having students privately or collaboratively identify their triggers and related strategies, which is in itself a disclosure activity, as we/they would need to decide how to discuss triggers. By positioning the internet as a space of embodied disclosure, a focus on trigger warnings allows for complex relationships of researcher and research that makes room for diverse engagements with disability, disease, and disorder.

Listening to Questions: A Final Disclosure

The irony of embodied research being what it is, I was struggling with a number of symptoms and no clear diagnosis during much of the writing of this

268 · *Negotiating Disability*

chapter. (On disclosing such diagnoses in academic writing, see Kerschbaum [2014].) In addition to many medical tests, I was spending time Googling my symptoms, reading about hard-to-diagnose diseases, and running various ideas by my husband (a veterinarian). A lot of this happened late at night, and it would appear that I was engaged in cyberchondria (though I'd also suggest that my research is/was useful). If I narrated my (many) online searches, as I asked my students to do, there would be quite a bit of me starting a search, then leaving to peruse social media or my email, then jumping back into the search with new (or repeat) symptoms. If I disclosed my emotions (many of my students did not), there would be many, because I don't want to try giving up dairy, or feel scared to eat popcorn at the movie theater, or miss tucking in my son because I am in pain.

When I go online to search health symptoms and diagnoses, I want information, but I also want to offer my questions and get a response (even an automated one), in this age when doctors have no time, when I'm wary of scaring my aging parents with questions, and when many in my age group quickly suggest "lifestyle changes" for what are often impenetrable chronic health issues. In her narrative, one of my students noted, "When I substitute the human interaction of a doctor to the machine-consciousness of a data-base, I should be prepared to accept cold data in place of a warm hug." But I'm not convinced it's that simple. The internet may not consistently give me useful information, but it "listens" to my tender disclosures, then forgets, then lets me ask again. In considering the intersections of disclosure, student research, and disability, I am reminded that online health research is not only a quest for answers, but a desire to be heard when asking questions. Identifying the internet as my closest health partner may be the most difficult disclosure of all, but one that leads me back to my assignment and to my students, so that I might recognize the power of the internet to disclose, cherish, and discomfort, share the story of what went wrong last time (in my search, in my class), and try again.

References

Aiken, M., and G. Kirwan. 2012. "Prognoses for Diagnoses: Medical Search Online and 'Cyberchondria.'" *BMC Proceedings* 6 (Supplement 4): P30.

Baumgartner, Susanne E., and Tilo Hartmann. 2011. "The Role of Health Anxiety in Online Health Information Search." *Cyberpsychology, Behavior, and Social Networking* 14 (10): 613–18.

Blaser, Art. 2003. "Awareness Days: Some Alternatives to Simulation Exercises." October. http://www.raggededgemagazine.com/0903/0903ft1.html

Brueggemann, Brenda Jo. 2001. "An Enabling Pedagogy: Meditations on Writing and Disability." *JAC* 21: 791–820.

Burgstahler, Sheryl, and Tanis Doe. 2015. "Disability-Related Simulations: If, When, and How to Use Them in Professional Development." *Review of Disability Studies 1.2 (2004): 4–17*. Accessed May 15. http://staff.washington.edu/sherylb/RDSissue022004.html

Dickson-Swift, Virginia, Erica L. James, Sandra Kippen, and Pranee Liamputtong. 2009. "Researching Sensitive Topics: Qualitative Research as Emotion Work." *Qualitative Research* 9 (1): 61–79.

Ellingson, Laura. 2006. "Embodied Knowledge: Writing Researchers' Bodies into Qualitative Health Research." *Qualitative Health Research* 16 (2): 298–310.

Finger, Anne. 2009. *Call Me Ahab: A Short Story Collection*. Lincoln: University of Nebraska Press.

Fox, Susannah, and Kristen Purcell. 2015. "Chronic Disease and the Internet." *Pew Research Center: Internet, Science & Tech*. Accessed July 30. http://www.pewinternet.org/2010/03/24/chronic-disease-and-the-internet/

Fox, Susannah, and Sydney Jones. 2009. "The Social Life of Health Information." *Pew Research Center: Internet, Science & Tech*. Accessed July 30 2015. http://www.pewinternet.org/2009/06/11/the-social-life-of-health-information/

Friedersdork, Conor. 2014. "What HBO Can Teach Colleges about 'Trigger Warnings' *The Atlantic*. Accessed July 30. http://www.theatlantic.com/education/archive/2014/05/what-trigger-warning-activists-and-critics-can-learn-from-hbo/371137/

Garland-Thomson, Rosemarie. 2009. *Staring: How We Look*. Oxford, New York: Oxford University Press.

Holmes, Martha Stoddard. 2009. *Fictions of Affliction: Physical Disability in Victorian Culture*. Ann Arbor, Mich.: University of Michigan Press.

Johnson, Angus. 2014. "Essay on Why a Professor Is Adding a Trigger Warning to His Syllabus | InsideHigherEd." Accessed May 15 2015. https://www.insidehighered.com/views/2014/05/29/essay-why-professor-adding-trigger-warning-his-syllabus

Kafer, Alison. 2016. "Un/Safe Disclosures: Scenes of Disability and Trauma." *Journal of Literary and Cultural Disability Studies* 10 (1): 1–20.

Kerschbaum, Stephanie L. 2014. "On Rhetorical Agency and Disclosing Disability in Academic Writing." *Rhetoric Review* 33 (1): 55–71.

Kleege, Georgina. 2007. "Blind Rage: An Open Letter to Helen Keller." *Sign Language Studies* 7 (2): 186–94.

Koford, Amelia. 2014. "How Disability Studies Scholars Interact with Subject Headings." *Cataloging & Classification Quarterly* 52 (4): 388–411.

Krummel, Miriamne Ara. 2001. "Am I MS?" In *Embodied Rhetorics: Disability in Language and Culture,* edited by James C. Wilson and Cynthia Lewiecki-Wilson, 61–77. Carbondale, IL: Southern Illinois University Press.

Lewis, Tania. 2006. "Seeking Health Information on the Internet: Lifestyle Choice or Bad Attack of Cyberchondria?" *Media, Culture & Society* 28 (4): 521–39.

Linton, Simi. 1998. *Claiming Disability: Knowledge and Identity.* New York: New York University Press.

Loos, Amber. 2013. "Cyberchondria: Too Much Information for the Health Anxious Patient?" *Journal of Consumer Health on the Internet* 17 (4): 439–45.

Lopes, Carla Teixeira and Cristina Ribeiro. 2011. "Comparative Evaluation of Web Search Engines in Health Information Retrieval." *Online Information Review* 35 (6): 869–92.

McElroy, Eoin and Mark Shevlin. 2014. "The Development and Initial Validation of the Cyberchondria Severity Scale (CSS)." *Journal of Anxiety Disorders* 28 (2): 259–65.

Muse, Kate, Freda McManus, Christie Leung, Ben Meghreblian, and J. Mark G. Williams. 2012. "Cyberchondriasis: Fact or Fiction? A Preliminary Examination of the Relationship between Health Anxiety and Searching for Health Information on the Internet." *Journal of Anxiety Disorders* 26 (1): 189–96.

Norr, Aaron M., Brian J. Albanese, Mary E. Oglesby, Nicholas P. Allan, and Norman B. Schmidt. 2015. "Anxiety Sensitivity and Intolerance of Uncertainty as Potential Risk Factors for Cyberchondria." *Journal of Affective Disorders* 174 (March): 64–69.

"On Trigger Warnings | AAUP." 2015. Accessed May 15 2015. http://www.aaup.org/report/trigger-warnings

Paré, Jean-Nicolas Malek, Claude Sicotte, and Marc Lemire. 2009. "Internet as a Source of Health Information and Its Perceived Influence on Personal Empowerment." *International Journal of Healthcare Information Systems and Informatics* 4 (4): 1–18.

Price, Margaret. "The Mail—The New Yorker." 2014. Accessed July 30 2015. http://www.newyorker.com/magazine/2014/06/30/the-mail-37

Reed, L. 2002. "Governing (through) the Internet: The Discourse on Pathological Computer Use as Mobilized Knowledge." *Communication Abstracts* 25 (6): 755–909.

Roff, Sarah. 2014. "Treatment, Not Trigger Warnings." *The Chronicle of Higher Education Blogs: The Conversation.* May 23. http://chronicle.com/blogs/conversation/2014/05/23/treatment-not-trigger-warnings/

Segal, Judy Z. 2009. "Internet Health and the 21st-Century Patient a Rhetorical View." *Written Communication* 26 (4): 351–69.

Shapiro, Joseph P. 1993. *No Pity: People with Disabilities Forging a New Civil Rights Movement.* New York: Times Books.

Shaw-Thornburg, Angela. 2014. "This Is a Trigger Warning." *The Chronicle of Higher Education,* June 16. http://chronicle.com/article/This-Is-a-Trigger-Warning/147031/

Siempos, I. I., A. Spanos, E. A. Issaris, P. I. Rafailidis, and M. E. Falagas. 2008. "Non-Physicians May Reach Correct Diagnoses by Using Google: A Pilot Study." *Swiss Medical Weekly* 138 (49–50): 49–50.

Singh, Karmpaul, and Richard J. Brown. 2014. "Health-Related Internet Habits and Health Anxiety in University Students." *Anxiety, Stress, & Coping* 27 (5): 542–54.

Sontag, Susan. 1990. *Illness as Metaphor; And, AIDS and Its Metaphors*. New York: Doubleday.

Starcevic, Vladan, and Elias Aboujaoude. 2015. "Cyberchondria, Cyberbullying, Cybersuicide, Cybersex: 'New' Psychopathologies for the 21st Century?" *World Psychiatry* 14 (1): 97–100.

Starcevic, V and D. Berle. 2013. "Cyberchondria: Towards a Better Understanding of Excessive Health-Related Internet Use." *Expert Review of Neurotherapeutics* 13 (2).

Tang, H., and J. H. Ng. 2006. "Googling for a Diagnosis—Use of Google as a Diagnostic Aid: Internet Based Study." *BMJ (Clinical Research Ed.)* 333 (7579): 1143–45.

Tindale, Christopher W. 2007. *Fallacies and Argument Appraisal*. Cambridge, New York: Cambridge University Press.

Tustin, Nupur. 2010. "The Role of Patient Satisfaction in Online Health Information Seeking." *Journal of Health Communication* 15 (1): 3–17.

Warnick, Barbara. 2007. *Rhetoric Online: Persuasion and Politics on the World Wide Web*. New York: Peter Lang.

White, Ryen W. and Eric Horvitz. 2009. "Cyberchondria: Studies of the Escalation of Medical Concerns in Web Search." *ACM Trans. Inf. Syst.* 27 (4): 23:1–23:37.

Wood, Tara. 2011. "Overcoming Rhetoric: Forced Disclosure and the Colonizing Ethic of Evaluating Personal Essays." *Open Words* 2 (1): 38–52.

Zehner, Jacquelyn. 2015. "Trigger Warnings Aren't Trivial—They're Necessary." *New York Times*. March 6. http://tsl.pomona.edu/articles/2015/3/6/opinions/6105-trigger-warnings-arent-trivial-theyre-necessary

Zickuhr, Kathryn. 2010. "Generations 2010." *Pew Research Center: Internet, Science & Tech*. Accessed July 30 2015. http://www.pewinternet.org/2010/12/16/generations-2010/

IV

Institutional Change and Policy

Access to Higher Education Mediated by Acts of Self-Disclosure

It's a Hassle

MOIRA A. CARROLL-MIRANDA

Institutions of higher education (IHE) are required to provide qualifying students access to services, programs, and activities offered to the public (Torkelson and Gussel 1996). Students living with disabilities are entitled to access these services and programs on equal grounds as students who do not live with disabilities. For instance, some students may require alternative means to access curriculum materials that are provided in written format, while others may require structural (physical) accommodations to access a building. However, students living with disabilities who have qualified for an academic program and enroll in an IHE may encounter contradictions among the above claims and their lived experiences. Often these students find that they cannot participate throughout an IHE on equal grounds.

With the intent to increase IHE accessibility in accordance with federal legislation such as the Americans with Disabilities Act of 1990 (as amended 2008) and Section 504 of the Rehabilitation Act of 1973, guidelines, parameters, and policies have been created to determine who qualifies and how to receive services (Albrecht 1992; Kafer 2013; Horejes and Lauderdale 2007). These services are often requested through disability services offices available in many IHE (Madaus 2011) that require students to disclose their disability. These processes respond to institutional bureaucratic structures that become a "hassle" for many students living with disability. In other words, the process of requesting services in this context becomes an ongoing struggle between how students experience disability and how the institution responds to disability.

Overview of the Study

This essay offers a glimpse into the stories of five students from Puerto Rico who are living with disability: Coral de Fuego, Nina, Abde, NMJ2, and Ariel.[1] Their stories emerged through a qualitative study guided by the tenets of disability studies (Kafer 2013; Linton 1998; Barnes 2012; Wendell 1996). The original purpose was to explore the process of inclusion and the role of assistive technologies from the perspective of students living with disabilities who were attending an IHE. The site was a public IHE in Puerto Rico (P.R.). Because of the political relationship between P.R. and the United States (U.S.A.), the IHE system and its characteristics are synonymous with the prevailing IHE system in the U.S.A. (Abreu-Hernández 2011). IHEs in P.R. follow the U.S.A. model in terms of legal obligations, educational levels, titles and degrees granted, student financial system, and so forth (Abreu-Hernández 2011).

The participants were a purposeful selection of students living with disability (SLWD). I use SLWD not as a homogenizing term but rather as an act of acknowledging the heterogeneity of human beings and our experiences. First, the word *living* is calling attention to the idea that as we live, we engage in experiences that may be unique as well as collective (Kafer 2013). Second, the term *disability* is used also as an experiential component that shapes the lives of individuals in different ways through the ongoing interaction between physical, mental, and physiological differences, with different physical spaces, social structures, and reactions to bodily differences (Longmore 2003; Wendell 1996). Third, although each participant in this study experiences disability in diverse ways, they have a commonality: the experience of discrimination centered on their disabilities (Kafer 2013; Linton 1998; Longmore 2003; Wendell 1996).

I was asked to disclose my experiences with disabilities by each of the participants. I am not a person living with disabilities within my body. My experiences with disabilities began as the daughter of a man that lives with disabilities. Growing up with different corporealities in my home became the root of my ontological and epistemological positions to disability. I did not see my father as having a problem within him; I did not see a problem at all. However, I did learn about how certain spaces could represent a limitation to people living with disabilities. I shared with the participants that learning about how individuals living with disability claim disabilities was critical to the person I am today as a daughter, mother, friend, professional, and intellectual.

I conducted semi-structured interviews with the participants during several encounters across seven months. Interviews were initiated with open-ended questions such as: *Could you describe your experiences with disabilities in your higher educational journey?* This technique allowed the participants and me to engage in dialogues, creating spheres of opportunities to learn from personal knowledge (Smith and Osborn 2003). Interviews were analyzed following the guidelines proposed by Smith and Osborn for interpretative phenomenological analysis, which emphasize an exploration of sense-making by the participant and researcher. During this phase the transcripts were transformed into what Connor (2008) refers to as *portraits-in-progress*, stories that present insider perspectives; in this case, becoming testimonies of living with disabilities and attending IHE.

The crafting of these *portraits-in-progress* began with the participants sharing their experiences. The interviews were then transcribed and shared with the participants for their approval. Once approved, I returned to the transcripts to carefully thread the participants' stories into a narrative text organized by themes identified during the analytical process. Each *portrait-in-progress* was sent to the participants asking them to read the text and to further validate that the stories represented their self-descriptions, experiences, stories, feelings, and voices. Their revisions, comments, and suggestions were included. The major suggestion was to present their stories as shared within the context of our encounters. One of the complex issues that surfaced repeatedly was the experience of disclosure that occurred during efforts to have equal access through institutional policies.

The following stories shared by Coral de Fuego, Nina, Abde, NMJ2, and Ariel are about disclosing their experiences with disabilities and how they confront, resist, struggle, and above all negotiate with social reactions to disabilities in the context of IHE.

Self-Disclosure: Positioning *Myself* Living with Disabilities

The act of self-disclosure of living with disabilities is related to how individuals position themselves in relation to their body vis-à-vis society's constructed identity of disability (Wendell 1996). The following words provide an insight into how each participant positioned themselves with disabilities.

CORAL DE FUEGO: I am twenty-five years old. I had a car accident. I have a spinal cord injury. I have paraplegia so I do not walk. This happened when I was eighteen . . . I believe that I am not an impaired person. I am a person with impairment. I mean, it is the same idea as "I'm not disabled, I have a disability." I identify with that philosophy.

NMJ2: I am a person in my forties and I am blind. My visual condition was a genetic one, so I have had several visual conditions since I was born. Although I could see before, a little but distorted, and some colors well, my condition was a progressive one, since I was young.

NINA: I am Nina. I am twenty-three years old. I am a resident of San Juan. I have muscular dystrophy. The specific condition . . . because muscular dystrophy has numerous neuromuscular conditions . . . mine is spinal muscular atrophic . . . I mean . . . it is not like a very tough condition.

ABDE: I am twenty-six years old and I live in Río Piedras, Puerto Rico. Well, I consider myself a person who loves to help others and to participate in different research projects and that's why I got excited and accepted to participate with you. I have a Bachelor's Degree in Social Work and Physical Education. I began to study at this university in the year 2005. . . . I have a desire to share experiences. My condition is known as Retinitis Pigmentosa. It is a visual condition that you can either be born with it or develop it later in the years of development. It is a condition where you can only see frontal or laterally. In my case, I can see laterally.

ARIEL: I am originally from C. R. I have been living in Puerto Rico for ten years now . . . towards the year 2003 I came here (P.R.). I was accepted here (the university) . . . to study. I finished my bachelor degree . . . I did not finish education. That is why I have to continue studying to get the teaching licensure. I entered the Hispanic Studies program, and they offered me the option of continuing my studies towards the master's degree without taking the admissions test. If I remained in Hispanic Studies, I could continue the master's program without additional major requirements . . . I came to realize that if I did not have a degree—at least as a person with disabilities, one of my shields is my degree. It is not the best of my shields, but it is one of them. Because the question always is "How do you do it?"

Coral de Fuego positions herself as an individual that experiences disability as part of her corporeality. She expresses how it is that her interactions with physical, social and institutional structures lead her to more disabling experiences than her body (Barnes 2012; Titchkosky 2011; Oliver 1996). She has lived the experience of living in a body without disability and living with an acquired disability. In the following words, she expresses instances when her disability positionality clashes with the social construction of disability.

> CORAL DE FUEGO: I also identify with the fact that sometimes it is not the people who are disabled; it is the structures that cause the impairment. I identify myself as a person that was born normal and was normal up until eighteen and then everything fucked up and now is learning to live fucked up. In this process, the person faces the necessity to be strong and realized how strong she was. The accident was like a way to prove and confirm that I am a strong person and that's how I perceive myself. I am not perfect, man, I am not perfect. I have a lot of flaws also.

Instances of self-disclosure require individuals to engage in the continuous act of positioning herself from within and from the outside (Wendell 1996). In the case of NMJ2, he positions himself embracing his corporeality with an assurance of who he is regardless of how society may see him. Nina embraces hers when she claims "mine is," referring to the medical categorization of her disability. In these words the participants claim their body and express some of their positionalities with disabilities. Abde and Ariel claim their positionality by presenting how they see themselves in relation to who they are prior to disclosing that they live with disabilities. Each presents their positionality related to how they see and perceive themselves in juxtaposition to how they are seen by others. Abde's expressions provide a further illustration of this in the following words:

> ABDE: Because sometimes the obstacle is not the person with disabilities, it is the other party. Sometimes a person . . . sees a person with a disability and people look as if we were an alien or something. As if we were something they had never seen in life . . . we are not the norm because we are abnormal . . . of course we are different . . . If you ask me, I consider myself abnormal. If the norm is not to study, if the norm is to be dependent, if the norm is being conformist, well that's not me. So, in that aspect I will be abnormal . . .

How the participants embrace their corporeality becomes an important factor that influences their interactions across different spaces within the IHE. One of the questions that arises through this process of interaction is "the degree of control" (Linton 2010, 224) that the individual has in embracing a terminology for their experiences with disabilities. In the expressions from Coral de Fuego and Abde, there is a constant struggle between their bodies being understood by society as their major life limitation and how their interaction with social structures becomes their major impairment and disability.

The degree of *control* the individual has in the process of embracing a terminology is often challenged by different situations such as requesting services and assistance to equitably participate in an opportunity in the IHE. Situations such as the above also entail moments where the individuals' identities are challenged and confronted by the social imaginary of disability that surfaces through institutional policies and practices (Martín-Baró 1985). For example, Abde struggles as he challenges the social notion of being considered *normal* vis-à-vis being *abnormal*. From his understanding, what is expected from SLWD is *not to study . . . be dependent . . . being a conformist.* He challenges what society expects from him by doing exactly the opposite.

Disability Identities and Institutional Policies: A *Clash* of the Titans

Living with disabilities and its effect on the experiences of the individual will vary depending upon cultural, social, and historical contexts (Linton 2010). However, as different as these experiences can be, there are commonalities. Among the commonalities are the experiences SLWD engage with as they struggle to access participation in an IHE on equal grounds as students that do not live with disabilities. These experiences, for the most part, are a constant struggle through which SLWD resist and challenge taken for granted assumptions related to living with disability in a society that not only rejects disability but often reacts negatively toward bodily differences. An instance when the identities of SLWD may clash with the institutional imaginary of disabilities is when they are held responsible to come forward and disclose their disability in terms established by the institutional policies. SLWD are required to disclose their disability in order to request accommodations in IHE services and programs (Madaus 2011). The act of agreeing to self-disclose or not is complex. The study participants claimed that these institutional requirements transformed the act of disclosure and self-disclosure into a bureaucratic institutionalized one. Coral de Fuego explains this experience in the following words:

> CORAL DE FUEGO: The experience is difficult. It is difficult because you have to make more effort to be the same as the rest. In . . . the office that serves students with disabilities, you go there and take a letter from your physician or evidence that you have any kind of disability so that they then give you a letter of reasonable accommodations. . . . From there on you let the professors know, well that you have a condition and you have to explain it yourself.

Greene and colleagues link disclosure to the act of revealing *private* information ". . . information about oneself that others might not normally have access to but that is not actively hidden from them . . ." (Greene, Derlega, Yep, and Petronio 2003, 5). When talking about disclosure and SLWD attending IHE, this act is transformed into a bureaucratic act further perpetuating different manifestations of institutionalized discrimination (Barnes 1991; Longmore 2003). Nina shares an experience that further illustrates the above claim:

> NINA: I went to the [disability services office] and requested a letter . . . the accommodations they write are standard and do not address my particular needs . . . they simply transfer the information from one student to another. *We give you the letter for you to identify yourself as a person with disabilities within the campus.*

The institutional practices of requesting services through disclosure engage in further acts of discrimination. First of all, Coral and Nina have to disclose a qualifying disability in order to receive *a letter* that certifies that they live with disabilities and are entitled to receive reasonable accommodations. The institutional policies become an instrument to further determine who qualifies to be protected under the established legal terms. SLWD need to present *evidence*, to receive relevant services that are intended to ensure sure them access to participate in IHE in equal grounds. Nina claims that the list of accommodations she receives through a letter from the institution do not respond to her *particular needs*.

The institution has determined a priori the needs of SLWD and how to address them regardless of how Nina describes her needs to the institution's representative. This experience is an example of how institutional discrimination takes place. Barnes argues that ". . . institutional discrimination becomes evident when the policies and activities of all types of modern organizations result in irregularity between disabled people and- nondisabled people . . . is apparent when they are ignoring or meeting inadequately the needs of disabled people" (1991, 3). Coral de Fuego claims that the experience of requesting services is difficult because *you have to make more effort to be the same as the rest.* Here is an explicit struggle SLWD face seeking to be treated on equal grounds as students that do not live with disabilities. This act of institutional discrimination could be understood as one of many unintentional consequences of their practices and policies. Although they may be unintentional, overlooking these consequences and not interrogating how and why they recur is problematic and reflects a dangerous tendency to normalize discrimination and its manifestations that needs to be brought into the forefront.

Coral de Fuego compares what it was like to attend and participate in the IHE living without disabilities and later living with disabilities in the following words:

CORAL DE FUEGO: The system of the University Access has this *come-mierdería* like "*We* [talking for the University] are the state's institution; so what do you have to offer to this institution so that you could be worthy of attending here?" [mocking an authoritarian figure through her voice]. This should not be like this. It should be that the institution opens up its doors to the students and lets them know that they are welcome. I was already in the system, but I had to withdraw when I was in [rehabilitation]. Then it was a mess to come back, a big bureaucracy. One of the things they do [the University] is block you out. Make it impossible, in a sense when all you want is to study.

These are very powerful claims in simple words. First, she claims that the institution should *open the doors* to all students and let them know they are welcome. Coral de Fuego once felt welcome to study, however when her corporeality changed, the institutional bureaucracy became a burden to return and continue her studies. Another claim present in these words is her sense of worthiness becoming undermined by the institution's practices and policies that regulate the participation of SLWD. After acquiring a disability, she feels that she has to demonstrate being *worthy* of attending the institution; that she has something to give. Moreover, she claims that the bureaucratic processes make it *impossible* to study. These might be considered unintentional consequences, which are rooted in the negative reaction to disability (Barnes 2010, Longmore 2003).

Struggling with IHE Disclosure Policies

Paul Longmore argued that the social recognition through governmental social service policies has "forced millions of us to the margins" (2003, 231). This claim is based on how the policies are rooted in the assumption that disability, from a biomedical perspective, is the only factor that "substantially limits one or more major life activities" (Americans with Disabilities Amendments Act of 2008). From this point of view, the limitation resides only within the individual, making invisible the myriad factors that interact across the lifespan of any individual with disabilities. Furthermore, Longmore claims "They give assurance that determination of eligibility for aid can be a fairly clean-cut process. Doctors and other professionals can reduce both impairment and disability to a set of numbers; numbers that will show who objectively qualifies to receive benefits" (2003, 238).

In the IHE where this study took place, the decision for an individual to qualify for aids and services needs to be certified by what is considered a professional judgment: first by a specialized doctor in medicine, a psychologist, among other health professionals and later by the IHE's employee that provides services to SLWD. IHE's policies are based on federal and local legislations that regulate postsecondary institutions in the United States of America and its territories. As a consequence of this, the determinations for eligibility are done from a pathological and medical perspective (Albrecht 1992; Longmore 2003). Among the issues that arise are how the individual defines her/himself, how society and its institutions understand disability, and how these collide in a relationship full of ongoing tensions (Wendell 1996). The act of disclosure becomes a contested site of struggle for many SLWD. The following extracts from the *portraits-in-progress* provide further insights to this struggle.

CORAL DE FUEGO: It is like a *hassle*, it is a problem like—What a burden!—I do not even do it anymore. I do not do it because it seems to me like a useless protocol sometimes. Sometimes it is for me something useless, a struggling burden that does not always have a result. Because if you do something, like you engage in the effort of doing something it is because in the long run you will benefit from it. Sometimes there are not that many benefits when compared with all the burdens faced, like all the difficulties that come with having to take the documents, that you have to get them here or there . . . it takes time and in the end it is not as effective for all the struggles you go through.

ARIEL: The majority of the students go to the students with disabilities services office when they are stuck up to their necks, facing a huge problem and go so that they can help them solve it . . . I do it . . . because it is a legal procedure. I mean, literally you arrive here thinking about the worst. I will have a professor that will not want to deal with me and therefore I will have to arrive with the legal steps. I got the letter, I signed it, he didn't want to comply, and then this is where I will move to. Then I will go to this other office and such. I am already thinking in that process; I do it but in that legal process. But it is not an office that I can say I have a problem with my tuition and they will me assist me, no.

NINA: In my case, I understand this to be of benefit because, due to my condition, I face some limitations for what I have explained previously related to the chair and mobility when writing and all that . . . Regardless if I need the letter or not, they see me and they know I have a particular condition and that I need some accommodations. Most of the time that letter is requested to receive the accommodations that they can offer and for the agreements met. For example, not all the professors allow the use of a tape recorder in their class even if the letter says so. I mean that even if I get the letter, the agreements will always be made between the professor and the student. At least in my case it is favorable because if I ever faced the situation where a professor . . . I need something right and the professor claims "I don't see that you need anything because I don't see you struggling . . ." There have been semesters when I didn't even register myself in the office simply because I realized that it stops being of significance. Because at least in my condition you can see it, you can see that I have a condition . . .

ABDE: [I]n the University it changes . . . you become your own advocate . . . given that the attitude at this University is—"We admit you and from now on you are on your own . . ." That, well in that point the University is a bit harsh because you have to do all the *gestiones* even if you want the minimum thing . . . The only reasonable accommodation I need is that if the professor wants to give me a test then arrange a time frame to take it, or what they truly do is that they let a person function as human reader and note-taker. What I do, here at the Center [for students with disabilities in the library], I reserve a person that is available to read to me the test and that's it . . . I mean, although at the [disability services office] they require you to hand each of the professors a letter, I came across few professors that requested the letter related to what kind of reasonable accommodations I needed. During the first day of class, at the end of the class as it says in the syllabus: Any student that needs any reasonable accommodation should communicate with the professor. I would stay and say—Professor, no worries I can do everything. The only thing I need is that when you give a test that you either give it to me or we make arrangements for a human reader or note-taker. For the rest, you keep on teaching that *¡vamos pa'encima!*—That way, of course, my case is not everybody else's case; everyone has a particular condition that requires reasonable accommodation to fulfill their specific needs. In my case, that's how they work.

NMJ2: In my case, at the beginning I did face many situations of disadvantage and because I was no longer in overprotected spaces I was in competitive spaces . . . and regardless, being in disadvantaged positions . . . it was hard and there were many times that I thought, this is like being a masochist . . . Each time you began a semester, it was beginning all over again with a disadvantage from zero. The professor without the materials, they not having the minimum idea of how to work with a blind student . . . explaining all over again . . .

Coral de Fuego, Nina Abde, Ariel, and NMJ2 engaged in the act of disclosure by requesting services in compliance with the institutional policies at some point in their university studies. As they initiated their higher educational journey, they felt the need to request services to ensure they would be granted access to the institution's activities. They believed that this process would guarantee them access and protect them from discrimination. However, after engaging in several acts of complying through the institutional requisite of disclosure, they learned that it is a daunting process that does not render the benefits they thought it would.

The act of self-disclosure following institutional policies becomes a bureaucratic institutionalized tool to address disability that continually clashes with who they are, what they want to achieve, and how they want to participate in the IHE. Moreover, they do not necessarily identify with having a disability as defined by the institution's policies for various reasons. Among the reasons is their claim that the major limitations are experienced through their interaction with physical and social spaces such as in the IHE they attend.

The participants mentioned how they stopped seeking services because they felt this service did not respond to their specific needs. In other words, they did not resist disclosing that they live with disabilities, but resisted the experiences of going through the bureaucratic disclosure processes. They preferred to challenge the process and struggle using whatever resources they have in hand, hoping to avoid "the energy-sapping, dehumanizing bureaucratic labyrinth" (Longmore 2003, 231) they faced through this process.

Abde expressed he does not need to ask for assistance in the disability services office and instead he seeks to establish agreements with professors beforehand. In other words, he prefers to self-disclose directly with the person he will be engaging in an academic relationship. He prefers to establish his own terms, resisting the institutional requirements to engage in the act of self-disclosure through bureaucratic procedures.)

On the other hand, some participants such as Ariel and NMJ2 expressed that they kept seeking the services for legal purposes. They felt they were in a position of never knowing with certainty what could happen given that the institution and its members were the ones to decide if the students would be given access. Because they constantly faced ambivalence from faculty and the possibility of discrimination hindering their participation, the students' acts of bureaucratic disclosure became an instrument of survival within the educational institution. The letter provided by the institution was a way for students to establish power relations among the institution's administration, the faculty, and the student. Although, as Ariel explained:

> ARIEL: This letter is a process that professors sign, but at the same time, they can do with what the letters say whatever they want . . . in the end, the professor rules. Look in the offices working with people with disabilities, not just in college but many, using the example of a university that is a reflection of society, are out of date and misinformed. They are not very aware of what the student lives.

In a contrasting approach, NMJ2 explained that due to knowledge gained through his life experiences, he engaged in exhausting other resources such as dialoguing with the professors before going to the disability services office.

NMJ2: I never go to that office . . . na, na, na. I learned how life is. Life is like that and sometimes you have to go to such offices; well if a professor says no to me I will do everything that is in my power to resolve it on my own, I will solve it directly with him/her. Because what I am interested in learning is how to solve it. If sooner or later I have to go to the system's formalism . . . but not without having searched other strategies to try to solve it myself. Even if he/she claims "No, because you need this . . ." "Well ok I will do it, but in the meantime, can we start with this other thing?" Yes, I will always try to be a step ahead . . .

NMJ2's approach did not deny that he might need to engage in a power struggle with the professors, but he preferred to establish a dialogue. He learned with his experiences that engaging in the act of dialogue becomes a way to create a space where he can directly establish his needs and negotiate his participation in the classroom. Developing a direct human relationship becomes a priority rather than the more daunting relationship represented by the act of bureaucratic disclosure.

Ariel claimed that institutional disclosure was a tiring struggle that in the end did not accomplish what the IHEs claimed to offer. It became an endless cycle that perpetuated a sensation of needing to comply in order to participate.

ARIEL: You begin to fight, with the system. It [IHE] says that it makes things accessible, but you realize that what they do is sell you the services; it is not given to me thinking about me as a person. Then you say this struggle is like the struggle that goes backwards . . . Then you begin to realize—Listen, how do I play this? Everything starts getting into this and then you realize that you are tired. But you are tired of dealing with the system, dealing with all of this stuff but you tell yourself, "I need this," if not I wouldn't even do it . . .

Ariel's experience illustrates how he struggled to comply with the institutional requirements to disclose in order to receive assistance, and in other instances, he resisted them. The major struggle in the process is not within the act of disclosure; it is how the institution sets the grounds for such an act to take place.

Not every SLWD finds the institutional practices of disclosure problematic. Some consider them the norm; just the way it is (Titchkosky 2011). These bureaucratic policies and protocols become the taken-for-granted process that an individual should face when seeking access to participation. In other words, they become mechanisms of inclusion that naturalize practices of exclusion while further institutionalizing acts of discrimination (Longmore 2003, Titchkosky 2011). The problem with naturalizing practices of exclusion is that they become a taken for granted reaction and interaction to bodily differences, perpetuating the notion that human beings are excludable from social participation because of their corporeality.

Concluding Thoughts

The participants described the process of disclosing their disability through institutional policies as being a "hassle," a "constant struggle," and even "useless." Although they described the process as a hindrance to access, they found themselves forced to submit. They found this process to be more about legal compliance than of actual help. The institutional practices not only became disabling devices but also became institutionalized obstacles. Paradoxically, the policies turned against those it was promising to protect. The message being *you are not worthy of protection unless you come out under our terms.* This is a dangerous position in a society that puts so much power over the lives of its members in the judicial system (Kumari Campbell 2005). The laws, policies, and regulations become a hollow rhetoric (*letra muerta*) when institutions fail to comply and the law fails to protect the individual, in this case, from acts of discrimination.

The experiences presented through this essay offer insight into how the process of disclosure through institutional policies represents an ongoing struggle between students living with disability and their identities as they are confronted with the social imaginary of disability. Moreover, the act of disclosure is not a single act; it is a continuous series of interacting situations experienced by the individual in a given context across multiple instances. While disclosure of living with disabilities, either public or private, could lead to stigmatizing consequences, it also remains an avenue toward access.

The participants claimed they had learned that it was more effective to establish a relationship with a professor and negotiate the terms of disclosure. This act represented resistance to bureaucratic disclosure processes that often clashed with the student's identity and disability positionalities. Such negotiation required students to self-disclose and initiate a dialogue with their professor, which became an opportunity to express their need to participate on equal grounds in the educational setting from their own positionality. The participants did not deny that there were moments when disclosure might entail negative reactions from their professors because of the stigma that accompanies living with disabilities. Nonetheless, they still preferred to take charge of the process as much as the circumstances permitted. It was a way for SLWD to claim their space in society. It fostered the opportunity to explore alternative ways of participating within a classroom setting established by the SLWD and the professor.

This kind of interaction suggests the importance of developing spaces where power relationships and identities are negotiated through dialogues (Freire 2001). The participants claimed the importance of shifting the act from talking *to*, to talking *with* professors bidirectionally. This meant that professor and student acknowledged the importance of negotiating their terms and their experiences with disabilities. Similarly, institutional policies, regulations, and programs that provide services to SLWD must respectfully recognize their voices. How the institution, its structures, policies, and practices react to SLWD should be brought to the forefront. Moreover, IHEs need to transform how the act of disclosure, in its multiple manifestations, is approached. Otherwise in Ariel's words: "Then I say, well, they are not thinking about the person."

References

Abreu-Hernández, Viviana. 2011. *La Educación Superior en Iberoamérica: La Educación Superior en Puerto Rico 2005–2009.* Consejo de Educación Superior de Puerto Rico. http://www2.pr.gov/agencias/cepr/inicio/publicaciones/

Albrecht, Gary. 1992. *The Disability Business: Rehabilitation in America.* Newbury Park, California: SAGE Publications.

Americans with Disabilities Act Amendments Act of 2008. Public Law 110–325. § 3406.

Barnes, Colin. 1991. *Disabled People in Britain and Discrimination: A Case for Antidiscrimination Legislation.* London, United Kingdom: Hurst and Company.

Barnes, Colin. 2010. "A Brief History of Discrimination and Disabled People." In *The Disability Studies Reader*, edited by Lennard Davis, 20–32. 3rd ed. New York: Routledge.

Barnes, Colin. 2012. "Understanding the Social Model of Disability: Past, Present, and Future." In *Routledge Handbook of Disability Studies*, edited by Nick Watson, Alan Roulstone, and Carol Thomas, 12–29. London, England: Routledge.

Connor, David. 2008. *Urban Narratives: Portraits in Progress; Life at the Intersections of Learning Disabilities, Race and Social Class.* New York: Peter Lang.

Freire, Paolo. 2001. *Pedagogy of Freedom: Ethics, Democracy, and Civic Courage.* Lanham, Maryland: Rowman and Littlefield Publishers.

Greene, Kathryn, Valerian Derlega, Gust Yep, and Sandra Petronio. 2003. *Privacy and Disclosure of HIV in Interpersonal Relationships*. Mahwah, New Jersey: Lawrence Erlbaum Associates Publishers.

Horejes, Thomas and Pat Lauderdale. 2007. "Disablism Reflected in Law and Policy: The Social Construction and Perpetuation of Prejudice." *The Review of Disability Studies: An International Journal* 3(3): 13–23.

Kafer, Alison. 2013. *Feminist Queer Crip*. Bloomington: Indiana University Press.

Kumari Campbell, Fiona. 2005. "Legislating Disability: Negative Ontologies and the Government of Legal Identities." In *Foucault and the Government of Disability*, edited by Shelley Tremain, 108–32. Ann Arbor, Michigan: University of Michigan Press.

Linton, Simi. 1998. *Claiming Disability: Knowledge and Identity*. New York: SUNY.

Linton, Simi. 2010. "Reassigning Meaning." In *The Disability Studies Reader*, edited by Lennard Davis, 223–36. New York: Routledge.

Longmore, Paul. 2003. *Why I Burned My Book*. Philadelphia, Pennsylvania: Temple University Press.

Madaus, Joseph. 2011. "The History of Disability Services in Higher Education." *New Directions for Higher Education* 154, 5–15. doi:10.1002/he.429

Martín-Baró, Ignacio. 1985. *Ideología y Acción: Psicología Social Desde Centro América*. 2nd ed. San Salvador, El Salvador: UCA Editores.

Oliver, Michael. 1996. *Understanding Disability: From Theory to Practice*. New York: Palgrave.

Smith, Jonathan, and Mike Osborn. 2003. "Interpretative Phenomenological Analysis." In *Qualitative Psychology: A Practical Guide to Research Methods*, edited by Jonathan Smith, 51–80. Thousand Oaks, California: Sage.

Titchkosky, Tanya. 2011. *The Question of Access: Disability, Space and Meaning*. Ontario, Canada: University of Toronto Press.

Torkelson-Lynch, Ruth, and Lori Gussel. 1996. "Disclosure and Self-Advocacy Regarding Disability-Related Needs: Strategies to Maximize Integration in Postsecondary Education." *Journal of Counseling & Development* 74(4): 352–57. doi:10.1002/j.1556–6676.1996.tb01879.x

Wendell, Susan. 1996. *The Rejected Body: Feminist Philosophical Reflections on Disability*. New York: Routledge.

Intellectual Disability in the University

Expanding the Conversation
about Diversity and Disclosure

BRIAN FREEDMAN

LAURA T. EISENMAN

MEG GRIGAL

DEBRA HART

The Higher Education Opportunity Act (2008) reauthorization included provisions for students with intellectual disabilities (ID); offering for the first time guidance on quality indicators for programs and eligibility for federal financial aid for students with ID. These provisions legitimized and drew attention to the small, but growing, number of such college programs across the United States, Canada, and Europe. Gaining access to a higher education brings people with ID into an environment they have historically been excluded from, resulting in a host of questions about diversity, belonging, and disclosure of a disability.

This chapter presents a brief overview of higher education programs for young adults with ID. Challenges related to academic disclosure for students with ID and their support mediators (e.g., program staff and families) are explored, including complications with how ID is defined, assigned, and disclosed by institutions and students themselves. Additionally, social disclosure issues that result from interactions of students' goals, program structures, and campus institutions are examined. Finally, policy and practice recommendations that facilitate inclusion of students with ID and address disclosure concerns are identified.

Postsecondary Education for Students
with Intellectual Disabilities

Historically, students with intellectual disability (ID) have not been included in higher education, but recent growth in both available programs and student access have been evident in the United States (Grigal, Hart, and Weir 2012; Papay and Bambara 2011). The Higher Education Opportunity Act authorized model demonstration programs for students with ID, defined as individuals with cognitive impairment characterized by significant limitations in intellectual functioning and conceptual, social, and practical adaptive behavior who must be or have been eligible for special education services. The Act also authorized a National Coordinating Center that provides technical assistance, evaluation, outreach, and recommendations for accreditation standards. The Act also created a new kind of Title IV program called Comprehensive Transition and Postsecondary programs that allow students with ID to apply for Pell grants, Supplemental Educational Opportunity grants, and the Federal Work-Study Program (*Student Eligibility* 2011).[1] From 2010 to 2014, model demonstration programs served 1,815 students across twenty-seven IHEs in twenty-three states. Students were supported to take both inclusive and specialized courses, participate in internships, and engage in paid employment as part of their program (Grigal et al. 2014).

Postsecondary programs for students with ID have adopted varying policies and practices. These differences may be based upon availability of funding for particular program activities, philosophy of program leadership, or access issues unique to the institution. As illustrated in table 4, institutional responses to students with ID often differ from institutional practices with students who have more prevalent disabilities, e.g., learning disabilities, orthopedic impairment (Grigal and Hart 2010a).

The most salient aspect of such programs is their approach to academic inclusion. Some may not provide any access to typical courses but instead offer a specialized curriculum for students with ID. Others may offer a mix of specialized curriculum (such as independent living skills) for students with ID and also offer students access to some inclusive courses and social opportunities in a two- or four-year IHE. Still, other programs offer inclusive opportunities in all aspects of college life, including a course of study related to a student's career goal(s), campus activities, and integrated competitive employment opportunities (Grigal, Hart, and Weir 2014). Each variation has implications for how intellectual disability is represented and disclosed in academic and social settings on campus.

Table 4. IHE practices for supporting students with intellectual and other disabilities

	More Prevalent Disabilities	Intellectual Disabilities
• Admissions	• Utilize standard admission procedures involving submission of test scores, high school credentials, and a standard application.	• Typically do not use the same entrance criteria • May have a different application procedure • May include behavior criteria, e.g., ability to follow code of conduct or specific academic functioning levels. • Different documentation requirements (e.g., high school diploma may be waived)
• Advising	• Advisors provide guidance on a course of study that helps them obtain their desired degree or certification. • Advisors often do not have a specialty in working with students with disabilities.	• Often do not rely on the existing academic advising system. • Often create their own system of advisement, combining traditional advising and person-centered planning. • Advisors often have previous disability experience.
• Accommodations	• Sought through disability services office • Communication of accommodations by disability services office to instructors • Modifications to course activities or materials is not offered.	• Some may use the disability services office and other programs may not. • Students with ID may also receive nontraditional supports such as peer mentors or educational coaches.
• Degrees and Credentials	• Two- or four-year degree is often the goal. • Wide array of credential, certificate and degree options available.	• Paths to the degrees or traditional certificate options often not available. • Often offer program-specific credentials only for students with ID. • Credentials may have limited recognition or meaning outside of the program.

Guiding Principles for Programs Serving Students with ID

When navigating disclosure issues across these different contexts, it is imperative that IHEs be guided by three principles: inclusion, self-determination, and person-centeredness.

Inclusion

Programs and practices need to be inclusive and therefore aligned with existing policy and practice established by the IHE for any other student, including accommodations sought from an institution's disability services office. A unique aspect of programs for students with ID is often the provision of additional supports via the use of education coaches, mentors, ambassadors, etc. (Grigal et al. 2014). These nontraditional supports may introduce unexpected disclosure issues, such as sharing information about disability with an undergraduate student and peer who is providing mentoring.

Self-Determined

Students with ID should be provided necessary supports to make informed decisions about disclosure based on self-awareness, personal goals, and knowledge of support options. Students may need to communicate about effective accommodations, learning strategies, or specific technologies with higher education personnel and disability services staff. This level of self-advocacy may require instruction, repeated practice, and support.

Person-Centered

Finally, staff who work with students with ID should be guided by a person-centered philosophy taking students' individual strengths, supports, and preferences into consideration and creating a reciprocal experience that positions students with ID in control of their course of study and their supports. This individualized approach will ultimately support the student in learning how to take responsibility for and direct their services and supports.

Disclosure of ID and the Academic Community

Historically, research on disclosure and people with ID has focused on issues of stigma and social identity (Ali, Hassiotis, Strydom, and King 2012; Cunningham and Glenn 2004; Paterson, McKenzie, and Lindsay 2012; Spassiani and Friedman 2014). People with ID are often aware of the negative stereotypes associated with intellectual impairments, and to the degree that they incorporate those negative assessments into their social identity, they may experience less psychological well-being and self-esteem. Research with the aging population has shown that internalization of stereotypes can have implications for individual outcomes (Levy 2009). By similar thinking, a person with ID who is consistently told that people with ID do not seek or do not do well in postsecondary education may be less inclined to attend college, have difficulty disclosing their ID if they attend college, and perhaps are at greater risk of failure. The experience of "passing" (Carey 2013) is also relevant to this group of students. Some may have more observable markers of ID, such as the common facial characteristics of a person with Down syndrome, which preclude them from hiding a disability identity from others. Some may have observable physical differences that may not be commonly associated with intellectual disability by the general public and choose to claim whichever disability identity they believe is more desirable on the disability hierarchy (Olney and Brockelman 2003). Still others have no immediately observable differences. They may recognize that the nature of their cognitive differences will be revealed only as they grapple with abstract concepts or complex processes not previously encountered, and which, depending upon with whom they interact, may result in negative judgments about them (Rapley, Kiernan, and Antaki 1998).

Stigma and Representation of ID at College

Pride in a disability label or identity is not at the forefront for people with ID as it might be for other disability groups (Spassiani and Friedman 2014). Students with ID enrolled in an IHE may experience social tensions similar to those experienced by others with ID as described by Carey (2013). Students may be keenly aware of the negative judgments made within schools about individuals who are perceived as having limited intelligence and, therefore, too often presumed academically incompetent. The decision to "hide" their disability may be a rational choice in the face of social stigma. They recognize that these negative judgments often extend into the social sphere, where some experienced bullying as children. Similar to others with ID (Siperstein, Pociask, and Collins 2010), they wrestle with the stigma associated with special education and derogatory terms such as the "R-word." Students with ID may struggle to construct a positive social identity, seeking to be deemed capable by others' standards even while calling for their differences to be accepted.

Disclosure and Prior Academic Experiences

To further understand the complex negotiations of social identity and disclosure that students with ID may experience in college, it is important to consider the influence of their prior school experiences. Research on the transition from school to postsecondary activities demonstrates the positive impact of higher levels of self-determination on students' with disabilities outcomes related to employment, further education, and independent living (Chambers et al. 2007; Cobb, Lehmann, Newman-Gonchar, and Alwell 2009). The secondary special education transition literature is replete with suggestions for developing student self-awareness and self-advocacy from an early age throughout high school and adult life (Wehmeyer, Field, and Thoma 2012). Grigal and Hart (2010b) recommend that before leaving high school students should be aware of the nature of their disability, know what types of accommodations they might need in postsecondary education settings, and have had supported practice in asking for accommodations.

However, due to the prevalence of negative discourse, stigma, and even silence about disability in schools, students with ID may not have had such preparation (Eisenman and Tascione 2002; Valle and Connor 2011). In high school settings, students do not have to disclose a disability in order to access academic accommodations or educational services. Adults make the diagnoses, suggest the label to be used to secure funding for special education services, and make the decisions about instructional interventions, academic accommodations, and curricular modifications. Although students may recognize they are receiving special services, they may not identify as disabled but rather as having difficulties with particular tasks (Ali et al. 2012). School IEP teams, faced with ambiguous psychoeducational assessment results for a student with low achievement scores, may choose the less stigmatized term "learning disability" over "intellectual disability" when assigning a label for Individuals with Disabilities Education Act (IDEA) funding purposes, further complicating dialog about the nature of a student's disability. Whether due to limited openness about disability, preference for less stigmatizing labels, or control of the disclosure process by adults, students with ID may exit high school unprepared for understanding the typical processes and implications of disability disclosure in higher education (Eisenman and Mancini 2010; Madaus 2010). Further, students with ID often have not had opportunities in general to practice making decisions about whether and how much to disclose, choosing the method and language of disclosure (e.g., framing and explaining differences), or considering the potential consequences of disclosure.

Potential Points of Disclosure

Unlike students with disabilities entering higher education through traditional admissions processes, students with ID who want to enter these specialized college programs must disclose documentation supporting an ID diagnosis and prior special education status in order to be determined eligible for admission. This begins a series of circumstances during the student's time at the institution in which disclosure of information about their disability and/or accommodation needs takes place. For traditional students with disabilities, this would likely involve the student and, at times, the disability services office (DSO). For students with ID, other members of their support network at the IHE might become mediators of the disclosure process (see table 5). Depending on the degree to which the postsecondary education program has been integrated into the institution, staff members from that program may counsel or teach students with ID on how to access accommodations through typical channels, intervene directly with DSO personnel on behalf of the student, or sidestep official mechanisms and provide accommodations through other means.

Families

Families of students with ID may expect to play a much larger role in their young adult's education than is considered acceptable—or legal under the Family Educational Rights and Privacy Act (FERPA)—in higher education. Having been central to the Individualized Education Program (IEP) team decision-making on behalf of their child for many years, they may not be prepared for the shift of primary responsibility for educational decision-making to students. Just as their children may have had limited opportunities to prepare for the realities of disclosure in college settings, families often report having been unaware of the need for transition planning and unprepared for navigating post-school environments, supports, and services (Kraemer and Blacher 2001; Martinez, Conroy, and Cerreto 2012). Additionally, even when families of students with ID release more decision-making responsibility to their young adults, the way in which families characterize ID and frame potential personal or social restrictions to their children has an influence on how those individuals describe their disability or label themselves (Cunningham and Glenn 2004). When agreed upon by the student, program staff can work with a parent in order to understand prior diagnoses and supports, foster the release of greater decision-making responsibility, and ultimately reduce disclosure of information by the parent.

Faculty and Coursework

Faculty's knowledge and perception of ID also may play a role in how or whether students with ID or program staff handle disclosure in academic settings. General public knowledge and attitudes about individuals with ID may be limited due to the varying terminology that is used to describe the disability and the long-standing misconceptions about its impact but malleable over time given interactions that promote perceptions of individuals with ID as capable (Morin, Rivard, Crocker, Boursier, and Caron 2013; Scior 2011). Similarly, the relatively few studies of faculty attitudes toward ID sug-

Table 5. Points of Disclosure of Intellectual Disability and/or Accommodations

Activity or People at IHE	Sources of disclosure of ID	Potential challenges
Application for admission	Submission of documentation of ID/ prior records; student/ parent via interview for admission	Prior documentation poorly reflects student's strengths and abilities; parent is uncomfortable with the role expected by the IHE; student is asked direct questions about disability and is unprepared to respond
Courses/faculty	Student/mentor/program staff/disability services office	Disclosure process may be different than for traditional student; instructor may react poorly to request
Mentors	Student/program staff	Student may feel uncomfortable disclosing to peer mentor
Classmates	Student/mentor/ program staff	Student may feel uncomfortable disclosing to peers; classmates may have insensitive reaction
Peers/Staff for Campus Activities	Student/mentor/ program staff	Peers/staff may be unaccustomed to receiving accommodation requests
Co-workers/ supervisors for internship/work	Student/mentor/ program staff	Requires proactive self-advocacy, which might be difficult; Supervisor may be unfamiliar/uncomfortable with accommodations requested (e.g., job coach).

gest that as a result of having experienced students with disabilities in their classes, faculty may form more positive attitudes toward diversity and disability; but a link to changed practices is not clear (O'Connor, Kubiak, Espiner, and O'Brien 2012). Faculty members' personal belief about the potential impact of having students with disabilities in the classroom has a stronger influence on their provision of accommodations than other factors, but knowledge of legal responsibilities and perceptions of institutional support also influences faculty's personal belief (Zhang et al. 2010).

What is less clear given the limited research to date is how these factors influence students' with ID decisions to disclose when given a choice. It may be the case that students in more welcoming, accommodating, and universally designed classes have less need to disclose or that they feel more comfortable with disclosing their support needs (Matthews 2009). Some courses, based on their structure, may not require accommodation requests beyond the typical institutional process (e.g., foundational courses). Work-based learning experiences (e.g., internships) require more proactive self-advocacy and can be challenging, and even those who self-disclose in college may choose not to disclose to their employers (Cunnah 2015; Madaus 2010).

Program Staff

Student disclosure can also be mediated by the program staff who support students with ID. Staff members' roles in facilitating student academic participation and their interactions with faculty may vary relative to the inclusive structure and purpose of the program. Staff in fully inclusive programs may have less direct involvement with faculty, instead supporting students with ID on self-advocacy skills and preparing for conversations regarding disclosure prior to the student's direct communication with the instructor. In other programs for students with ID, staff may take on a mediating role such as identifying faculty who have a reputation of being welcoming of students with disabilities, approaching faculty to determine their openness to incorporating "non-traditional" students into their courses, or negotiating the nature of student involvement in course activities (Eisenman and Mancini 2010). These opportunities may allow staff to emphasize how a student's interests and goals align with a course and de-emphasize their differences from other students, which may in turn allow faculty to be more receptive than if approached directly by a student with an ID. Educational coaches and mentors, typically supervised by program staff, typically also offer support for students with ID in academic settings across various program environments.

Academic Peers

Findings from research on academic peers' attitudes toward students with ID mirror that of research on faculty (Griffin, Summer, McMillan, Day, and Hodapp 2012; May 2012). Peers' knowledge and prior experiences with people who have ID influence their attitudes toward inclusive postsecondary education for students with ID. Further, having opportunities to interact with students who have ID and learn about their capabilities can promote peer acceptance of diversity. The physical presence of students with ID as part of inclusive college programs can create opportunities for more positive appraisals of the capabilities of people with ID (Piepmeier, Cantrell, and Maggio 2014). Reciprocally, positive interactions with others and experiences of success on campus can support students' with disabilities positive reframing of their identity (Cunnah 2015). As suggested by Spassiani and Friedman (2014), peer association has an impact on students' perception of community. However, they may still be wary of revealing the specifics of ID due to fear of negative judgments often associated with that particular disability.

Disclosure of an ID and Campus Experiences

Campus life represents a critical component of the postsecondary education experience. Through opportunities to use campus resources, engage in extracurricular activities, and connect with peers with similar interests, college students develop a sense of community that complements and extends beyond the academic experience. Students who are more connected to their institution and have stronger social ties exhibit higher self-esteem (Booth, Travis, Borzumato-Gainey, and Degges-White 2014), have greater academic persistence (Shepler and Woosley 2013), and have higher retention rates (Woosley and Miller 2009). Participation in campus activities (e.g., joining student-run organizations) also creates opportunities for students with ID to increase social relationships with their peers, pursue personal interests, and connect with others who have similar career goals, all of which may increase independence and expand their social network (Eisenman, Farley-Ripple, Culnane, and Freedman 2013; Ross, Marcell, Williams, and Carlson 2013). Access to campus life, availability of supports, and overall campus participation may hinge on the way in which information about a student's disability and support needs are disclosed, as well as the reaction to that disclosure from others at that institution.

Differences in Social Disclosure Processes for Students with ID

The disclosure process and availability of accommodations in higher education can be quite different for campus activities. First, leaders of campus organizations will often be students, many of whom may be unfamiliar with supporting students with disabilities in general. As a result, they may feel uncomfortable with disability disclosures and may purposely or inadvertently convey negative perceptions and stereotypes in response. Second, even student leaders who are familiar with typical supports for college students with disabilities may be unfamiliar with the types of accommodation and support requests made by students with ID (e.g., explicit step-by-step instructions, support regarding communication processes, and social boundaries). This may result in confusion or, even worse, active minimization of opportunities for students with ID to participate.

The informal process through which a student with ID would make accommodation and support requests for participation in campus activities, versus an academic course, may also impact their level of participation. Disclosure of disability may be more comfortable and easier for some students, requiring only brief discussions with fellow college students. Students with ID may also not feel it necessary to initially disclose, since the nature of many activities requires few or no supports. As a result, the student with ID may feel like they have more control over the process and require less support from a mediator (program staff or mentor). Others may still prefer to have a mediator support them through the disclosure process and perhaps provide some initial support. Ideally, the student with ID and/or the student's program staff can work with campus activity leaders on creating a system of natural supports so that the student with ID can eventually fully participate without external support.

Disclosure of disability and requesting support/accommodations for campus activities can prove more challenging for some students with ID. The informal accommodation request process may be uncomfortable for students who prefer and perhaps rely upon more explicit procedures. Students may not be sure who to approach or what supports to request if it is their first time at an event. Students with ID will often benefit from discussion or explicit instruction from program staff prior to attending campus activities. Some students with ID may also request a mediator (e.g., mentor) to go with them in order to support them in becoming acclimated, identifying their accommodation needs for this particular setting, and determining whom is the best contact to discuss accommodations. Training for student organization and campus activity leaders on methods for responding to students' disclosure of all disabilities and request for accommodations and supports can be beneficial in order to create a trusting atmosphere for the student with ID, as well as allow the student leader to immediately be aware of resources.

Legitimacy within Institutional Systems

Participation in campus life also may be dictated by the enrollment or matriculation status of the students with ID. Some higher education programs for students with ID are administratively categorized as a "Continuing Education" programs. Students who attend such programs may not be identified as full-time, matriculated students in the enrollment data systems for that institution, despite spending full-time equivalent hours on campus. These students may have limited institutional access to certain types of resources, supports, and opportunities, including attendance at campus events, access to student clubs, and participation in recreational activities. These limitations can significantly minimize opportunities for developing peer relationships. Students who want to participate in campus life may need to disclose information about their program status and, therefore, their disability to their undergraduate peers. Students may feel uncomfortable disclosing this information because they may not have planned to do so or otherwise need to disclose. This discomfort may result in some students avoiding campus activities altogether. Providing non-matriculating students with ID access to the full array of campus activities that are offered to matriculating students may help to minimize disclosure dilemmas. If this is not possible, program staff may need to offer support to students on how to navigate these restrictions in a way that makes them comfortable.

The Who/What/When of Disclosure in Campus Life Activities

Decisions about disclosure of disability in campus activities may be based on multiple variables. First, the student may not need or want accommodations for a particular activity. The student may decide to participate on a trial basis to determine whether any accommodations or disclosure is required. Alternatively, a student may request and/or require more formal support during the activity from a mediator, like program staff or a mentor. This support is often made available to the student in order to help that student acclimate to the campus activity, remember certain tasks (who to connect with, important questions the student wanted to ask), or to be reminded of behavioral expectations (e.g., related to social engagement). The support person may initially reach out to the event coordinator in order to introduce the program and offer any general information that the event leader(s) may desire. While this can be helpful in offering background information on students with intellectual disabilities, it can also be problematic since it can establish an immediate hierarchy and power differential in which the student with ID is assumed to not be able to self-advocate and is left out of subsequent conversations between the event coordinator and the support person.

University staff and event leaders should work with the student with ID to delineate clear roles and understandings about communication, and ensure that they are following the student's lead about their desire for disclosure of information, request of supports, and general communication. Preferences regarding disclosure may then evolve over time, and it is critical to be responsive to these changing student preferences. Decisions about support provisions, both who will provide support and the type of support provided, should be guided by the desires of the student with ID. This ensures a programmatic focus on building student self-determination, as students can become stronger at articulating their own goals and advocating for themselves (Paiewonsky et al. 2010). In doing so, students are more likely to be successful in postsecondary education and have a positive adjustment (Getzel and Webb 2012; Murray, Lombardi, and Kosty 2014). An approach that values the opinion of students with ID would also maintain a person-centered philosophy, embedding flexibility and an individualized support structure into the IHE.

Disclosure and Relationships with Peers

Traditional college students tend to be very open to having students with ID be a part of campus life. Griffin et al. (2012) found that undergraduates were very comfortable with students with ID joining their classes and many formed friendships. Hafner, Moffat and Kisa (2011) found that a majority of students felt comfortable taking classes with their fellow students who had ID, as well as living with them in the dorms. In these studies, students who had more exposure to students with ID (e.g., in their college courses) also had a greater comfort level with students with ID, suggesting that inclusive programs may facilitate more accepting environments.

Proactive social disclosure may be helpful at times for a student with ID. For example, there may be instances when a student with ID is having trouble communicating with peers or has issues understanding a social boundary. Instead of the student being perceived as being difficult or not following social etiquette, they can be supported to offer explanations about the challenges they have in understanding social relationships and advocate for straightforward feedback from peers when interactions go awry. The student with ID may even choose to share contact information about their program or support staff if the difficulties they or their peers are facing require extensive support.

Training and communication is vital to successful inclusive higher education programs for students with intellectual disability. Some students, faculty and staff may be taken aback by the idea of a college student needing the types of accommodations and support that are required by students with ID. Campus event and student organization leaders may not understand why accommodations are necessary for their activity. Some student groups also may not understand the types of accommodations that would be helpful for a student with an intellectual disability. For example, they might get frustrated with having to offer more concrete instructions, provide information in multiple formats, or overall having to provide more support than they are accustomed to with their traditional members.

This experience could be similar to a faculty member who may feel unprepared for having a student with ID attend their course, unsure of the types of supports that may be helpful. For this reason, embedding training on universal design and providing accommodations and support for students with disabilities, including ID, into the typical orientation/training process for faculty, staff and student leaders (e.g., presidents of student-run organizations) can promote a greater success for students with ID and a smoother disclosure process.

Recommendations for Policy and Practice around ID Disclosure

College campuses can create an inclusive atmosphere that is respectful of the rights of students with ID and fosters open disclosure and communication of support needs. Students with ID can be successful in higher education if they experience an inclusive learning environment, are provided opportunities to develop and express self-determination, and programs and practices emanate from a person-centered approach. The opportunity to support the creation of such an environment is held by multiple groups: IHE administration; program staff who support students with ID; campus faculty, staff, and student leaders; and secondary education professionals who prepare students for entry into postsecondary education. By focusing on policies and practices that promote inclusion, person-centeredness and self-determination, students with ID can have successful postsecondary education experiences in which they further develop their career goals, sense of self-identity, and decision-making abilities regarding self-disclosure. Recommendations for policies and practices in each of these three areas and the agency that can support this development include the following.

Fostering an <u>Inclusive</u> Atmosphere

- Create clear mechanisms for students with ID to have the same access as other students without the need for them to disclose how/why they were able to achieve that access. This includes IHE-wide information systems, student services and supports, and financial aid.
- Include "intellectual disability" in all definitions of nontraditional students and references to students with other disabilities to facilitate campus-wide knowledge of their legitimacy as students.
- Include students with ID in disability and diversity initiatives.
- Offer services to students with ID through the Disability Services Office in order to identify accommodations and communicate this to instructors.
- Create openness among campus organizations and activities that students with a variety of abilities and disabilities may be participating.
- Offer easy-to-access resources for student leaders who are unsure of how to provide appropriate accommodations.
- Ensure that resources and support are available for faculty (e.g., training in Universal Design for Learning).
- Create natural supports across the campus in a variety of settings.
- Offer coursework (e.g., undergraduate mentoring course), internships, or other formal mechanisms to facilitate connections to other students.
- Encourage and support the inclusion of students with ID in high-exposure situations, such as through student leadership opportunities.
- Create opportunities to expose students, faculty, and staff to people with ID who have been successful in college and their careers.

Supporting the Development of <u>Self-Determination</u>

- Develop standards for program staff to support the process of self-disclosure, and outline processes and describe supports available.
- Create mechanisms to support students with ID in determining their disclosure preferences and communicating these to the appropriate people.
- Incorporate student-directed coaching supports across college activities (e.g., coursework, campus life) that can facilitate disclosure of information at a pace and level that is comfortable for the student with ID.
- Embed opportunities for self-advocacy when disclosure might be necessary.
- Make resources available to students so that they can disclose information about their program of study.
- Support students in understanding when and how to share contact information about their program or support staff when circumstances require more extensive support.

Maintaining a <u>Person-Centered</u> Approach

- Engage with the students with ID to delineate clear roles and understandings about communication, and ensure that professionals and peers follow the students' lead about their desire for disclosure of information, request of supports, and general communication.
- Encourage faculty and campus staff to support the presence of mediators (e.g., peer mentors) who can facilitate discussions about disclosure, accommodations, and student success across a variety of academic and social activities.
- Ensure that campus life staff and student leaders follow the student with ID's lead in disclosing information and have clear communications regarding desired supports.
- Respect the desires of students with ID who may feel sensitive to their specific diagnosis and prefer only specific information to be disclosed.

Students with intellectual disabilities are increasingly seeking higher education. While college opportunities can promote positive growth, there are also unique challenges related to the disclosure of ID for these students. Federal legislation has promoted strong expectations for college campus inclusion and research suggests a very positive impact across the college campus when students are included. However, negative stereotypes of people with ID and programmatic differences compared to typical college processes require a nuanced approach for disclosure of ID. In general, a person-centered approach is recommended for supporting students with ID in all facets of their program, including related to disclosure. Natural contexts across college settings foster important opportunities for students with ID to further develop their identity and make decisions about disclosure. As this occurs, steps can be taken by program staff, administrators, and instructors in order to promote a campus environment that is accepting of people with intellectual disabilities.

References

Ali, Afia, Angela Hassiotis, Andrea Strydom, and Michael King. 2012. "Self Stigma in People with Intellectual Disabilities and Courtesy Stigma in Family Careers: A Systematic Review." *Research in Developmental Disabilities* 33 (6): 2122–40. doi:10.1016/j.ridd.2012.06.013

Booth, Nathan, Sterling Travis, Christine Borzumato-Gainey, and Suzanne Degges-White. 2014. "Social Involvement: Helping Students Find Their Place in Campus Life." In *College Student Mental Health Counseling: A Developmental Approach*, edited by Suzanne Degges-White and Christine Borzumato-Gainey, 69–79. New York: Springer Publishing.

Carey, Allison. 2013. "The Sociopolitical Contexts of Passing and Intellectual Disability." In *Disability and Passing: Blurring the Lines of Identity*, edited by Jeffrey A. Brune and Daniel J. Wilson, 142–66. Philadelphia: Temple University Press.

Chambers, Cynthia, Michael Wehmeyer, Yumiko Saito, Kerry Lida, Youngsun Lee, and Vandana Singh. 2007. "Self-Determination: What Do We Know? Where Do We Go?" *Exceptionality* 15(1): 3–15.

Cobb, Brian, Jean Lehmann, Rebecca Newman-Gonchar, and Morgen Alwell. 2009. "Self-Determination for Students with Disabilities: A Narrative Meta-synthesis." *Career Development for Exceptional Individuals* 32 (2): 108–14.

Cunnah, Wendy. 2015. "Disabled Students: Identity, Inclusion and Work-Based Placements." *Disability & Society* 30 (2): 213–26. doi:10.1080/09687599.2014.996282

Cunningham, Cliff, and Sheila Glenn. 2004. "Self-Awareness in Young Adults with Down Syndrome: I. Awareness of Down Syndrome and Disability." *International Journal of Disability, Development and Education* 51 (4): 335–61. doi: 10.1080/1034912042000295017

Eisenman, Laura, Elizabeth Farley-Ripple, Mary Culnane, and Brian Freedman. 2013. "Rethinking Social Network Assessment for Students with Intellectual Disabilities in Postsecondary Education." *Journal of Postsecondary Education and Disability* 26 (4): 367–84.

Eisenman, Laura, and Karen Mancini. "College Perspectives and Issues." 2010.

In *Think College! Postsecondary Education Options for Students with Intellectual Disabilities*, edited by Meg Grigal and Debra Hart, 161–87. Baltimore: Paul H. Brookes.

Eisenman, Laura, and Linda Tascione. 2002. "'How Come Nobody Told Me?' Fostering Self-Realization through a High School English Curriculum." *Learning Disabilities Research and Practice* 17 (1): 35–46.

Getzel, Elizabeth, and Kristine Webb. 2012. "Transition to Postsecondary Education." In *Handbook of Adolescent Transition Education for Youth with Disabilities*. Edited by Michael L. Wehmeyer and Kristine W. Webb, 295–311. New York: Routledge.

Griffin, Megan, Allison Summer, Elise McMillan, Tammy Day, Robert Hodapp. 2012. "Attitudes toward Including Students with Intellectual Disabilities at College." *Journal of Policy and Practice in Intellectual Disabilities* 9 (4): 234–39. doi: 10.1111/jppi.12008

Grigal, Meg, and Debra Hart, eds. 2010a. *Think College! Postsecondary Education Options for Students with Intellectual Disabilities*. Baltimore: Paul H. Brookes.

Grigal, Meg, and Debra Hart. 2010b. "Critical Components for Planning and Implementing Dual Enrollment and Other Postsecondary Education Experiences." In *Think College! Postsecondary Education Options for Students with Intellectual Disabilities*, edited by Meg Grigal and Debra Hart, 229–58. Baltimore: Paul H. Brookes.

Grigal, Meg, Debra Hart, and Cate Weir. 2012. "A Survey of Postsecondary Education Programs for Students with Intellectual Disabilities in the United States." *Journal of Policy and Practice in Intellectual Disabilities* 9 (4): 223–33.

Grigal, Meg, Debra Hart, and Cate Weir. 2014. "Postsecondary Education for Students with Intellectual Disabilities." In *Equity and Full Participation for Individuals with Severe Disabilities*, edited by Martin Agran, Fredda Brown, Carolyn Hughes, Carol Quirk, and Diane Ryndak, 275–98. Baltimore: Brookes Publishing.

Grigal, Meg, Debra Hart, Frank Smith, Daria Domin, Jennifer Sulewski, and Cate Weir. 2014. *Think College National Coordinating Center: Annual Report on the Transition and Postsecondary Programs for Students with Intellectual Disabilities (2012–2013)*. Boston, MA: University of Massachusetts Boston, Institute for Community Inclusion.

Grigal, Meg, and Frank Smith. 2014. "Current Status of Meaningful Credentials for Students with Intellectual Disabilities Attending TPSID Model Demonstration Programs." *Think College Fast Facts* 5. http://www.thinkcollege.net/images/stories/CredentialFF5_F.pdf

Hafner, Dedra, Courtney Moffat, and Nutullah Kisa. 2011. "Cutting-Edge: Integrating Students with Intellectual and Developmental Disabilities into a 4-Year Liberal Arts College." *Career Development for Exceptional Individuals* 34 (1): 18–30.

Higher Education Opportunity Act of 2008, Public Law 110–315, 2008.

Kraemer, Bonnie and Jan Blacher. 2001. "Transition for Young Adults with Severe

Mental Retardation: School Preparation, Parent Expectations, and Family Involvement." *Mental Retardation* 39 (6): 423–35.

Levy, Becca. 2009. "Stereotype Embodiment: A Psychosocial Approach to Aging." *Current Directions in Psychological Science* 18 (6): 332–36.

Madaus, Joseph. 2010. "Let's Be Reasonable: Accommodations at the College Level." In *Preparing Students with Disabilities for College Success*, edited by Stan Shaw, Joseph Madaus, and Lyman L. Dukes III, 37–63. Baltimore: Paul H. Brookes.

Martinez, Donna, James Conroy, and Mary Cerreto. 2012. "Parent Involvement in the Transition Process of Children with Intellectual Disabilities: The Influence of Inclusion on Parent Desires and Expectations for Postsecondary Education." *Journal of Policy and Practice in Intellectual Disabilities* 9 (4): 279–88. doi: 10.1111/jppi.12000

Matthews, Nicole. 2009. "Teaching the 'Invisible' Disabled Students in the Classroom: Disclosure, Inclusion and the Social Model of Disability." *Teaching in Higher Education* 14 (3): 229–39. doi: 10.1080/13562510902898809

May, Cynthia. 2012. "An Investigation of Attitude Change in Inclusive College Classes Including Young Adults with an Intellectual Disability." *Journal of Policy and Practice in Intellectual Disabilities* 9 (4): 240–46. doi: 10.1111/jppi.12013

Morin, Diane, Melina Rivard, Anne Crocker, C. P. Boursier, and Jean Caron. 2013. "Public Attitudes towards Intellectual Disability: A Multidimensional Perspective." *Journal of Intellectual Disability Research* 57 (3): 279–92. doi:10.1111/jir.12008

Murray, Christopher, Allison Lombardi, and Derek Kosty. 2014. "Profiling Adjustment among Postsecondary Students with Disabilities: A Person-Centered Approach." *Journal of Diversity in Higher Education* 7 (1): 31–44. doi: 10.1037/a0035777.

O'Connor, Barrie, John Kubiak, Deborah Espiner, and Patricia O'Brien. 2012. "Lecturer Responses to the Inclusion of Students with Intellectual Disabilities Auditing Undergraduate Classes." *Journal of Policy and Practice in Intellectual Disabilities,* 9 (4): 247–56. doi: 10.1111/jppi.12009

Olney, Marjorie, and Karin Brockelman. 2003. "Out of the Disability Closet: Strategic Use of Perception Management by Select University Students with Disabilities." *Disability and Society* 18 (1): 35–50.

Paiewonsky, Maria, Kristen Mecca, Tim Daniels, Carla Katz, Jim Nash, Ty Hanson, and Stelios Gragoudas. 2010. "Students and Educational Coaches: Developing a Support Plan for College." *Think College Insight Brief* 4. Boston, MA: University of Massachusetts Boston, Institute for Community Inclusion.

Papay, Clare, and Linda Bambara. 2011. "Postsecondary Education for Transition-Age Students with Intellectual and Other Developmental Disabilities: A National Survey." *Education and Training in Autism and Developmental Disabilities* 46 (1): 78–93.

Paterson, Lucy, Karen McKenzie, and Bill Lindsay. 2012. "Stigma, Social Comparison and Self-Esteem in Adults with an Intellectual Disability." *Journal of Applied Research in Intellectual Disabilities* 25 (2): 166–76. doi: 10.1111/j.1468-3148.2011.00651.x

Piepmeier, Alison, Amber Cantrell, and Asley Maggio. 2014. "Disability is a Feminist Issue: Bringing Together Women's and Gender Studies and Disability Studies." *Disability Studies Quarterly* 34 (2). http://dsq-sds.org/article/view/4252/3592

Rapley, Mark, Patrick Kiernan, and Charles Antaki. 1998. "Invisible to Themselves or Negotiating Identity? The Interactional Management of 'Being Intellectually Disabled.'" *Disability & Society,* 13 (5): 807–27.

Ross, Jeffery, Jamia Marcell, Paula Williams, and Dawn Carlson. 2013. "Postsecondary Education Employment and Independent Living Outcomes of Persons with Autism and Intellectual Disability." *Journal of Postsecondary Education and Disability* 26 (4): 337–51.

Scior, Katrina. 2011. "Public Awareness, Attitudes and Beliefs Regarding Intellectual Disability: A Systematic Review." *Research in Developmental Disabilities* 32 (6): 2164–82. doi:10.1016/j.ridd.2011.07.005

Shepler, Dustin, and Sherry Woosley. 2013. "Understanding the Early Integration Experiences of College Students with Disabilities." *Journal of Postsecondary Education and Disability* 25 (1): 37–50.

Siperstein, Gary, Sarah Pociask, and Melissa Collins. 2010. "Sticks, Stones, and Stigma: A Study of Students' Use of the Derogatory Term 'Retard'." *Intellectual and Developmental Disabilities* 48 (2): 126–34. doi:10.1352/1934–9556–48.2.126

Spassiani, Natasha, and Carli Friedman. 2014. "Stigma: Barriers to Culture and Identity for People with Intellectual Disability." *Inclusion* 2 (4): 329–41. doi: 10.1352/2326–6988–2.4.329

"Student Eligibility." 2011. 20 U.S. Code 1091, 1140.

Valle, Jan, and David Connor. 2011. "Contemplating the (In)visibility of Disability." In *Rethinking Disability: A Disability Studies Approach to Inclusive Practices,* 16–38. New York: McGraw-Hill.

Wehmeyer, Michael, Sharon Field, and Colleen Thoma. "Self-Determination and Adolescent Transition Education." 2012. In *Handbook of Adolescent Transition Education for Youth with Disabilities,* edited by Michael L. Wehmeyer & Kristine W. Webb, 171–90. New York: Routledge.

Woosley, Sherry, and Angie Miller. 2009. "Integration and Institutional Commitment as Predictors of College Student Transition: Are Third Week Indicators Significant?" *College Student Journal* 43 (4): 1260–71.

Zhang, Dalun, Leena Landmark, Anne Reber, HsienYuan Hsu, Oi-man Kwok, and Michael Benz. 2010. "University Faculty Knowledge, Beliefs, and Practices in Providing Reasonable Accommodations to Students with Disabilities." *Remedial and Special Education* 31 (4): 276–86.

Accommodations and Disclosure for Faculty Members with Mental Disability

STEPHANIE L. KERSCHBAUM

AMBER M. O'SHEA

MARGARET PRICE

MARK S. SALZER

In[1] 2012, the American Association of University Professors (AAUP) released a report titled "Accommodating Faculty Members Who Have Disabilities" (2012). Aimed at helping colleges and universities comply with the 1990 Americans with Disabilities Act (ADA) and implement sorely needed changes in higher education as a workplace, "Accommodating Faculty Members" sought to explain the law regarding faculty workplace accommodation and sketched out a procedure that institutions might follow to comply with the law. The procedure described in the AAUP report begins with the faculty member's disclosure of a disability to the appropriate administrators or human resources professionals, includes the identification of the essential functions of the faculty member's position, and concludes with negotiations that determine and implement reasonable accommodations that are needed.

This process may seem straightforward, but it is difficult, if not impossible, to implement in actual practice. The paucity of institutional structures in place for faculty accommodation, the lack of general awareness around disability in general and mental disability[2] in particular, not to mention legalistic maneuvering around "essential functions" and "reasonable accommodation" all contribute to the difficulty of following the procedure outlined by the AAUP (see, e.g., Kerschbaum et al. 2013; Price 2011a; Anderson 2007). Disclosure is in fact one of the key challenges behind ensuring needed accommodations are in place. When mental disability comes into the equation, disclosing a disability and negotiating accommodations can be particularly difficult. Many mentally disabled faculty members report being unfamiliar with accommodation procedures—if they exist at all—on their campuses (Price, O'Shea, Salzer, and Kerschbaum), and when a disability is not easily identified or named (see, e.g., Avinger, Croake, and Miller 2007; Bolaki 2011; Hirschmann 2015; Price 2011a) or when needed accommodations are not already available as options on a checklist, negotiating accommodations can feel scary, be risky, or altogether fail to meet faculty members' needs. These accounts also indicate the importance of understanding processes for disclosure and accommodation for faculty with mental disabilities, who are dramatically understudied in research on faculty life and work in higher education. Studies of faculty life (e.g., Blackburn and Lawrence 1995; Teichler, Arimoto, and Cummings 2013) often do not mention disability, and in what research does exist on disability and faculty life, mental disability has been shown to be significant where disclosure is concerned (Price et al. 2017; Horton and Tucker 2014).

Existing knowledge about faculty with mental disabilities has largely come from autoethnographic or interview research as well as personal essays and memoirs about disability and academic life (see, e.g., Cvetkovich 2012; Jamison 1995; Myers 2007; Pryal 2014a, 2014b, 2015; Saks 2007; Skogen, 2012; Smith 2013; Vance 2007). These accounts of mentally disabled faculty members' experiences are valuable because they offer examples of ways that faculty have shaped their work lives to achieve access, and they call attention to pervasive systems of inequity. But these studies do not have the data to explore broader patterns and trends in mentally disabled faculty members' experiences with disclosure and accommodation.

The knowledge we have about disability accommodation in higher education is overwhelmingly about students' experiences (see, e.g., Hitt 2015; Lightner, Kipps-Vaughan, Schulte, and Trice 2012; Marshak, Van Wieren, Raeke Ferrell, Swiss, and Dugan 2010; Wolf 2001; Wood 2014). Some studies within this body of work do specifically examine students with mental disability (usually operationalized within this literature as mental illness, psychiatric disability, or psychiatric disorder), and among the best-known are Kessler, Foster, Saunders, and Stang (1995), which examined data from the U.S. National Comorbidity Survey Replication, and a survey by Collins and Mowbray (2005), which gathered data from 275 U.S. colleges and universities. Recent studies by Salzer and colleagues (Salzer, Wick, and Rogers 2008;

Salzer 2012) have investigated the experiences of college students with mental illness in a more granular way, exploring topics such as retention issues, possible sources of distress, types of accommodation used, and how helpful students found their accommodations.

Student-focused research can usefully inform research on faculty accommodation in some ways, as faculty and students share some common concerns, including logistical challenges and considerations of stigma (see Wood, this volume). However, these concerns resonate quite differently among these groups. For example, students and faculty are not always—perhaps not even usually—served by the same office at a given college or university. While many students may work with an institutional Office for Disability Services, there is no consistent or easily identifiable office where faculty accommodations are handled: faculty are sometimes sent to Human Resources, sometimes to their department chairs, sometimes to a school's ADA coordinator, and sometimes to the Office for Disability Services. Even just asking where to go for accommodation can be tantamount to disclosure. Thus, faculty who are unclear on how to navigate their school's disability-accommodation procedure (assuming one even exists) may have to disclose that they need disability accommodations to multiple parties in order to even find the right channel to make a formal request.

To better understand the nature of higher education as a workplace and the ways that disclosure and accommodation work in tandem for faculty members, we conducted an anonymous survey of faculty members who identified as having a mental disability. In what follows, we report on data regarding faculty members' disclosure and negotiation of accommodations for a mental disability.

Study Design and Methods

The data reported in this article are drawn from an anonymous online survey of a national sample of faculty members with mental disability. For the purposes of the study, a "person with a mental disability" was defined as someone who has been the recipient of a mental health diagnosis or who has received mental-health care; this definition was provided on the first page of the survey. Participants were also informed that they did not have to identify as "disabled" to participate in the survey. Our survey defined "faculty member" as "someone who is employed (part- or full-time) at an institution of higher education and is not a graduate student. Faculty members may have titles including 'instructor,' 'lecturer,' 'professor,' or another title."

When recruitment began, we initially contacted human resource departments, disability offices, and professional associations in colleges and universities. Due to a lack of response from human resources and disability offices, we then reached out to faculty senates at colleges and universities, including HBCUs, since survey participation from those who identified as African American were low. Invitations to participate were also sent to various LISTSERVs of faculty members (e.g., Disability Studies in the Humanities, Association on Disability and Higher Education, Writing Program Administrators LISTSERV) working in institutions of higher education across the United States. Approximately 16,000 recruitment emails were sent out, not including the LISTSERV announcements.

The survey was designed using the web-based software SurveyMonkey, and the survey link was live from November 1, 2012, to October 31, 2013. Two of the chapter authors, Salzer and Price, developed the survey, in consultation with a multidisciplinary team of researchers as well as people with mental health histories. The survey consisted of four sections. The first section included eleven questions aimed at gathering demographic information (e.g., rank as a faulty member, field or discipline, age, gender, etc.). The second section asked about mental health background. This section included eight closed and open-ended questions such as "What is your primary diagnosis?" The third section of the survey consisted of twenty-four questions that asked about work modifications[3] related to mental disability. The format of these questions varied and included Likert-type questions (e.g., "How familiar are you with accommodations that you may be entitled to under the law?" with responses ranging from *Not at all familiar* to *extremely familiar*); questions in which participants were able to select multiple responses (e.g., "At your institution, who/what is responsible for managing faculty accommodation requests related to disability?"); and closed questions (e.g., "Have you ever formally or informally requested modifications to your work process related to your mental disability at your current institution?"). Additionally, a list of twelve specific workplace modifications were presented, and participants were asked to indicate whether or not they had received these modifications. Participants were asked to use a five-point Likert scale (ranging from "*Not at All*" to "*Extremely*") to indicate either how helpful the modification was or how helpful the modification would be. The final section of the survey included eight questions that examined barriers and support. Demographic information and descriptive results are presented below.

Survey Results

A total of 323 surveys were submitted online. Of the 323 surveys, 28 were not used in the analysis because they represented an international sample,[4] 5 were missing more than 10 percent of the data, and 23 were excluded because their self-reported diagnosis did not fall into the following disorder categories: mood, anxiety, psychotic, or attentional; those that we excluded for this analysis were not mental health disabilities (e.g., learning disabilities). Finally, 59 did not respond to questions regarding the use of accommodations. Demographic variables for the remaining sample (*n* = 208) are presented in table 6.

Requests for Modifications

Participants were asked to report whether or not they had ever formally or informally requested modifications to their work process related to their mental disability at their current, primary institution. Of the 208 participants, 15.9 percent (*n* = 33) reported that they had requested modifications while 84.1 percent (*n* = 175) reported they had not. Data on the percentage of employees with any disability who seek workplace accommodations is not readily available. While the rate for those with observable impairments is likely high, we suspect that it is relatively low for those with hidden impairments, especially those with mental health issues where workplace stigma remains a serious issue. Therefore, the percentage of faculty in our survey who reported seeking accommodations seem in line with our expectations. In addition to reporting whether they requested modifications, participants were asked to indicate how helpful specific modifications were that they received. Finally, those who did not receive each specific accommodation were asked how helpful it would have been if they had received it. These results are presented in table 7.

Discussion

Our survey results show that a relatively small proportion of faculty members reported requesting accommodations—15.9 percent. While we cannot report why accommodation requests were made (our survey only asked why accommodations were not requested), we do know that at least some of the accommodation requests were connected to decisions faculty members made to disclose their disabilities—or not to disclose. Elsewhere, we have written about why faculty members with mental disabilities chose not to request ac-

Table 6. Frequency and percent for demographic variables

Variable	N	%
Faculty Rank		
Non tenure track professor in permanent position	18	8.7
Non tenure track professor on a contract > one year	17	8.2
Non tenure track professor on a contract < year	33	15.9
Assistant professor	61	29.5
Associate professor	48	23.2
Full professor	29	14.0
Professor emeritus/a	1	0.5
Institution Type		
Community college	17	8.2
4-year undergraduate granting primarily associate's	2	1.0
4-year undergraduate granting primarily bachelor's	35	16.8
University granting doctorates and master's	145	69.7
University granting master's degrees only	8	3.8
Tribal college or university	0	0.0
Historically Black college or university	3	1.4
Specialized school	2	1.0
Other	9	4.3
Gender		
Woman	153	73.6
Man	53	25.5
Genderqueer	4	1.9
Transsexual	2	1.0
Transgender	3	1.4
Other	1	0.5
Race		
White	192	92.3
Black and/or African American	9	4.3
Latino and/or Hispanic	4	1.9
American Indian	3	1.4
Native Hawaiian or other Pacific Islander	0	0.0
Asian	6	2.9
Other	3	1.5
Primary Diagnosis		
Attention-deficit/hyperactivity disorder	8	3.8
Depression	101	48.6
Bipolar disorder	16	7.7
Anxiety disorder	76	36.5
Other	7	3.4

commodations: because making an accommodation request would be risky or dangerous in some way, because they felt their mental health disabilities were private matters, and/or because accommodations were not needed or not relevant to their work (Price et al.). While not listed in our survey, a fourth reason that faculty members with mental disabilities may not request accommodations is because—for many people in academia—there is little imagination of the possibilities of accommodation for mental disability in academic workplaces. In interviews conducted with some of the survey respondents afterwards, we asked participants what accommodations they wish they had but do not. In response to that, one interview participant with mental health disability said, "Yeah, what <u>could</u> they do" (Price and Kerschbaum 2015).

Few people have paid close attention to accessibility issues for mentally

Table 7. Use and perceived helpfulness of modifications

Variable	Received modification			Modification was very or extremely helpful			Modification would be very or extremely helpful		
	N	Total N	%	N	Total N	%	N	Total N	%
Extended time to complete work	200	25	12.5	25	18	72	175	45	25.7
Extended advance notice of work assignments	196	9	4.6	9	6	66.7	187	46	24.6
Adjusted proportion of responsibilities	201	11	5.5	11	7	63.6	190	59	31.1
Modified but not reduced teaching schedule	198	11	5.6	11	7	63.6	187	47	25.1
Change of modality for work-related events	194	6	3.1	6	1	16.7	188	40	21.3
Alternative or additional modes of processing information	196	7	3.6	7	4	57.1	189	7	3.7
Alternative or additional work equipment	195	12	6.2	12	7	58.3	183	8	4.4
Memory cues	195	8	4.1	8	3	37.5	187	28	15
Availability of quiet space	199	20	10.1	20	14	70	179	74	41.3
Natural or incandescent lighting	198	12	6	12	6	50	186	65	34.9
Virtual attendance	195	12	6.2	12	4	33.3	183	47	25.7
Additional mentoring or feedback sessions	198	12	6	12	7	58.3	186	51	27.4

disabled faculty. As Price has noted (2011a; 2011b), the sorts of accommodations that mentally disabled faculty might need are often not listed along with the standard or typical accommodations most often referenced when talking about workplace accessibility and the ADA, such as ramps into buildings, elevators, sign language interpreting, or screen-reading software. To find out more about accommodations that mentally disabled faculty might want or need, Price and Salzer generated a list of potential accommodations, many of which were pulled from Salzer (2012), to help identify accommodations that would be viewed as most useful. Of the twelve accommodations listed on the survey, the two that faculty members most commonly reported requesting were "extended time to complete work" (n = 25, 72 percent) and "availability of quiet space" (n = 20, 70 percent). Note that this does not mean that only twenty-five out of the 208 faculty members in this sample received extended time to complete work or that only twenty had quiet space available—but rather, that these faculty members reported receiving them as a workplace accommodation. We make this point because our research has repeatedly reinforced for us that for mentally disabled faculty members, the accommodation process described by the AAUP ("Accommodating")—when it does exist on campuses—by and large does not fit the needs of faculty with mental disabilities nor does it account for the ways that those faculty members receive needed workplace accommodations.

In addition to asking about accommodations that faculty members actually did receive, the survey asked faculty members to predict which—if any—accommodations from the list might be important or useful to them. Results show that survey respondents named several accommodations that would be "very or extremely helpful" to them. More than fifty respondents pointed to "availability of quiet space" (n = 74, 41.3 percent), "natural or incandescent lighting" (n = 65, 34.9 percent), "adjusted proportion of responsibilities" (n = 59, 31.1 percent) and "additional mentoring or feedback sessions" (n = 51, 27.4 percent). More than forty people indicated that the following accommodations would be "very or extremely helpful": "virtual attendance" (n = 47, 25.7 percent); "modified but not reduced teaching schedule" (n = 47, 25.1 percent); "extended advance notice of work assignments" (n = 46, 24.6 percent); "extended time to complete work" (n = 45, 25.7 percent); and "change of modality for work-related events" (n = 40, 21.3 percent).

As we reviewed these results, we were struck by the number of negotiated and desirable accommodations that dealt with the themes of *time* and *physical environments*. For example, receiving extended time and having opportunities to readjust, balance, or reallocate work responsibilities involve the timeframes of faculty life, while quiet spaces, lighting, virtual attendance, and modalities for completing work deal with the physical spaces and materials people use in their work. We also want to acknowledge that a large majority of our sample (84.1 percent) did not report negotiating any accommodations to their work. Some aspects of faculty life are inflexible, such as the tenure clock or mandated office hours and teaching schedules, but many other aspects are indeed flexible. Faculty members at many institutions can choose whether to complete work at home or in a campus office, and have varying degrees of autonomy. It is also important to acknowledge the contingent conditions under which a growing majority of faculty work (see, e.g., Adjunct 2008) as well as the different stresses experienced by faculty members who regularly experience racial and other microaggressions (Sue et al. 2007). Contingent employment can contribute to the physical and mental stress that faculty members experience. These stresses can exacerbate mental health issues or lead to new physical and mental conditions.

At least since Zola's (1988) use of "crip time," disability-studies scholars have been aware that time takes on unpredictable, sometimes paradoxical shapes, for those who are disabled. Although at times this is assumed to be simply an addition of time to a particular situation (such as offering "extended time" for a task), crip time is more complex than that; in Kafer's phrase, crip time is not merely extended, "but exploded." The term refers to a full "reorientation" to the notion of time and associated concepts such as *future* or *healing* (2013, 27). Among responses to the survey, results were mixed in terms of how helpful faculty said the accommodations of extra time for tasks, or advance notice for tasks, had been (if they received this accommodation) or would be (if they did not receive this accommodation). Theories of "crip time" (Baril 2016; Dalke and Mullaney 2014; Price 2011a; Samuels; Titchkosky 2011) further reinforce that there is no simple answer to the question of time as a possible accommodation, or as a problem to be solved, in academic work.

Along with issues of time, physical environments were highly significant for many of the faculty members in our study. Having quiet space available, for example, is important for faculty who deal with ADD/ADHD. Other faculty may have mental disabilities that are exacerbated when their physical environment does not include regular access to natural light: working under fluorescent lighting can produce migraines or exacerbate a seizure disorder, and faculty who experience depression benefit from access to natural light. Faculty members may need ways to manage or arrange their physical environment to make it most conducive to their daily work lives and to ensure that it does not create additional barriers to their success and thriving.

As noted above, faculty members with mental disabilities do not often experience the accommodation process detailed by the AAUP or outlined by their institutions as an effective means for procuring accommodations. There are numerous reasons for this. For one, the unpredictability of many mental disabilities makes disclosure extraordinarily complex. The current accommodation model tries to make a specific match between identifying a "problem" as well as a corresponding accommodation that will fix the problem. However, for a faculty member whose mental disability symptoms are intermittent or episodic, it is often impossible to predict exactly when accommodations need to be in place or even which accommodations would be helpful at which times. Finally, the stigma of mental disability and the risks of disclosing—ranging from negative perceptions, retaliation, losing one's job, being deemed unqualified for the position, or being treated differently—make the prospect of opening one's disability as a topic for discussion deeply frightening. This sentiment was reinforced in interviews, as when one participant said, in response to a question about whether she has disclosed to colleagues in her workplace, "absolutely not" and "no way."

All of these factors—the complexity of disclosure, unpredictability of mental health issues, and stigma of mental disability—combine to make the relationship between disclosure and provision of accommodations for these faculty tenuous and uneasy at best. In both the anonymous online survey and the interview study, faculty members with mental disabilities most often reported pursuing accommodations via channels outside of the formal procedure delineated at their institution. Examples of these nonlinear paths to accommodation include asking for accommodations for a mental health disability by identifying a more readily apparent physical disability or health condition and participating in informal negotiations that result in the necessary accommodations, such as by volunteering for a less-plum teaching schedule in exchange for being able to work from home at needed times.

Survey Limitations

This survey has several limitations. Our sample size and the self-selection of survey participants prevent us from making any representative claims about faculty members with mental disabilities. Thus, our findings are suggestive and need to be more fully substantiated across a broadly diverse population and across myriad institutional settings. Of particular note is that our sample is predominantly white, despite specific efforts to recruit faculty of color, including directly contacting historically Black and tribal colleges and universities when publicizing the survey. This limitation emphasizes the need for research that is welcoming to faculty of color and centers their experiences. In continuing research, such as Price and Kerschbaum's interview study, those needs are given strong priority. Finally, twenty-eight survey respondents in our original sample came from countries outside of the United States. While we did not include these twenty-eight responses in the analyses performed for this article, we believe it is important to explore the relationships between U.S. higher education and postsecondary systems across the world (see, e.g., Alshammari, this volume). Thus, we understand the relationship(s) between mental disability and the situational, environmental, and identity factors that are significant to faculty members' experience as an unaddressed need for further research.

Conclusion

What does it mean to work as a faculty member with mental disability? What are the costs, the nuances of interpersonal interactions, and the potential advantages of living with a mental disability in academia? What structural supports are needed to ensure that mentally disabled faculty lead successful (defined capaciously) work lives? In asking these questions, we also hope that others will take up questions branching out from this investigation. For example, what might be learned about the process of accommodation for graduate students, who are often in the fraught position of being both students and employees of one college/university at the same time? What are the experiences of academics with mental disability who *do* ask for accommodation, an area our survey did not explore in depth? How do the stories of faculty with various kinds of disabilities differ across intersectional experiences including differences of class, gender, race, institutional type, rank, and geographical location?

From the present study, at least one critical point comes clear: the nonlinear paths to accommodation described in our "Findings" section indicate the severity of injustice at work in higher education's "business as usual" model with regard to mental disability. If it were emotionally, professionally, and logistically simple to request accommodations through an easily findable Office of Disability Services, presumably, faculty members would be doing that. The fact that mentally disabled faculty are *not* often using the official (and reportable) route to accommodation—indeed, according to our survey, are avoiding that route in droves—inspires the question, "Why?" While our survey raises the possibility that many mentally disabled faculty do not need accommodations, research reporting high levels of attrition among psychiatrically disabled students (Collins and Mowbray 2005) suggests that similar attrition rates may be possible or likely for faculty, too. We offer that the system for accommodation in U.S. higher education is itself a barrier to access. The ADA is usually interpreted according to a highly problematic "minimum standards" and "compliance" model (see, e.g., Abram 2003; "Supporting" 2012). When considered alongside the additional difficulty of working in academe as a person with mental disability, these problems are compounded.

It may be that mental disabilities were never a good fit for the ADA as it was written. The ADA works on the assumption of a predictable series of events: identify a problem (imagined to be located in the body of a disabled person), figure out an accommodation, then retrofit existing systems to put this accommodation in place. As the authors in "Faculty Members, Accommodation, and Access in Higher Education" (Kerschbaum et al. 2013) explain in depth, such linearity doesn't work well for any kind of disability, no matter how stable that disability might seem to be. And if the disability in question is highly stigmatized (e.g., autism, borderline personality disorder) or unpredictable (e.g., many chronic illnesses that affect energy and cognition), it is not simply a poor fit for the ADA model; it doesn't fit at all.

Drawing upon Garland-Thomson's concept of the "misfit," disabilities that are highly stigmatized or strongly unpredictable are problematic in higher education because their appearance exposes the "incongruent relationship between two things . . . [and] the awkward attempt to fit them together" (2011, 592–93). Academic work requires a mind that can fulfill the "essential functions" of the job. But it's unclear whether the ability to fulfill these functions can include, say, traits such as intermittent major depression, panic attacks, migraines, or unpredictable changes in cognitive processing speed. Attempting to "solve" such problems via individual accommodation quickly exposes the "misfit" at work. First, simply disclosing this sort of "unfitness" can put one's job at risk—not only for untenured faculty, but even for tenured faculty, all of whom work under the requirement of being able to fulfill the essential functions of their jobs. Second, even if the problematics of disclosure are not an issue (a big if), asking for an individual accommodation for a disability that involves being unable to teach, probably at short notice and at unpredictable intervals, would sound absurd in most departments. Yet we all know of departments where this sort of accommodation does work, fairly smoothly and without much discussion—*if* it is a department that already works on principles of interdependence, and in which colleagues pitch in for each other as needed. "Accommodations" like these can be achieved through environmental and systemic changes; as Garland-Thomson empha-sizes, the misfit forces us to "recognize that bodies are always situated in and dependent upon environments through which they materialize as fitting or misfitting" (598).[5] In summary, although the presence of mental disability in the academic workplace seems to confound the linear, individual ADA model of accommodation, if we imagine the ways that mental disability is *al-ready* accommodated in the academic workplace, we can envision an alternate landscape: one that is characterized by interdependence, shared vulnerability (see Fineman 2008; Siebers 2010), and collective moves toward access.

How might such moves be carried out? There is no easy recipe, particu-larly since a mutually supportive, interdependent academic unit can be diffi-cult to sustain in an atmosphere of competition, individual achievement, and scarce resources. Yet it is possible to create such spaces—*not*, we emphasize, through individual heroics, but through institutional support, both material and attitudinal, that lessens the tendency of faculty members to compete against each other and creates spaces that are more open and welcoming of differences of all kinds. The "how" of access is usually mandated through broad policy, but it is enacted at the local level. We hope this article conveys the importance of both those levels of institutional change, as well as some of the layers in between.

References

Abram, Suzanne. 2003. "The Americans with Disabilities Act in Higher Education: The Plight of Disabled Faculty." *Journal of Law and Education* 32 (1): 1–20.

"Accommodating Faculty Members Who Have Disabilities." 2012. American As-sociation of University Professors. http://www.aaup.org/report/accommodat-ing-faculty-members-who-have-disabilities

Adjunct, Alice K. 2008. "The Revolving Ramp: Disability and the New Adjunct Economy." *Disability Studies Quarterly* 28 (3). http://dsq-sds.org/article/view/110/110

Alshammari, Shahd. This volume.

Anderson, Robert L. 2007. "Faculty Members with Disabilities in Higher Edu-cation." *Disabled Faculty and Staff in a Disabling Society: Multiple Identities in Higher Education,* edited by Mary Lee Vance. Huntersville, SC: Association of Higher Education and Disability. 183–200.

Avinger, Charles, Edith Croake and Jean Kearns Miller. 2007. "Breathing Under-water in Academia: Teaching, Learning and Working with the Challenges of Invisible Illnesses and Hidden (Dis-)Abilities." In *Disabled Faculty and Staff in a Disabling Society: Multiple Identities in Higher Education.* Edited by Mary Lee Vance, 201–15. Huntersville, NC: AHEAD.

Baril, Alexandre. 2016. "'Doctor, Am I an Anglophone Trapped in a Francophone Body?' An Intersectional Analysis of Trans-Crip-t Time in Ableist, Cisnormative, and Anglonormative Societies." *Journal of Literary and Cultural Disability Studies* 10 (2): 155–72.

Blackburn, Robert T., and Janet H. Lawrence. 1995. *Faculty at Work: Motivation, Expectation, Satisfaction*. Baltimore, MD: Johns Hopkins University Press.

Bolaki, Stella. 2011. "Challenging Invisibility, Making Connections: Illness, Survival, and Black Struggles in Audre Lorde's Work." In *Blackness and Disability*, edited by Christopher M. Bell, 47–74. East Lansing: Michigan State University Press.

Collins, Mary Elizabeth, and Carol T. Mowbray. 2005. "Higher Education and Psychiatric Disabilities: National Survey of Campus Disability Services." *American Journal of Orthopsychiatry* 75 (2): 304–15. doi: 10.1037/0002–9432.75.2.304

Cvetkovich, Ann. 2012. *Depression: A Public Feeling*. Durham, NC: Duke University Press.

Dalke, Anne, and Clare Mullaney. 2014. "On Being Transminded: Disabling Achievement, Enabling Exchange." *Disability Studies Quarterly* 34 (2): n.p. http://dsq-sds.org/article/view/4247

Fineman, Martha Albertson. 2008. "The Vulnerable Subject: Anchoring Equality in the Human Condition." *Yale Journal of Law & Feminism* 20 (1): 1–23.

Garland-Thomson, Rosemarie. 2011. "Misfits: A Feminist Materialist Disability Concept." *Hypatia* 26 (3): 591–609. doi:10.1111/j.1527–2001.2011.01206.x

Hirschmann, Nancy. 2015. "Invisible Disability: Seeing, Being, Power." In *Civil Disabilities: Citizenship, Membership, and Belonging*, edited by Nancy J. Hirschmann and Beth Linker, 204–22. Philadelphia: University of Pennsylvania Press.

Hitt, Allison. 2015. *From Accommodations to Accessibility: How Rhetorics of Overcoming Manifest in Writing Pedagogies*. PhD diss., Syracuse University. Communication with author.

Horton, John, and Faith Tucker. 2014. "Disabilities in Academic Workplaces: Experiences of Human and Physical Geographers." *Transactions of the Institute of British Geographers*, 39: 76–89. doi:10.1111/tran.12009

Jamison, Kay Redfield. 1995. *An Unquiet Mind*. New York: Vintage.

Kafer, Alison. 2013. *Feminist, Queer, Crip*. Bloomington: Indiana University Press.

Kerschbaum, Stephanie L., Rosemarie Garland-Thomson, Sushil Oswal, Amy Vidali, Susan Ghiaciuc, Margaret Price, Jay Dolmage, Craig Meyer, Brenda Brueggemann, and Ellen Samuels. 2013. "Faculty Members, Accommodation, and Access in Higher Education." *Profession*. https://profession.commons.mla.org/2013/12/09/faculty-members-accommodation-and-access-in-higher-education/

Kessler, Ronald, Cindy Foster, William Saunders, and Paul Stang. 1995. "Social Consequences of Psychiatric Disorders, I: Educational Attainment." *American Journal of Psychiatry* 152: 1026–32. doi:10.1176/ajp.152.7.1026

Lewiecki-Wilson, Cynthia. 2003. "Rethinking Rhetoric through Mental Disabilities." *Rhetoric Review* 22 (2): 156–67.

Lightner, Kirsten L., Deborah Kipps-Vaughan, Timothy Schulte, and Ashton D. Trice. 2012. "Reasons University Students with a Learning Disability Wait to Seek Disability Services." *Journal of Postsecondary Education and Disability* 25 (2): 145–59.

Marshak, Laura, Todd Van Wieren, Dianne Raeke Ferrell, Lindsay Swiss, and Catherine Dugan. 2010. "Exploring Barriers to College Student Use of Disability Services and Accommodations." *Journal of Postsecondary Education and Disability* 22 (3): 151–65.

Myers, Kimberly Rena. 2007. *Illness in the Academy: A Collection of Pathographies by Academics.* West Lafayette, IN: Purdue University Press.

Price, Margaret. 2011a. *Mad at School: Rhetorics of Mental Disability and Academic Life.* Ann Arbor: University of Michigan Press.

Price, Margaret. 2011b. "It Shouldn't Be So Hard." *Inside Higher Ed* (February 7). https://www.insidehighered.com/advice/2011/02/07/margaret_price_on_the_search_process_for_those_with_mental_disabilities

Price, Margaret. 2015. "The Bodymind Problem and the Possibilities of Pain." *Hypatia* 30 (1): 268–84. doi:10.1111/hypa.12127

Price, Margaret, Mark Salzer, Amber M. O'Shea, and Stephanie L. Kerschbaum. 2017. "Disclosure of Mental Disability by College and University Faculty: The Negotiation of Accommodations, Supports, and Barriers." *Disability Studies Quarterly* 37 (2) http://dsq-sds.org/article/view/5487

Price, Margaret, and Stephanie L. Kerschbaum. 2015. "Disabled Faculty" (unpublished interview data).

Pryal, Katie Rose Guest. 2014a. "Disclosure Blues: Should You Tell Colleagues about Your Mental Illness?" *Chronicle of Higher Education Vitae*, June 13, 2014, https://chroniclevitae.com/news/546-disclosure-blues-should-you-tell-colleagues-about-your-mental-illness

Pryal, Katie Rose Guest. 2014b. "Rough Accommodations." *Chronicle of Higher Education Vitae*, November 20, 2014, https://chroniclevitae.com/news/809-rough-accommodations

Pryal, Katie Rose Guest. 2015. "Revisiting Disclosure." *Chronicle of Higher Education Vitae.* June 26, 2015. https://chroniclevitae.com/news/1047-revisiting-disclosure

Saks, Elyn R. 2007. *The Center Cannot Hold: My Journey through Madness.* New York: Hyperion.

Salzer, Mark S. 2012. "A Comparative Study of Campus Experiences of College Students with Mental Illnesses Versus a General College Sample." *Journal of American College Health* 60 (1): 1–7. doi:10.1080/07448481.2011.552537

Salzer, Mark S., Lindsay C. Wick, and Joseph A. Rogers. 2008. "Familiarity with and Use of Accommodations and Supports among Postsecondary Students with Mental Illness." *Psychiatric Services* 59 (4): 370–75. doi:10.1176/ps.2008.59.4.370

Samuels, Ellen. "Crip Time: Undoing the Normative Future." Unpublished manuscript. Last updated January 2015. Microsoft Word document.

Siebers, Tobin. 2010. "In the Name of Pain." *Against Health: How Health Became the New Morality*, edited by Jonathan M. Metzl & Anna Kirkland, 183–94. New York: New York University Press.

Skogen, Rochelle. 2012. "'Coming into Presence' as Mentally Ill in Academia: A New Logic of Emancipation." *Harvard Educational Review* 82 (4): 491–510. doi:10.17763/haer.82.4.u1m8g0052212pjh8

Smith, Phil, ed. 2013. *Both Sides of the Table: Autoethnographies of Educators Learning and Teaching with/In Disability*. New York: Peter Lang.

Sue, Derald Wing, Christina M. Capodilupo, Gina C. Torino, Jennifer M. Bucceri, Aisha M. B. Holder, Kevin L. Nadal, and Marta Esquilin. 2007. "Racial Microaggressions in Everyday Life: Implications for Clinical Practice." *American Psychologist* 62 (4): 271–86. doi:10.1037/0003-066x.62.4.271

"Supporting Accommodation Requests: Guidance on Documentation Practices." 2012. Association on Higher Education And Disability. https://www.ahead. org/learn/resources/documentation-guidance

Teichler, Ulrich, Akira Arimoto, and William K. Cummings. 2013. *The Changing Academic Profession: Major Findings of a Comparative Survey*. Dordrecht, Netherlands: Springer.

Titchkosky, Tanya. 2011. *The Question of Access: Disability, Space, Meaning*. Toronto: University of Toronto Press.

Wolf, Lorraine E. 2001. "College Students with ADHD and Other Hidden Disabilities." *Annals of the New York Academy of Sciences* 931: 385–95. doi:10.1111/j.1749-6632.2001.tb05792.x

Wood, Tara Kathleen. 2014. *Disability and College Composition: Investigating Access, Identity, and Rhetorics of Ableism*. PhD diss., University of Oklahoma. Communication with author.

Vance, Mary Lee, ed. 2007. *Disabled Faculty and Staff in a Disabling Society: Multiple Identities in Higher Education*. Huntersville, NC: AHEAD.

Zola, Irving Kenneth. 1988. "The Language of Disability: Problems of Politics and Practice." *Australian Disability Review* 1 (3): 13–21.

An Initial Model for Accommodation Communication between Students with Disabilities and Faculty

TONETTE S. ROCCO

JOSHUA C. COLLINS

The disability rights movement in higher education began in the fall of 1962 when Ed Roberts chose a school based on his academic needs not his disability (Shapiro 1993). At the time, only four university campuses were accessible to individuals with disabilities. He needed the university to accommodate his iron lung, the technology of the time that helped him breathe. He also needed a way to get into buildings and to classes. These were major considerations. Prior to the 1970s, children with disabilities were not guaranteed a public education, nor did nonveterans with disabilities have a legally protected right to an accessible education. Section 504 of the Rehabilitation Act of 1973 (P. L. 93–112) changed that, making it illegal for any federal agency, public university, or recipient of federal funds to discriminate against an individual on the basis of a disability. The Americans with Disabilities Act of 1990 (P. L. 101–336) (ADA) expanded the protection provided by Section 504 into the areas of employment, state and local government services, public accommodations and commercial facilities, and telecommunications. The ADA Amendments Act of 2008 (ADAAA) further expanded the definition of "disability" to be more broad and inclusive (Bowman 2011). The foundation of the ADA is based on Section 504 and the Civil Rights Act of 1964 with the intent to "protect against institutionalized and structural discrimination while simultaneously fostering social inclusion across all domains of public life" (Parker Harris et al. 2014, para 1).

Both the ADA and ADAAA define a disability as "a physical or mental impairment that substantially limits one or more of the major life activities of such individual; a record of such an impairment; or being regarded as having such an impairment" (P. L. 101–336; §3). Learning is considered a major life activity and students can request reasonable accommodations. Academic accommodations include a range of strategies that provide equal access to course materials, academic programs, and student services without compromising quality or content (Hadley 2007). These strategies are often determined through consultations between the students and the staff in an office serving students with disabilities, who then inform the faculty member who works with disability services to implement the accommodations.

Students have the right to choose whether or not to consider themselves disabled. If a student considers her- or himself disabled and in need of accommodations, then the student must disclose and request accommodation—a task which requires skills in self–advocacy, self-disclosure, navigating higher education student services, and managing faculty expectations (Rocco and Fornes 2010; Rocco 2001a). Institutions have the right to verify the disability and discuss reasonable accommodations. This begins the obligation of the postsecondary institution to accommodate the individual with the disability (Jarrow 1993).

The number of students with disabilities who are academically prepared and capable of earning four-year degrees is growing. Five years after passage of the Rehabilitation Act of 1973, 2.6 percent of first-year college students reported a disability; by 1994, the number of students had increased to 9.2 percent (Henderson 1995). According to the National Center for Education Statistics (2015), 11 percent of undergraduate students in the 2007–8 and 2011–12 academic years had disabilities. While this percentage has held relatively steady since 1996, students have an increased awareness of their rights due to several generations benefiting from the federal special education law (IDEA) and Section 504 protection. Veterans and others who became disabled in high school or later are more knowledgeable about their rights. While the environment for people with disabilities has not changed enough, there is more awareness of disability and more familiarity with common accommodations such as ramps and restrooms than existed five decades ago. Understanding the process of communicating accommodation needs and the potential pitfalls for students, faculty, and the institution is important to the success of students with disabilities seeking undergraduate degrees.

This chapter describes a model for the accommodation communication (AC), which focuses on the communication process between faculty and students with disabilities in higher education. Before this communication occurs, the student must report to the office that serves students with disabilities on campus in order to be certified as disabled. Often, this office advises students on how to talk to faculty, sends a notice of a need to accommodate to faculty, and works with students and faculty to ensure compliance and understanding. All steps in the process are important; however, an experience students have with faculty can overshadow other experiences in college, positively or negatively. The standards of the Association on Higher Education And Disability (AHEAD n.d.) that guide disability services are concerned with the disability services interactions with the institution, students, and faculty. While the standards promote self-determination of students, the actions taken by the office of disability services are unique to the institution and between the office and the student or the office and the instructor (Dukes and Shaw 2008).

The model presented in this paper is focused primarily on the interaction between the student and faculty member. The disclosure relationship between a student and faculty member closely mirrors the same forced disclosure the student will have to make to a prospective employer. We use the phrase forced disclosure to acknowledge that disclosure is mandated by law as a first step to securing accommodation. Many accommodations afforded college students with disabilities are taken for granted activities by students without disabilities. This is consequential. For instance, a student with a disability must disclose and ask for an accommodation to record audio of a classroom discussion; a student without a disability audio records the discussion without asking permission from anyone. It is disturbing, and ironic, that a system intended to equalize the playing field can actually create such inequalities and injustices.

Relevant to the AC are the notions of self-advocacy and self-disclosure. Self-advocacy can be defined as individuals "speaking up and speaking out for themselves, solving their own problems and making their own decisions, knowing and exercising the full rights and responsibilities of citizenship" (People First of Washington 1986, 2). According to Gadbow and DuBois (1998), "Self-advocacy encourages individuals with disabilities to advocate for the accommodations that they require, but it also stresses that little is gained when demands and requests are viewed as unreasonable" (101). Other aspects important to successful self-advocacy are: (a) providing a rationale, (b) understanding different perspectives, (c) stressing the importance of academic standards and mastery of material, and (d) resolving problems while building rapport (Gadbow and DuBois 1998). Self-disclosure involves the verbal presentation of information to another person about the nature or cause of a personal experience. Self-disclosure is "any information exchange that refers to the self, including personal states, dispositions, events in the past, and plans for the future" (Derlega and Grzelak 1979, 152). Disclosure is the most important element in AC. Four factors are involved in the decision of a person with a disability to disclose voluntarily: (a) weighing the positive and negative reactions of others, (b) determining its value to the relationship, (c) reducing uncertainty and tension for adults with disabilities, and (d) reducing the tension and uncertainty of adults without disabilities (Rocco 2001a).

Accommodation Communication Model

The AC model presented in this chapter emerged from the authors' dissertation research and subsequent research around disability and disclosure, especially a study where faculty and students with invisible and visible disabilities were interviewed about their experiences with accommodations (Rocco 1997). The model has been further informed by the authors' institutional-level service (e.g., disability task force, founding member of student organization); working relationships with disability services at two universities (Midwest, Southeast); work with students with disabilities as faculty members at three large, research-focused institutions (Midwest, Southeast, and South); mentoring students with disabilities; and listening to faculty concerns, as well as insights from the literature. The literature that informs this work comes from adult education, disability studies, and disclosure. The ADA specifies that a person with a disability must **request** an accommodation, before there is any **responsibility** to accommodate (bold elements in figure 1). The process starts with a legal mandate that forces disclosure regarding disability status, accessibility needs, and often presentation of documentation of the disability. Disclosure is accompanied by validation of the information, which can occur as a formal request for documentation or by tacit acceptance of the disclosure. After a request for accommodation occurs, it creates the responsibility to provide reasonable accommodations on the part of the instructor, institution, or employer. The responsibility to accommodate exists once the request has been made and the institution and/or instructor is satisfied that the student's claim is legitimate. The importance and credibility of the disclosure is based upon the timing of the request and the way negotiations proceed. As the student and instructor negotiate, the student communicates his or her needs, and the instructor imparts her or his expectations of academic performance; this negotiation process, when successful, produces mutually acceptable goals.

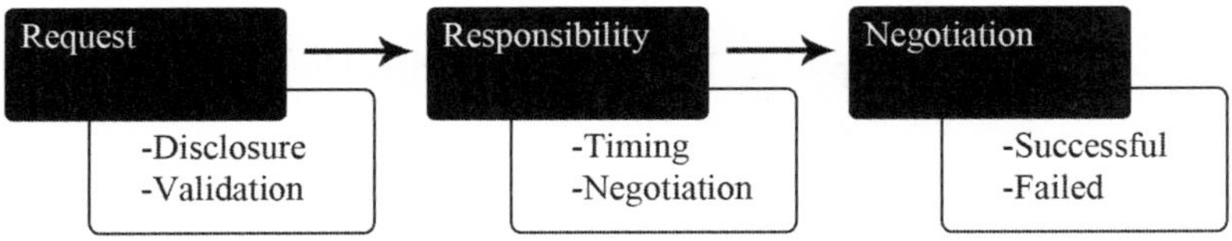

Fig. 1. Accommodation and communication model

The accommodation communication is the act of requesting access to the materials, documents, and information provided by an instructor that facilitate or enhance learning the course content. The model is presented here in an effort to help faculty and students improve their communication about accommodation needs and is based on our views of this process as it is. The elements of the accommodation communication are: (a) requesting accommodations, (b) disclosure, (c) validation, (d) the responsibility to accommodate, (e) timing of request, (f) negotiating accommodations, and (g) failed negotiations.

Requesting Accommodations

A student who needs the accommodation initiates the process by making the request, which can be directed towards an individual, a department, or an institution. This usually begins when the student reports to disability services to be certified as a person with a disability and to determine possible, appropriate accommodations. Students usually make their original requests at the institutional level by notifying disability services. In most postsecondary institutions, notification of disability services is required before any accommodations are provided.

Once the student has been certified by disability services, the next step is to contact the instructor. In the experience of the two authors, this has played out differently depending on the institution. At the Midwestern university, after connecting with disability services, students would contact the instructor to discuss accommodations in the course, bringing documentation to verify the claim. Counselors worked with students individually and in workshops to develop self-advocacy skills. At the Southeastern university, instructors were notified via email that an accommodation was needed and how to carry it out. Students might never speak directly to the instructor about the accommodation. At the Southern university, students would contact the instructor to discuss accommodations in the course, and instructors would communicate with disability services to verify the claim and strategize appropriate accommodations.

There are many issues with these scenarios. Some disability rights advocates suggest that disability services should handle such communication. However, this extends the dependence of the student with a disability on an agency to take care of an issue for him or her. Other advocates suggest students should not have to deal with faculty because faculty can be skeptical, rude, and discriminatory or prejudiced against the student (Rocco 1997; Rocco 1999). The ADA forces this communication and gives the power to the temporarily able-bodied person. If students practice this communication while pursuing higher education, maybe they will be better able to counter the negative attitudes of potential employers when they seek employment.

Another issue arises when students, for a variety of reasons, do not contact disability services for accommodations. They may decide to deal directly with the instructor, struggle in a class until they realize they need help and approach the instructor, or the instructor senses something is wrong and speaks to the student. Two issues arise when students discuss accommodations with their instructors: disclosure and validation.

Disclosure

Disclosure is not a benign or neutral act. In fact, there are two classifications of people who are required to disclose in higher education: people with disabilities and people with felony convictions (Rocco, Collins, Meeker, and Whitehead 2012). We believe this is an important distinction when contemplating how the process of communicating accommodation needs unfolds.

Several issues exist surrounding disclosure: (a) making people feel more comfortable, (b) the negative impacts of attitudes and stereotyping, (c) the issue of power in the disclosure relationship, (d) reactions to disclosure, and (e) the process of understanding and articulating the disability (Rocco 1997). The amount of personal information necessary for disclosure varies according to type of disability, length of time the person has lived with the disability, and the comfort level with disclosure. On the other side, recipients of the disclosure vary according to their knowledge of disability, attitudes about persons with disabilities, and willingness to find the disclosure credible.

Students with visible disabilities often disclose to put the recipient of the disclosure at ease (Rocco 2001b), believing it is their responsibility to do so. Students with disabilities disclose more personal information than students without disabilities to lay the groundwork for asking permission to do things that students without disabilities take for granted such as recording class lectures. Students with invisible disabilities, such as cognitive or mental disabilities, may have trouble understanding what to say to an instructor and how to say it. This can sometimes be a manifestation of the disability and sometimes not. However, instructors are rarely trained to understand general or specific manifestations of disabilities and may look upon this fumbling as dishonesty. If a student has difficulty with disclosure, it is likely the student will also have difficulty with the other steps in the model.

Validation

The disclosure and request for accommodation can be made by an individual with a disability, but if it is not believed, an accommodation might not be made. How a disability is validated is not defined by law. Section 504 and the ADA require verification of the disability, which is made through assessment procedures determined by disability services and the administration (Schuck and Kroeger 1993). The ADAAA does not specify documentation of disability status (Bowman 2011). Guidelines have been suggested by the Educational Testing Service (ETS) and AHEAD (Shaw, Keenan, Madaus, and Banerjee 2010), but their implementation is at the discretion of the institution. Administrations are often concerned with cost containment and providing accommodations only to officially diagnosed students.

Validation is the process a student goes through with an institution or instructor to establish a right to accommodation. Validation of the claim is made (a) upon registration of the student with disability services, (b) when written documentation verifying the disability is received by the instructor, (c) by calling disability services to verify information with a counselor, and/or (d) by accepting the word of the student. This is accomplished only when the instructor is satisfied the disability exists and the student is not trying to take advantage of the system (Rocco 2000). In some institutions, disability services informs an instructor that a student needs an accommodation. There are problems with this approach. It takes the responsibility away from the adult college student to negotiate with the instructor, and there are issues with timing. For example, at institutions where notifications from disability services may not come until a week or two into the semester, students may be forced to go without accommodation for a considerable amount of time.

Either the desire to follow procedure or skepticism can motivate a request for documentation. Instructors who trust and respect students are more likely to take at face value the disclosure and accommodation request. Some instructors have expressed dismay with instructors who think anyone might claim a disability if they do not have one; this concern echoes the sentiments of students with invisible disabilities who may feel no one wants the negative stereotyping that comes with disability disclosure (Rocco 1999; 2000).

When the instructor is satisfied that the disclosure and request for accommodations are valid, acceptance of the disclosure has occurred. The institution, through disability services, controls this element if the student registers with the office. In the end, though, the instructor's control over this element is more meaningful to the student's future. Even if the notification comes from disability services, the instructor can choose not to implement the accommodation or can simply forget to implement it each class session. Or the instructor can be skeptical that a disability exists, questioning the student's veracity and capability (Rocco 1999).

Responsibility to Accommodate

The responsibility to accommodate begins with the accommodation request, creating a legal and financial obligation to make accommodations. The responsibility to accommodate is usually seen first as an institutional responsibility, even though the institution, disability services, the department, instructors, and students should share it. Faculty sometimes feel they would like to help, but believe accommodations really are within the purview of disability services (Rocco 2000). Faculty may feel their home departments do not have the resources or time to provide accommodations, such as securing an audio or digital version of a textbook. Faculty can also struggle with knowing what to do for the student. Some faculty have described self-directed learning projects they engaged in to inform them about particular disabilities when they felt a personal connection to someone with the disability (Rocco 2000), but it is rare for faculty to understand disability status.

Other faculty may consider accommodations one more burden the institution places on them. Because of this, some faculty may think they have the right to deny an accommodation. The right to deny an accommodation often comes from the faculty members' beliefs that they know what is fair to the instructor and other, non-disabled students. The sentiment of fairness and personal rights is usually directed toward students with invisible cognitive disabilities, such as attention deficit or learning disabilities, more often than those with visible disabilities. These disabilities are "suspect disabilities," meaning faculty at times express doubts as to whether they should be classified as disabilities (Rocco 2000).

Students utilize disability services for all accommodation needs until the office fails to ensure the accommodations happen. Students have reported scribes for exams not being capable of writing mathematical symbols or of books not being audio recorded well or in time. When disability services fails to provide meaningful accommodations, students can respond in a number of ways. Some do nothing, others go to another school; ask the academic department for assistance; or recruit classmates, friends, relatives, or pay people to help them (Rocco 1997; 2001b). Thus, a major issue related to the responsibility to accommodate is that when that responsibility has not been met by the appropriate party(ies), people with disabilities often assume the onus of responsibility and may become less likely to disclose in the future.

Timing of the Request

The timing of the request can be guided by the student's personality, the type of accommodation needed, external support, and self-discovery. Instructors influence the timing of the request by their availability, understanding, and willingness to comply. Students who want to communicate accommodation needs to the instructor before the first day of class can only do so if they can reach the instructor by phone, in person, or by e-mail. Instructors may not always be available and sometimes forget to return phone calls or reply to messages.

The timing of the request for accommodation affects credibility and the ability to facilitate the accommodation. Timing can affect the reception of the disclosure, the accommodation request, and the responsibility to accommodate. The earlier a student discloses in the term, the more credible and "doable" the request is perceived to be. Disclosure timing ranges from before the term begins to the last weeks of the term. Faculty usually favorably remember students who request accommodations prior to the beginning of the term and on the first day of class but are suspicious of those who disclose later in the term (Rocco 2000).

Students might disclose near the end of a term because of recent diagnosis or when compensation skills have failed. Faculty might become frustrated and question the ability of the student. A recent diagnosis creates other difficulties. The diagnosis does not create an instant and complete understanding in an individual of the disability, its manifestations, and needed accommodations. Without adequate knowledge and experience, articulating accommodation needs concisely and with assurance is difficult and can make a student appear incompetent and full of excuses for inadequate performance. This is particularly acute when the student has an invisible disability, as noted by one faculty participant in Rocco's (2000) study:

> When she came in and almost had a look of ecstasy on her face because she had been diagnosed and that sort of explained it all—But this person was sort of like using it as an excuse for—suddenly there was all the answers why things weren't working for her. . . . Maybe I could understand that up to a point because she was having some problems getting things done and so suddenly she sort of had a label or a reason but it's as I've always said to my oldest son [who is hard of hearing] that might be an explanation but it's not necessarily an excuse. What you do is find ways to compensate. I didn't say any of this to her because it was the end of the quarter. (p. 388)

This situation raises several issues. First, the student did not know enough about the disability to speak convincingly about accommodations. Her words sounded to the instructor like rambling. Second, the student's work in the course had been unsatisfactory to the point that the instructor wondered if she was capable of doctoral level work. When she disclosed a disability she only recently discovered and didn't know much about, her credibility suffered. A common misperception is that individuals with attention deficit disorder are not very bright. It was easy for the instructor not to move from this belief, especially when the student could not articulate why she was disclosing and what, if anything, he could do for her so late in the quarter other than give her an incomplete for the course. The instructor would have given any student an incomplete with a reasonable explanation. In this case, this student's disability interfered with her accurate assessment of the situation and when to disclose.

Third, the counselor failed to provide the student with adequate information about the disability and accommodations needed. In this case, this counseling deficit contributed to a strained relationship between a doctoral student and an instructor. For undergraduate students, a loss of credibility produces discomfort for the term. For a graduate student, and particularly a doctoral student, the instructor may be encountered repeatedly and serve on the exam or dissertation committees and can influence the opinions of other faculty.

An instructor can delay and hinder a requested accommodation in other ways as well. Students sometimes describe instances where the instructor did not provide an initial reading list, or loan a book, or send in a book order in time to have it audio recorded. Students without disabilities can access the material on the reading list the same day they receive the list, if they choose to do so. It can take several weeks before a student can have a book recorded, depending on the availability of a digital or audio recording from the publisher and on the backlog at disability services. On occasion, instructors have refused to accommodate students with invisible disabilities because they did not believe their disclosure. This reaction increases the time delay before accommodations are started because students must turn to disability services, which will advocate on their behalf. If the instructor does not believe the student, then the accommodation communication has not been finalized or has failed. This usually results in intervention by disability services, or the student may choose to withdraw from the course. The timing of the accommodation request is critical to any future relationship between the instructor and student. If the student has to take multiple classes with an instructor who is skeptical and wonders if the disclosure is accurate or honest, the ramifications are serious for the student's learning and overall wellbeing.

Negotiating Accommodations

Negotiating accommodations is the act of determining to what degree the instructor and the student each find the request and its compliance reasonable and adequate (Rocco 2000). The phrase "reasonable accommodations" lays the groundwork for negotiations between parties to determine what is reasonable. Negotiation is thought of as a process that people engage in who each have something to offer to the other party. In this case, instructors may usually be more concerned with losing something such as academic freedom, decision-making control, academic standards, or time. For example, some instructors feel that accommodating a student will take time away from their other duties, time they do not want to waste. One instructor in Rocco's (2000) study spoke about students with cognitive disabilities as needing more guidance on writing assignments and believed this to be time taken away from other students. Rarely do instructors consider the benefits to other students in the class when certain accommodations are made universally available (Torkelson-Lynch and Gussel 1996). Some instructors have reported that changing teaching styles for a student with vision impairment has helped them to become more aware of different senses (Rocco 2000).

Effective communication involves assigning each party responsibility, which is understood as such by both. The student is usually requesting an academic accommodation and providing the instructor with the necessary documentation. Instructors usually believe that the student is the primary source of information about the disability and accommodations. Some instructors may express the idea that accommodations are negotiated between the student, who knows how the disability manifested itself, and the instructor, who knows the course material. For other instructors, additional information about the necessary accommodations is seen as the responsibility of an agency. The idea of negotiating is lopsided. Instructors often consider it much more a reality than do students. Instructors see accommodation as a negotiation process because they feel a need to find compromises between their time (and other) constraints and a student's needs (Rocco 2000). Student responses to the negotiation can vary from waiting patiently for compliance, or when instructors do not comply for whatever reason, attempting to secure the accommodation in another way.

Part of the dynamic between instructor and students negotiating accommodations includes the fact that the student is trying to communicate needs and the instructor is trying to communicate expectations. The student whose student-instructor negotiation failed does not have access to the course material in the same manner as students without disabilities. This may affect the student's grade in subtle or not so subtle ways. If the instructor fails to communicate his or her expectations, the instructor's attitude toward this student or students with disabilities may be negatively impacted. The instructor may believe the failed communication is because of some deficit on the student's part rather than assume responsibility for being vague. A failed negotiation rarely affects the instructor in a meaningful way.

If the student fails to communicate needs so that the instructor understands them or the instructor fails to comply with the request, the negotiations fail and the student must take an alternative action, which varies in intensity and impact. The student's experience, attitude, coping ability, and the number and severity of similar failed negotiations determine the intensity of the response. These student responses (see table 8), from least resistant to most resistant, are to become: (a) withdrawn, (b) passive, (c) an advocate, or (d) an adversary. The student's response affects the student and the university more than the faculty member.

Withdrawn

Perhaps the most alarming response a student with a disability may have to failed negotiation is to become withdrawn. A student may withdraw socially and isolate herself or himself in effort to cope with disability alone, relying only on the self. Becoming withdrawn in such a way may influence the student to refrain from disclosure in the future. A student may also withdraw from the environment altogether, meaning exiting a particular course, department, major, or the university over a failed negotiation experience.

Passive

A passive response occurs when the student excuses their own or an instructor's behavior or ignores the difficulty. When a student ignores the difficulty and waits until the information is provided to the entire class, the student might make up for lost time by trying to encourage others to do their part quickly, or just wait patiently, pretending it does not matter. Another tactic

Table 8. Student reactions to the breakdown of negotiations

Type of Response (from least to most resistant)	Level or Direction of Response	Examples of Internal-External Responses
Withdrawn	(a) Into oneself	
	(b) From the environment	1. Class 2. Major/department 3. University
Passive	(a) Ignore difficulties	1. Make up for lost time 2. Go around the instructor
	(b) Excuse the behavior	1. Being nice is expected 2. Feelings of helplessness 3. Afraid of • Curtailed services • Offending the instructor • Affected grades
Advocacy	(a) On behalf of oneself	
	(b) On behalf of others	1. For support 2. Coalition of students 3. Interactions with management
Adversary	(a) File complaint with the university	1. Disability Services 2. President, Vice Presidents, Deans 3. Board of Trustees
	(b) File external complaint	1. State or Federal Agencies 2. Public Opinion 3. Media

would be to go around the instructor by going to a former student to get the reading list or to disability services for intervention.

A passive student starts out by excusing the behavior of the instructor for three reasons: (a) being nice is expected, (b) feelings of helplessness, and (c) fear (Rocco 1997; 1999; 2001b). The student is afraid that (a) the instructor will be offended, (b) the grade might be affected, or (c) services will be curtailed. Feelings of helplessness are often prevalent with students who do not know how to articulate their needs or feel the more they push the instructor, the less they will be liked. For graduate students who interact with the same instructor many times, this can create an ongoing problem.

Most instructors believe themselves to be fair-minded and able to control the effect of their attitude on the grade a student earns. An instructor with a negative attitude about a student's disability may believe she or he can fairly grade the work and that the student did not know about the negative attitudes. However, students have reported being aware when instructors have negative attitudes toward them or their disability (Rocco 1997; 2000), and often feel powerless to say anything.

Advocate

Advocacy is the proactive, firm, and responsible pursuit of reasonable accommodations. Students advocate for accommodations on behalf of themselves and other students, and sometimes form groups to work with the administration. Advocating involves persistence in dealing with the instructor to get a reading list or syllabus prior to the term starting. The first request for the accommodation includes a time frame for the instructor. When the instructor does not have the material(s) ready when discussed, more information can be provided to the instructor either about the importance of time, the steps involved in carrying out the accommodation, or information about the disability and its impact on learning and accessing information. This information might encourage the instructor to meet the next negotiated deadline. If this tactic does not work, disability service providers can be asked to call the instructor to advocate on behalf of the student. Sometimes fellow students can become advocates on behalf of other students with disabilities by accompanying them to visit the instructor to discuss accommodations.

Students may organize student groups to advocate on behalf of students with disabilities, to provide moral support, and to have greater strength when discussing issues with the administration. Moral support includes listening to other students, discussing ideas, and finding their own solutions such as supporting disability services on grant applications or volunteering in the office. Advocacy groups can make positive contributions to campus life. The administration can learn from the innovative ideas and practical solutions offered by students. If the administration encourages the students to help, an additional source of volunteers to assist with the work of disability services is available, saving the university money. If the students in the advocacy groups are not listened to and given positive outlets for their frustration, they may become adversarial in their dealings with the university.

Adversary

The breakdown of negotiations can become adversarial after the student has tried the other approaches without results. Students do not enter a university believing they are going to have to fight for every accommodation they receive. On the contrary, this reaction comes about over time, accompanied by much frustration. Formal and informal testimony can be made with the university through the ombudsperson, the board of trustees, the President, and other high-level administrators. Legal action starts with filing a complaint with the appropriate state or federal agency.

Legal actions can cost the university real money, not estimated dollars from the loss of a potential market. This real money is spent on lawyers, extra security when protests ensue, combating negative publicity, and to rectify the situation. If the court orders a university to rectify the situation, the terms, conditions, and time frame for making program adjustments will no longer be at the sole discretion of the university.

Implications for Higher Education

With growing numbers of adults with disabilities on college and university campuses, it is important to know and understand the process of communicating accommodation needs. Students who do not know how to effectively communicate these needs may experience increased discrimination and limited education and employment opportunities. Educators who react negatively to disclosure may find that these students leave their programs or take legal action.

Frequently, disability is glossed over if mentioned at all in conversations about diversity and multiculturalism (Rocco and Delgado 2011). Educators can assist students with disabilities by providing increased opportunities for discussion of disability issues. First, by including an accommodation statement on all course syllabi (Rocco 1995); instructors can then discuss this statement as they cover the syllabus during the first class. This may create a friendlier atmosphere for students with disabilities in the classroom, possibly encouraging a discussion of the differences in accessing information among all students. Students with and without disabilities may benefit from learning about different ways to access information. Second, instructors that strive to include material on gender or race in course packets should also consider including relevant material on disability issues or experiences. Third, once a disclosure has been made to an instructor, the instructor can take this opportunity to practice the accommodation communication. This may be particularly helpful to students with invisible disabilities whose opportunities to practice disability disclosure and the accommodation communication are often limited (Rocco 1997). Disability disclosures done ineffectively, without ready suggestions for accommodation and poorly timed, increase the likelihood of further stereotyping and discrimination (Torkelson-Lynch and Gussel 1996). Implementing these suggestions, accommodation statements, readings on disability, and encouraging discussion, will provide opportunities to make the experience of this minority group more visible, which may change attitudes and stereotyping behaviors of other members of the class or faculty.

Many faculty assume that the way their institution handles accommodations is the correct and only way to act; however, disability services procedures vary across the country. AHEAD and ETS have standards to guide processes and procedures of disability services offices (Shaw et al. 2010). These standards cover advocacy efforts, disability awareness, and working with faculty in a number of ways. For example, disability services offices that teach students self-determination and self-advocacy skills as well as the skills necessary to learn about the students' own disability also enable students to share information with instructors in a meaningful way. Disability services that send notices to instructors and do not encourage the students to speak to instructors may be doing these students a disservice. Providing students opportunities to practice disclosure for accommodation purposes can help them to confidently ask for reasonable accommodations in employment situations. Also, disability services can help make faculty aware of hidden biases such as sympathizing with a person who has a visible disability while finding someone with an invisible disability less credible. Many universities have centers that work to improve the teaching effectiveness of faculty. Disability services can work with these centers to infuse through their curriculum information on learning styles and needs that include students with disabilities. When faculty think about different ways to learn, incorporating techniques that make their teaching more accessible can improve learning for all students.

References

AHEAD. *AHEAD Program Standards and Performance Indicators*. Retrieved from: https://www.ahead.org/uploads/docs/resources/Final-Program-Standards-with-Performance-Indicators.doc

Americans with Disabilities Act of 1990. Public Law 101–336. § 1.

Americans with Disabilities Act Amendments Act of 2008. Public Law 110–325. § 3406.

Bowman, Lorenzo. 2011. "Americans with Disabilities Act as Amended: Principles and Practice." *New Directions for Adult and Continuing Education* 132: 85–95. doi:10.1002/ace.434

Derlega, Valerian J., and Janusz Grzelak. 1979. "Appropriateness of Self-Disclosure." In *Self-Disclosure: Origins, Patterns, and Implications of Openness in Interpersonal Relationships*, edited by G. J. Chelune, 151–76. San Francisco: Jossey-Bass.

Dukes III, L. L., and Stan F. Shaw. 2008. "Using the AHEAD Program Standards and Performance Indicators to Promote Self-Determination in the Daily Practice of Office of Disability Services." *Journal of Postsecondary Education and Disability*. 21(2): 105–8.

Gadbow, Nancy F., and David A. Du Bois. 1998. *Adult Learners with Special Needs. Strategies and Resources for Postsecondary Education and Workplace Training*. Malabar, FL: Krieger.

Hadley, Wanda M. 2007. "The Necessity of Academic Accommodations for First-Year College Students with Learning Disabilities." *Journal of College Admission* 195: 9–13.

Henderson, Cathy. 1995. *College Freshmen with Disabilities: A Triennial Statistical Profile*. Washington, DC: American Council on Education, Heath Resource Center.

Jarrow, Jane. 1993. "Beyond Ramps: New Ways of Viewing Access." *New Directions for Student Services* 64: 5–16. San Francisco: Jossey-Bass.

National Center for Education Statistics. 2015. *Digest of Education Statistics*. U.S. Department of Education. https://nces.ed.gov/programs/digest/d13/tables/dt13_311.10.asp

Parker Harris, Sarah, Robert Gould, Patrick Ojok, Glenn Fujiura, Robin Jones, and Avery Olmstead IV. 2014. "Scoping Review of the Americans with Disabilities Act: What Research Exists, and Where Do We Go from Here?" *Disability Studies Quarterly* 34 (3).

People First of Washington. 1986. "People First of Washington." *The U. T. Quarterly* 2–3.

Rehabilitation Act of 1973. Public Law 93–112.

Rocco, Tonette S. 1995. "Academic Accommodation: Meaning and Implications for Adult Education Practitioners." *Midwest Research-to-Practice Conference in Adult, Continuing, and Community Education*. Chicago, IL.

Rocco, Tonette S. 1997. "Hesitating to Disclose: Adult Students with Invisible Disabilities and Their Experiences with Understanding and Articulating Disability." *Midwest Research-to-Practice Conference in Adult, Continuing, and Community Education*. East Lansing, MI.

Rocco, Tonette S. 1999. "Aren't You Glad You're Not Stupid?" In A. Austin, G. E. Hynes, and R. T. Miller, eds.. *Proceedings of the 18h Annual Midwest Research-to-Practice Conference in Adult, Continuing, and Community Education*, 226–31. St. Louis, MO: University of Missouri at St. Louis.

Rocco, Tonette S. 2000. "Making Assumptions: Faculty Responses to Students with Disabilities." In *Proceedings of the 41st Adult Education Research Conference*, edited by Thomas J. Sork, Valerie-Lee Chapman, and Ralf St. Clair, 387–91. Vancouver, BC: University of British Columbia.

Rocco, Tonette S. 2001a. "Helping Adult Educators Understand Disability Disclosure." *Adult Learning* 12(2): 10–12.

Rocco, Tonette S. 2001b. "'My Disability Is Part of Me:' Disclosure and Students with Visible Disabilities." In *Proceedings of the 42nd Adult Education Research Conference*, edited by Regina O. Smith, John M. Dirkx, Pamela L. Eddy, Patricia L. Farrell, and Michael Polzin, 319–24. East Lansing, MI: Michigan State University.

Rocco, Tonette S., Joshua C. Collins, Carolyn Meeker and Chaundra Whitehead. 2012. "Disclosing 'Deviance' in the Workplace: Understanding the Relationship between Disclosure, and Stigmatized Identities." In *Proceedings of the LGBTQ Preconference* edited by J. Gedro, M. Eichler, and R. Mizzi, 22–26. Saratoga Springs: Empire State University.

Rocco, Tonette S. and Antonio Delgado. 2011. "Shifting Lenses: A Critical Examination of Disability in Adult Education." *New Directions for Adult and Continuing Education* 132: 3–12.

Rocco, Tonette S., and Sandra Fornes. 2010. "Perspectives on Disability in Adult and Continuing Education." In *The Handbook of Adult and Continuing Education*, edited by A. Rose, C. Kasworm and J. Ross-Gordon, 379–88. Thousand Oaks: Sage.

Schuck, Judy, and Sue Kroeger. 1993. "Essential Elements in Effective Service Delivery." *New Directions for Student Services* 64: 59–68.

Shapiro, Joseph P. 1993. *No Pity: People with Disabilities Forging a New Civil Rights Movement*. New York: Three Rivers Press.

Shaw, Stan, Walter Keenan, Joseph Madaus, and Manju Banerjee. 2010. "Disability Documentation, the Americans with Disabilities Act Amendments Act and the Summary of Performance: How Are They Linked?" *Journal of Postsecondary Education and Disability* 22(3): 142–50.

Torkelson-Lynch, Ruth, and Lori Gussel. 1996. "Disclosure and Self-Advocacy Regarding Disability-Related Needs: Strategies to Maximize Integration in Postsecondary Education." *Journal of Counseling & Development* 74(4): 352–57. doi:10.1002/j.1556–6676.1996.tb01879.x

I Am Different / So Are You

Creating Safe Spaces for Disability Disclosure (A Conversation)

DAISY L. BRENEMAN

SUSAN GHIACIUC

VALERIE L. SCHOOLCRAFT

KERI A. VANDEBERG

Entering the Conversation

Like many collaborations, ours started with a combination of luck and intentionality: two faculty members, the director of the Office of Disability Services and a peer access advocate at James Madison University, decided to answer the Disability Disclosure conference call for papers. Through a series of professional and personal connections, we ended up in the right space to begin conversations. We joined together for this project to provide an example of individuals in different institutional roles stepping into conversation, trusting each other, and building relationships and understanding. Within institutions, hierarchical and horizontal barriers—such as the division between Student Affairs and Academic Affairs—can prevent such conversations, or cause them to occur predominantly in the context of personal, legal, or educational contention. We sought to be proactive and open up welcoming spaces for talking about the processes and experiences of disability disclosure in a campus community. We crossed the boundaries to realize the potential of partnerships in creating inclusive spaces for disability disclosure, not only to facilitate access but to work together to bring about larger campus and social change. By listening to each other, we opened up possibilities for confronting ableism and other forms of power and resource inequalities that can make the process of disclosure so charged.

Drawing on Margaret Price's idea of kairotic spaces, which she describes as "the less formal, often unnoticed, areas of academe where knowledge is produced and power is exchanged" (2011, 21), we recognize such spaces most frequently involve an unequal distribution of power. We extend her ideas to include examples of disclosure on campus across a wide spectrum of bodies residing in kairotic spaces. Our exploration includes not only disclosure between students and faculty but also the multiple other disclosures that take place within a campus community, such as between a faculty member and human resources.

Building on explorations of disability disclosure in higher education, we chose to capture one moment in an ongoing conversation, to demonstrate the nuanced, powerful, and meaningful insights and understanding that can be created in a shared safe space. The project affirms the value of collaboration, perspective taking, and listening. Telling our stories and creating collective ones can be powerful because, as Tobin Siebers (2008, 14) notes, "Identities, narratives, and experiences based on disability have the status of theory because they represent locations and forms of embodiment from which the dominant ideologies of society become visible and open to criticism." With an awareness of the value of relationships, the relational nature (Gilligan 2011) of disclosure, and our interconnectedness as we work to build opportunities for disability disclosure from positions of empowerment and authenticity, we explore the complex social, cultural, and autobiographical forces that influence our perspectives on disability, including how our early experiences bring us to this space.

Individual and Personal Entrance to Disability Disclosure

VALERIE: My first meaningful memory with disability is from childhood. My grandfather had acquired throat cancer and he had surgery. As he was left with no voice box, interactions were emotional and he was frustrated in communication. I remember trying to encourage him: "it's okay; we'll write back and forth." Looking back, we were missing education or tools to work around the challenges. It had tremendous impact on the dynamics of the family and how people were functioning together.

SUSAN: In third grade, I had a classmate who was separated by a cardboard box on three sides. You weren't supposed to talk to him.

However, since I sat next to him, when he would punch his pencil through the cardboard I couldn't ignore him. He was my good friend's brother. I'm still not sure to this day what he had. And I was told to stay away from him for whatever reason—not to interact, but I did.

DAISY: My younger sister was diagnosed with a hearing impairment when she was a year and a half old, when my mother started noticing she wasn't responding to sounds. And I remember it being a sort of tragic disclosure. My mom talks about grieving the loss of a "normal life" for my sister. So the encounter with disability disclosure that shaped my early attitudes was one of loss. It wasn't until college when I started learning about disability, and celebration of Deaf culture, that I realized it doesn't have to be this way.

KERI: My earliest memory of disability and disclosure would be when my older brother got diagnosed with a learning disability— specifically a word processing disorder. At the time, I didn't understand. I had no idea what was really happening. But I remember my mom going to the IEP meetings and complaining to and fighting against the teachers and principals to get him appropriate accommodations. It was a constant battle.

DAISY: Once we start thinking about it, there are these, as you've said, Valerie, unfolding stories about family members and friends with disabilities. It has always been part of our lives. For me, it wasn't until college, when I started getting a vocabulary for it, that connections started happening.

Encountering Issues of Disability and Disclosure on Campus

VALERIE: Our experience, collectively, spans different types of educational settings, different campuses, different issues. It is important to talk about it in terms of the entire campus community. There are all kinds of campus community members—from your folks working in dining halls and your ground staff to your administrative team, right on through all levels of faculty, staff, students, campus visitors, and alumni. People are coming to events in our theaters, attending conferences, and things like that. I'm often encouraging others to remember the wider community complexity in terms of access and inclusion.

DAISY: It's a reminder, too, of the intersections with other issues and identities. Socioeconomic status and cultural capital make a difference in people feeling secure, or not, when disclosing.

SUSAN: One of the first times I encountered disability in the context of teaching writing was at a university where I did graduate work. One of my students had visual and auditory impairments. Since none of my teacher training had covered how to provide accommodations in class, my assignment on the film *Traffic*, ended up putting my student in a really awkward position because she was unable to see any of the subtitles when the characters were speaking in Spanish. In essence, she actually ended up missing one of the major narrative threads occurring in the film.

Nobody told me, "Oh, you could do this or that with the screen." In fact, nobody even told me if we had the technology to do that. I still don't know if I had that option. That's what I remember about the university itself not helping to facilitate disability accommodations on campus. I think you do a great job here with the Office of Disability Services (ODS).

DAISY: I was lucky enough to have been a grad student and new teacher here; we have resources available, so I've always felt supported. But I think the times I've been trying the hardest might be the times when I've made the most mistakes. It's challenging, for example, to give students opportunities to write about disability but also options to say yes or say no to those opportunities.

I immediately think of two students in particular, ones close to my heart, who at first didn't want to write about their disabilities because they didn't want to be defined by them. I pushed, and they eventually decided while they didn't want, they *needed*, to write their stories. Both had good outcomes, but it meant struggle and emotional pain. I recognize the emotional cost. Which is hard. But I saw them both, as they explored, start to become not defined by but owners of, their disability identity—agents. That was amazing. Both now identify as disability advocates.

But I still I wonder if it was the right thing. For some students, I imagine, it's not the right thing, or right time. We have to stay aware of the emotional complexity, to step both carefully and bravely as allies.

KERI: When I was an incoming freshman to James Madison University (JMU) and found out who my roommate was, I knew I needed to disclose because I wanted to pick the side of the room where

I could see her and the other half of the room; it's just personal preference. It makes me feel less blind when I can see the entire space and everyone in it. There's always a moment of hesitation when I am deciding to disclose. I always feel better afterwards, especially with people I would like to have a close relationship with. It's going to be revealed eventually and is a big part of myself, so afterwards I feel like it's out in the open and we can move on. I had a positive experience registering with the ODS. My experience goes onto working with my professors, disclosing to them, and giving them my access plans. Disclosing to professors involves a lot of self-advocacy. As a student, you're hoping the professor is going to be willing to meet you halfway. There have been times, not as many as good times, when I've had bad experiences with professors as a result of disclosing. In my work as a peer access advocate I get to support other students in their struggles coming to terms with disclosure and working with professors.

DAISY: Thank you. Keri, if this question is too personal, just tell me to shut up.

KERI: No, go for it.

DAISY: What are your concerns in the moment of disclosure?

KERI: With professors, it's about how proactive they are because a lot of them are like, "All right, whatever." And they'll take your access plan and forget it exists so it's a constant dialogue of, "Hey, did you remember? I need this accommodation before a test . . ." Which is fine because it is also my job to advocate for my own needs. But if they don't know a lot about your disability, there can be distrust because they don't understand why you need certain accommodations.

Sometimes, they will be unaware of how to create safe spaces for students with disabilities. A professor recently came up to me and a large group of my peers and said, "Which one of you has a visual impairment?" It forced me to disclose in front of everyone but thankfully . . . I'm in a comfortable place. But some students are not and an experience like that could be traumatizing.

DAISY: Do you ever feel like you have to be the voice of disability in classes?

KERI: Most definitely. I think it has less to do with my disability and more that I'm a peer access advocate. It's what I want to do with my career. When the subject comes up, professors might ask me to give a little spiel about the ODS. But I do have one professor I have recurring issues with who will call me out in front of the entire class. We had miscommunication about what preferential seating meant. She wanted me to sit in the front row—but I need to sit on a certain side of the room, not necessarily right up front. On the first day of class, I chose to sit about three rows back on the left side of the room, where I could see most comfortably. After I sat down, my professor looked at me and pointed at a seat in the first row. I proceeded to tell her that I was fine where I was and again she insisted that I move to the front row. We went back and forth a few times until I was incredibly embarrassed—since this was happening in front of my entire class—and just decided to move to the front row.

DAISY: Would you feel comfortable going to talk to that professor?

KERI: Yes and no. In that situation, it was nice to have ODS to come to knowing that I had people I could confide in who would give me advice and support. Valerie and I met and talked for an hour. We decided what I was going to do and how to talk to the professor about the situation.

VALERIE: And I think the concern Keri is mentioning is always relevant for me. Regardless of what point in the situation the student has come into the ODS to talk to me, I remember that this is a unique conversation for this person. What measure of emotion is attached to it? I want to leave that conversation with the student feeling empowered and ready to be a self-advocate because working with students at the collegiate level is to work with them and respect their agency and independence. We're really trying to meet that person wherever they are and walk with them through the next steps of the journey to a more positive outlook and way of talking about it together.

DAISY: I think faculty who disclose deal with some of those hurdles, too.

SUSAN: Yes, when I filed my multiple sclerosis diagnosis with Human Resources (HR), it didn't really feel welcoming. It didn't seem like the process that you're talking about that the students go through in order to say, "Hey, I really need accommodations. I need to talk to somebody." For me, it felt much more sterile and very problematic because I worried I might be fired. At the initial point that I filed, I wasn't asking for any accommodations—instead I was literally re-establishing who I was and am as an employee, which left me in a somewhat vulnerable space. It makes me happy that there's that level of acceptance and support for students.

DAISY: It sounds like relationships are making a world of difference.

VALERIE: Yes, I agree. Years ago, my professional perspective was more legalistic; I have come to understand how relationships influence that moment of disclosure. Over time, I kept hearing things from faculty, asking "Why are these students waiting until after they've flunked a test? Why are they shoving those access plans under my door?" Now when I go into conversations with faculty, I ask them to bear with the student. Understand that "the law" and some policies and procedures may be asking people to do difficult things that they may or may not be emotionally ready to do. This behavior may occur if it is the first time that this person has had to negotiate accommodations with an authority figure. And students will say: "I don't want this to be the first thing a faculty member hears from me: 'Oh, here's something that's going to mean more work for you.'" Or if a faculty member wants the student to repeat the entire story—how was the disability acquired or what they've gone through. Do students need that? Five classes, two semesters, four years—do they have to do that with forty people on campus? Recognizing the multiple perspectives influences the way I welcome students to my office. I try never to ask them about disability first. I always start the conversation to establish a relationship. I might ask, "What excites you about college?—What is it that you hope to do with your major?" Welcome the whole person and then try to help make it a more comfortable place. I encourage faculty members and students to establish a working relationship, recognizing mutual concerns that may contribute to the behavior in delaying the disclosure. Hopefully, we can have empathy and move toward a more empowered moment and encourage the student—recognizing what it took to get there.

SUSAN: This reminds me of when you, Valerie, said how when students disclose it's frequently not coming from a position of empowerment. Instead, it's often at that crucial moment when it's like, "oh, my goodness, I failed this and I need to go talk about this with someone."

DAISY: We need to find ways to help get students to that position of power, such as incorporating disability into the curriculum and allowing students to choose to explore their relationships to disability through coursework. If students have opportunities to read and write about disability, on their own terms, as opposed to being compelled to disclose through an access plan letter, they define themselves.

SUSAN: Also, kind of what you're asking is can you show me what you can do or what you hope for instead of asking students to fill out the kind of form I had to fill out at HR, which essentially asks: What's wrong with you? How long is it going to last? What do you need from us?

VALERIE: I've made the same mistake in form design. A student completed the registration form, which had a question about the nature of the disability with a black and white dichotomy: Is this permanent or is it temporary? The student was living with AIDS and cancer, going through treatment—and didn't have an answer for that. He pointed out to me how the question made him feel. With that awareness, I revised it to respect the student's perspective and ask simply for the information relevant to the discussion of accommodations. I thanked the student for being candid with me about how my form influenced how he felt. Since then, I've been more mindful about multiple perspectives on designs and questions.

DAISY: That's why feedback is so important. Keri, I was happy when you said you could go to the professor and have that conversation, because that kind of feedback is helpful to allies (Evans, Assadi, and Herriott 2005). When people point out that something we say is insensitive, or reinforces ableism, we can learn from it and be grateful. Making mistakes is part of the process of growing as allies (Myers, Lindburg, and Nied 2014, 72). Sometimes we say things trying to be supportive that have another effect entirely. I think there's that question of how to express care. I care about my students. And I care about you and I don't know how to express that without—because you said sometimes you get annoyed with "are you okay?"

SUSAN: Sometimes this question is really aggravating, especially if the person asking it knows a bit about your health history. Sometimes when a person expresses such concern, it might feel like they're staring at you to the point of it becoming uncomfortable.

DAISY: Keri, do you encounter that sort of smothering friend or smothering—

KERI: Mother. Yes. I lost my eye in an accident. I also have a rare bleeding disorder. I was not allowed to do anything at all, ever. It was overbearing. It pushed me to the point of wanting to do reckless things. My mom would not let me go sledding one year, and I went to Baltimore with a friend and her family was going sledding. So, of course, I went sledding with them. I ended up sledding across a frozen lake into a bunch of trees and getting a concussion. So, yes, people being overbearingly helpful can definitely be a bad thing. I have a lot of great friends who experienced my years of eye surgeries and struggling with me. They're very subtle and quiet about their help. If we're walking on the street, and there are cars on my blind side, they'll make a point to walk on that side of me. They are aware of my limitations. They don't say anything. They just quietly assist me, which, in my opinion, is the best way to do it.

VALERIE: So I am hearing you say it just becomes a part of how you are together.

KERI: Right. Yes.

VALERIE: It's no longer, necessarily, what we might frame in our school world as an accommodation?

KERI: Right.

VALERIE: But it just becomes a part of how you function together? And you have your strengths. My girlfriend—who is blind—will tell me jokingly and half seriously, "You're better at your job because of being friends with me; aren't you?" Well, actually, yes, we teach each other things all the time. It becomes a part of the relationship. She feels free to tell me when I'm overstepping or when I'm offering something of value. We appreciate our great friendship—being willing to challenge each other to be our best selves and knowing when to back off.

DAISY: I'm thinking about how that translates into a classroom space—how professors could more quietly do things, and have that comfortable back and forth feedback. At Bubba Gump restaurants, a sign on the table allows customers to communicate with the waiter: "run, Forest, run" if everything is okay, and "stop, Forest, stop" when you need attention at your table. I mean, I hate to compare a classroom to Bubba Gump. But the quiet kinds of ways to communicate without having to disrupt anything . . .

Perspectives and Contexts Surrounding Disclosure

DAISY: Some of the things bubbling up are flexibility and awareness of each person as an individual. Sometimes, we don't take the time we need to have these conversations. As Jim Corder (1985, 31) said, we have to teach the world to want time to care. Students want a quick response, but faculty are so busy; and faculty want the quick, basic answer to "what do I have to do?" And sometimes faculty might think "these are the best things for my classroom," and don't practice the flexibility needed for all learners with unique strengths, needs, and backgrounds.

SUSAN: I had one student who needed a particular type of chair, and as a result, we needed to move the same chair from room to room when she went to different classes. I kept wondering why the building manager or the university couldn't put a chair like that in every room?

DAISY: Yes, and talk about calling somebody out! It was a production to get her to class.

VALERIE: This is a fascinating moment for me, because you, as faculty members, are having the perception, from your side, that someone said we couldn't put a chair in every room. I had a different experience of that. It occurs to me we could have had a deeper conversation. I received a message that people were handling it and didn't necessarily want me to find a chair for every room. There may have been some assumption about cost. I don't know. But it is an intersection with disclosure because faculty members hauling chairs back and forth (right?) was an obvious visible reminder and redisclosure with every class. A goal in a disability services office, when considering processes and procedures, is to create a situation that allows the student, faculty member, or whomever to participate in that community as seamlessly as everyone else without making it apparent that anything had to happen—that anything had to be manipulated or changed to make it accessible.

DAISY: This is one of the reasons it is so important for us to get out of our bubbles. I'll hear misperceptions on the part of the faculty members about Disability Services. "Well, they want this ridiculous accommodation. I can't do that." I think some faculty perceive disability services as this sort of police, rather than as a partner. What faculty could do is listen and ask questions.

VALERIE: I try to listen to all sides of the story: faculty have reasons for designing an experience to facilitate learning. It is about relationships. I find, sometimes, that the student may have a notion about how a legitimate need should be met and the faculty member may be teaching in a way for which that particular accommodation won't work. For example, a student who's visually impaired came to me very upset that a faculty member would not accommodate with slides in advance. I didn't really understand. I don't know very many faculty members who, knowing the student was blind, would not support such accommodations. There's some piece missing. I called the faculty member to ask for an appointment and shared that the student was so unhappy she wanted to drop the class. It was that kind of reaction that Daisy mentioned: "I'm not talking to you until I know what the charges are." I said, no, this is not about charges. I'm not coming for that reason. I'm seeking to understand. I meet with the faculty member and find out that for this person, this is a new prep class. On top of that, the professor responds extemporaneously to student questions, doing some math in front of the classroom using an old overhead projector; and the reason he won't give the students slides in advance is that they don't exist in advance. And I said, thank you very much for letting me talk to you, because now I understand where you're coming from. Had I been able to be a part of the conversation before the two of you were so angry with one another, together we could have pursued another solution, perhaps hiring an upper level student to sit beside the student with a large piece of paper and a Sharpie to copy what you were writing on the board. The student would be accommodated and you wouldn't have to change your teaching. I mean, that story is all about finding some way to both address the student's legitimate need due to disability and think about why the instructor is teaching the way he or she is. And looking for a way to bring those things together without huge burden for either one, so that they can move on to the content of the class.

SUSAN: I wonder if there's a degree of embarrassment for him because sometimes when you get asked to teach a new class, or if you're teaching three different classes or however many preps you have—it's going to take a lot of preparation to get your act together and to get this done ahead of time.

VALERIE: Well, in that case, it wasn't about getting his act together. It was a part of the dynamic nature of addressing and responding to students' questions in class. Which is an interesting parallel. I've heard it asked, are we in ODS giving the same answers all the time? Well, no, we aren't. It's more about going through an effective dialogue and deliberative process rather than arriving at an identical answer. The solution for a particular academic situation is going to be potentially unique to that setting.

SUSAN: Here you have these two different conversations going on, one with a student and one with a professor. The professor might be feeling numerous stresses, and we also have a student asking "Why is this guy being such a jerk?"

VALERIE: They needed this office for the mediation.

DAISY: I wonder, Susan, going back to HR. Something is going on in the person in human resources' mind—maybe "I need to get this form. I need to get this done." But if you could have a conversation with HR about the process, what would be happening is breaking down barriers and—going behind the curtain.

SUSAN: Not sure how or when that could happen, but I worry that they'd be concerned by the work I am publishing since it calls out their office on this very issue.

DAISY: But don't you think that's an important step that you're speaking up and offering a perspective and maybe they'll have a perspective, too?

SUSAN: Yes, I think it's possible.

VALERIE: That brings a story to mind. A few years ago, a student felt wronged that a faculty member made some disclosures that the student would have preferred had not happened. The student wrote about it and it was published and the department found out. Retaliation cases are increasing because people have emotional reactions to stories being published. But that was her story. With that in mind, I'm respectful about how we bring students into the employment role as peer access advocates in the ODS and what that means for their resumes. Even during the interview, we talk about what that might mean down the road. When students request a reference, I will ask, specifically, what about your experience do you hope I'll highlight?

DAISY: Keri, are you concerned about outing yourself with your resume?

KERI: No. My ultimate career goal is to be an advocate for people with disabilities. So this is the perfect thing to have on my resume.

DAISY: So—no?

KERI: I was like, wahoo!

VALERIE: But I always ask about it and talk about it along the way.

DAISY: Doesn't it point to the problem that there is still stigma attached to the disability? That we haven't gotten to the point where we see it as human variation or diversity, but as something else. We say that, "What's wrong?" (see Dolmage 2014, 38).

Campus Strategies for Creating Safe Spaces for Disability Disclosure

DAISY: One of the ways I came into an interest in disability was through LGBT rights and social justice. Another disclosure story in the family is when my father came out as gay, though he never told me—I found out from a friend in middle school. (I lived in a small town). The ways that disability and sexuality intersect (Sherry 2004) fascinates me, and Susan and I have done some other work on that, joining a growing field of interest in those intersections. But while sharing certain features of oppression—stigma, shame, the very fact of having to "come out"—we can also learn from others, become allies, and work together. For example, Safe Zone, a campus group designed to help create safe spaces for LGBTQ individuals, can serve as a resource as we think about ways to create inclusive spaces for all. In looking at disability as diversity and a social justice issue, we tap into ally networks. It's everyone's responsibility, and we can all work together (Myers, Lindburg, and Nied 2014, 64).

VALERIE: I came into this work just after the ADA was passed. In those earlier days of disability services, ODS and faculty were not in this place together. I would call faculty with an authentic need for information and the faculty member would say "I don't want to talk to you until I know what I'm accused of." And to be received with that arm's length, "I'm not talking to you because we're adversaries," was tough (Goodin 2014).

SUSAN: Many university diversity conversations are about race or gender or sexual orientation (Davis 2011). So to be able to talk to you, and to others who pick up the baton, is good. As part of this, I designed and taught an undergraduate class on disability rhetorics and a graduate course that addresses the ways disability is represented and discussed across an array of normative public, institutional, technological, and social occasions.

DAISY: And I'm developing a course on Justice and Disability—disability is such an important part of the conversation (Nussbaum 2006).

SUSAN: Disability Studies history is everybody's history, so it should permeate the discussion. In terms of intellectual development, it should be part of the framework of an education. It should be part of the academic environment and culture: in curriculum design, in every discipline.

VALERIE: I've seen that it is critical to be in conversation with faculty and students. We do a variety of things such as focus groups, workshops, and departmental meetings, building in time to listen deeply and be responsive. With Disability Awareness Week, our intention is to partner with others and establish a reputation as approachable people. It's important for us to be out there and help others on campus also create that safe community. Students may not disclose to Disability Services first, so we want to ensure that others can make good referrals. Where there have been conversations before challenges arise, it's much easier to reach understanding and navigate to a good resolution, bringing varied perspectives and different needs together.

As much as we've worked on our relationships, reputation, and building allies across divisions and departments, we will continue to focus on that because it helps, making it easier for students to seek the services that are needed. With these conversations, the campus is more open and receptive to seeing disability as one aspect of diversity and building in principles of universal design to reduce the need for specific accommodations. For example, we partnered with the Institute for Visual Studies to host an interdisciplinary class and series of workshops and events focusing on representations of disability. Students worked with people with disabilities in a process-oriented, human-centered approach to co-creation, culminating in a closing reception to share their work; one particularly resonant project featured the phrase "I am different / so are you." The experience was collaboratively designed to open up safe spaces, create ally networks, and serve as a catalyst for deeper conversations about disability and sustainable change.

KERI: When I walked into ODS as a freshman, I was blown away by the level of comfort and acceptance. Overall, JMU is an accepting community. I think the problem is awareness—a lack of acknowledgement that we are here and motivation to make our campus more accessible. What we have done, in my job, is organize focus groups with registered students. In these groups, we ask questions like how the office is doing and what we can do to improve. We had a freshman focus group last year with the goal of creating an environment where students knew they were not alone on campus, that there are other students going through the same challenges of navigating through college with a disability. Through our annual Disability Awareness Week, we have come so far in creating a week where people can go to events and celebrate disability while also experiencing what our office is really about. We've had people say to us that they thought our office was more of a "talk at you" kind of office, but then when they came to Disability Awareness Week, they realized what we are actually all about, which is raising disability awareness, embracing diversity and creating accessible, inclusive environments at JMU.

DAISY: And good job on that! Many of my students who participate in Disability Awareness Week say it changes the way they think about everything.

VALERIE: And then you reinforce it in the classroom, right?

DAISY: Susan, you're the one who introduced me to many of the readings and you're willing to share articles and resources. And you're generous with your time and coming to talk to classes. It really comes down to the connections and relationships. Sometimes the informal conversations can be the most meaningful. Valerie, I'm glad we bumped into each other in D.C. (at the Composing Disability Conference) and had dinner. The official meetings and workshops are important, but so are the "let's chat" moments.

KERI: I totally agree. The dialogue that I engage in and the relationships that I've been fortunate enough to have within the office, especially with my fellow peer access advocates, has changed my life. Having people to talk to that understand is incredibly important.

VALERIE: For all of us, it was in a university setting where we gained the language and the tools for (re)shaping our approaches to disability. As a profession, if students graduate without this understanding, we do our students and our communities a disservice. It is important to confront and change stereotypical thinking, to expand thinking on disability and diversity.

DAISY: Keri, not everyone would feel comfortable sharing their story. What do you think makes you so comfortable being out?

KERI: I've been open about my disability from the beginning. Since I see myself as an advocate personally and professionally, being open is necessary to create more awareness on campus. Having difficult conversations and, for example, being willing to let the campus paper run a personal article about my disability, is a campus strategy in itself to create safe spaces.

You NEED advocates on campus. You need students who are willing and able to speak out and openly have conversation about inclusion, accessibility, and diversity to create a safe environment for ALL students with disabilities. Especially for the ones who are still finding their voice and navigating the process of identifying with their disabilities. Having student volunteer or employment positions, such as our peer access advocates, is one way to ensure that there are disability advocates on campus.

VALERIE: When we think back to our stories about our first encounters with disability, we can notice how our first encounters with disability influence our perceptions (Myers, Lindburg, and Nied 2014, 1), and much of our work is in response to those encounters. We now have a more sophisticated understanding of the emotions that people bring into these conversations about disability. It might be more polished, now, but our hearts are still there. What's underneath still holds.

DAISY: I realize I wanted to change the narrative. My family was only able to access the story of disability we knew at the time. So much of my work on campus has been about opening up spaces for new stories to emerge, more options that more authentically express the diversity and uniqueness of human beings. In my classes, we explore texts and authors, like Georgina Kleege or Eli Clare, who challenge those old narratives and speak from places of pride, dignity, and celebration. New stories open up new possibilities.

VALERIE: You can hear in my story about my granddad a lack of tools and strategies. For me, it's still about the tools—tools to carry on the activities of life and learning and communication.

SUSAN: One strategy that I hope campuses and society in general will adapt over time is fully incorporating disability narratives—not to teach us how to categorize bodies or embodied experiences, but to experience how such narratives are crucial to our larger questions about inclusion.

KERI: Witnessing my mom fighting the good fight for my brother influences my current passion for disability advocacy, especially since I see people encountering the same challenges today. My ultimate goal is to help create communities that are diverse, inclusive, and accessible for all people.

Conclusion

As we reflect on our stories and conversations, we highlight the importance of relationships, interconnectedness, and working across institutional and social barriers to listen to each other's perspectives and acknowledge the human as we bring our whole selves to our campus communities. Because each campus community is its own unique and dynamic entity, each must work together to develop strategies. A key strategy is working together to create opportunities and spaces for authentic conversations about disability, while considering that our autobiographies, positions, and a complex web of variables interact to create the *selves* we bring to such conversations—and the selves that others bring. We caution, too, that disclosure is intellectually, socially, and emotionally complex. Opening up opportunities for disclosure and the sharing of stories cannot be done without deliberate, thoughtful approaches to disclosure and an awareness of power and privilege. As Robert McRuer (2006, 152) argues, we must "continue to develop a rigorous vigilance as we struggle (in coalition) against interrelated systems of oppression."

None of the cautions, though, should prevent the conversations. The relationships that foster, and are in turn nurtured by, the conversations can become solid bases for action within the community. Just as sharing painful experiences serves as testimony to ableism and injustice, sharing experiences of positive access and inclusion celebrates progress and humanity. As David Bleich (1998, 12) notes, disclosure "asks us to take notice of the historically grounded suppressions, denials, and lies that accompany received cultural traditions and received knowledge." Disclosure itself is a political act that can create opportunities for social action and change. We encourage not only individual conversations, but campus- and community-wide conversations about diversity and disability. Social justice ally-hood requires both the willingness and the opportunities to work toward more just arrangements (Broido 2000). We encourage others to not only seize but intentionally create opportunities to work together to open up inclusive spaces for disability disclosure, to discover new possibilities for access, inclusion, and justice.

References

Bleich, David. 1998. *Know and Tell: A Writing Pedagogy of Disclosure, Genre, and Membership*. CrossCurrents. Portsmouth, NH: Boynton/Cook.

Broido, Ellen. 2000. "The Development of Social Justice Allies during College: A Phenomenological Investigation." *Journal of College Student Development* 21 (1): 3–18.

Corder, Jim. 1985. "Argument as Emergence, Rhetoric as Love." *Rhetoric Review* 4 (1): 16–32. *JSTOR*. http://www.jstor.org/stable/465760

Davis, Lennard J. 2011. "Why Is Disability Missing from the Discourse on Diversity?" *The Chronicle of Higher Education*. http://chronicle.com/article/Why-Is-Disability-Missing-From/129088/

Dolmage, Jay. 2014. *Disability Rhetoric*. Syracuse: Syracuse University Press.

Evans, Nancy J., Jennifer L. Assadi, and Todd K. Herriott. 2005. "Encouraging the Development of Disability Allies." *New Directions for Student Services* 110 (Summer): 67–79. doi:10.1002/ss.166

Gilligan, Carol. 2011. *Joining the Resistance*. Cambridge, UK: Polity Press.

Goodin, Sam. 2014. "Musings of Someone in the Disability Support Services Field for Almost 40 Years." *Journal of Postsecondary Education and Disability* 27 (4): 409–14.

McRuer, Robert. 2006. "We Were Never Identified: Feminism, Queer Theory, and a Disabled World." *Radical History Review* 94 (Winter): 148–54. doi: 10.1215/01636545-2006-94-148

Myers, Karen A., Jaci Jenkins Lindburg, and Danielle M. Nied. 2014. *Allies for Inclusion: Disability and Equity in Higher Education: ASHE* 39 (5). San Francisco: Jossey-Bass.

Nussbaum, Martha C. 2006. *Frontiers of Justice: Disability, Nationality, Species Membership*. Cambridge, MA: Belknap Press of Harvard University Press.

Price, Margaret. 2011. *Mad at School: Rhetorics of Mental Disability and Academic Life*. Ann Arbor, MI: University of Michigan Press.

Sherry, Mark. 2004. "Overlaps and Contradictions between Queer Theory and Disability Studies." *Disability and Society* 19 (4): 669–783. doi:10.1080/0968759042000284231

Siebers, Tobin. 2008. *Disability Theory*. Ann Arbor, MI: University of Michigan Press.

Notes

Chapter 1

1. The 2014 survey found that 47.8 percent of undergraduate respondents felt things were hopeless, 54.7 percent reported having felt overwhelming anxiety, and 33.2 percent reported having been too depressed to function.

2. For foundational work on disability and representation, see Longmore (2003); Garland-Thomson (1997); Mitchell and Snyder (2000); and Osteen (2010).

Chapter 3

1. For more information about the full survey and results, contact the second author.

Chapter 4

1. Borrowing from queer theory, several scholars have discussed disability disclosure as a process of "coming out." See Garland-Thomson (1997, ix, 14) and Swain and Cameron (1999, 68–78). For a critique of using the language of "coming out" as means of describing disability disclosure, see Samuels (2003).

2. For a feminist formulation on classroom authority, see Luke (1996).

3. Kerschbaum (2014) importantly acknowledges how disability disclosures are often met with less-than-desirable reactions from others.

4. In Fall 2013 at Saint Louis University, I taught a course titled "Disability Theory" (POLS 393). After students completed the course, I solicited anonymous feedback by asking students the following questions via a non-random Qualtrics survey: (1) In the "Disability Theory" course, did you feel comfortable disclosing personal narratives about your lived experiences with impairment and disability in class discussions about the academic material? Why, or why not?; (2) Reflecting on your experience this semester, how did the instructor's and/or students' disclosure of personal narratives impact your understanding of the course material, if at all?

Explain your reasoning; (3) In your view, how did the disability/ability status of the instructor impact your educational experience, if at all? Explain your reasoning; (4) Do you think it is important for the voices of people with disabilities to be represented in various spaces of academia? Why, or why not? Seven out of ten students responded to the voluntary survey.

5. O'Toole (2013) notes that once an academic comes out, there are many practical professional benefits as well. For instance, social networking allows for the information sharing of strategies for successfully handling discrimination barriers, locating disability positive professional services, finding support, and sharing culture.

6. For more on the importance of trigger warnings, see Johnston (2014). For an alternative critical viewpoint on trigger warnings, see Freeman et al. (2014).

7. For more on intersectionality, see Berger and Guidroz (2009).

8. For instance, as a class we watch the documentary *Sound and Fury* (2000) and discuss internal divisions in the Deaf community about the issue of cochlear implants.

Chapter 5

1. Sympathy is problematic for disabled people because it relies on an equation between misfortune and disability. Historically, the oppression of people with disabilities has often relied on such an equation. See Shapiro (1994) and Longmore (2013).

2. For more on disability rhetoric as cunning intelligence, see Dolmage (2014) and Walters (2014), both of whom theorize such rhetorical craftiness as *mētis* or *mētic-ethos*, respectively.

Chapter 6

1. In this chapter, we have chosen to speak from a collective "we" in order to foreground the similarities of our four experiences, express solidarity, and write in unison against the violences of ableism. We do not claim to speak for all graduate students with disabilities, nor do we aim to represent people with our disabilities at large. Rather, regardless of recognition or identification, we hope that our "we" can lead to solidarity and the forming of other "we's" that recognize intersectional difference and oppression, while still coming together for collective resistance and action.

Chapter 9

1. The authors gratefully acknowledge Ms. Denize Stanton-Williams and Ms. Tranesha Christie of the University of the District of Columbia for their contributions to the discussion that initiated this chapter.

2. The HBCU Disability Consortium (blackdisabledandproud.org) and this chapter is possible thanks to a grant from the Fund for the Improvement of Postsecondary Education (FIPSE), U.S. Department of Education (Project #P116B100141).

3. In this chapter, we use the term "African American" to refer to members of the African diaspora who identify as part of African American culture in the United States, particularly those descended from slaves in the U.S. The term "Black" is used as a more inclusive term to not only refer to African Americans but also those who may be perceived as "Black" in the United States, including some immigrants of Haiti, Africa, the Dominican Republic, and other countries. For example, HBCUs have a mission of preserving African American culture, but the student population is usually described as being predominantly Black.

Chapter 13

1. Another classic account of finding a non-self-punitive narrative in the social model occurs in the movie *Examined Life: Philosophy Is in the Streets* (2008), where Sunaura Taylor explains that learning of the social model allowed her to overcome her shame over her nonnormative tactics for negotiating the world, such as using her mouth to lift a cup of coffee.

2. Significant critiques and revisions of the social model appear in the work of Crow (1996), Mollow (2006), Morris (1991), Shakespeare (2013), and Siebers (2001), among others.

3. The availability of alternative models, however, is an urgent issue. The Sex Wars in feminism found a major point of contention in the question of whether society has instilled bad desires in us that we must be healed of, or whether there's no whole self to be "restored," since we are all socially constructed—each side tends to see the other as complicit in oppression, hence the intensity of Patrick Califia's response to Clare (Jones 1999). See Koyama (2013) for a recent critique of the "healing from trauma" model.

4. I would characterize the feeling I get thanks to having survived desperate and annihilating circumstances as hope rather than pride.

5. I have in mind Halperin's, "We would come home from the parade, collapse from our heroic efforts to sustain unflinching pride in our homosexuality before a skeptical public over the course of an entire six hours, and wonder whether we could now go back to the relative comfort zone of sexual shame which we were used to inhabiting" (2009, 43), which implies an interesting distinction between public pride and private shame.

6. Negrón-Mutaner speaks of the shame of the unprivileged as "associated with what Carl D. Schneider calls 'discretion-shame,' an affect that delimits sacred spaces that are proscribed to us not only as Puerto Ricans but also as workers, women, queers, and/or migrants" (2009, 91).

7. Perhaps in a more literal sense than Sedgwick uses the term.

8. I am influenced in this account of my relation to literature by Cameron's (1962) "Poetry and Dialectic."

9. I adopt the term from Baldwin (1974): upon reconnecting with her father, the heroine of *If Beale Street Could Talk* says, "In loving someone, I was loved and released and verified" (1974, 47). Interestingly, Sedgwick's account of the parent reciprocating the child's gaze seems applicable there.

10. Gotkin (2015) has suggested that science fiction may be particularly suited to the rendering of disability because of its literalism. Indeed, the literalization of metaphor that Ursula Le Guin (1993) and Samuel Delany (2009, 2010) have found to characterize science fiction resonates with the suspicion of metaphor (as a common tool for erasing the reality of bodies) that Finger (2013) and Clare (2008) have expressed.

11. Kafer (2013) observes that crip time "requires reimagining our notions of what can and should happen in time, or recognizing how expectations of 'how long things take' are based on very particular minds and bodies. . . . Not only might [illness and disability] cause time to slow, or to be experienced in quick bursts, they can lead to feelings of asynchrony or temporal dissonance" (27, 34). Samuels has observed that crip time can include "grief time" and signify "loss and its crushing undertow" (see Price 2013). See also Price (2011) and Kuppers (2009).

12. Moore (1950a, 1950b) and Sturgeon (1949, 1953a, 1953b), two authors who took a strong and sympathetic interest in anomalous bodies and minds, were among the pioneers in dramatizing these issues science fictionally.

13. One reason science fiction such as Dick's works so well as an alternative to the pride/social model story is that it's a deliberate rebuttal to the old science fictional cliché of a hero whose stigmatized condition or victimhood gains him or her admission to an elite body of fighters for justice: disability movement memoir and disability protest fiction sometimes have a similar "Yay I have joined the X-Men!" resolution.

14. Chandler (2010) has written movingly on the trouble with compulsory pride and the impossibility of erasing disability shame, explaining that "the task of 'taking one's place' by identifying as disabled with pride does not always follow a one-way, disappearing path. The arrival at a sense of 'being-in-the-world' as disabled with pride does not necessarily erase all markings of shame" and proposing that we seek "a place where a pride can exist in togetherness with shame." Chandler's (2013) experience of shame is very different from my own in that it is largely associated with being taunted in public for her visible disability; but her account of shame's ineradicability—"Pride needs shame as its taken-for-granted ground from which it can be distinct" (85)—recalls Sedgwick's account of the way pride movements operate.

Chapter 14

1. I extend my heartfelt thanks to the editors of this volume for their assistance. I also would like to publically thank Drs. Susan Burch, Brandon Man-

ning, Miriam Petty, and Michelle Wright for their keen editorial work and friendship.

2. There are a wide variety of documents in which these explanations about tenure can be found. Some include the faculty handbooks of small liberal arts colleges. One document explains the general rules and some unwritten rules regarding tenure. See Rockquemore and Laszloffy (2008).

3. Here, I intend to invoke Rosemarie Garland Thomson's (2011) ideas about misfitting. She understands it as a feminist materialist concept that confers agency on disabled subjects. I use it to point out how Chris's misfitting at the institution is not provoked by him, but since it is temporally and socially contingent, it clarifies that his ability to fit depends upon a particular set of social expectations.

Chapter 15

1. We read about logical fallacies (Tindale 2007), online rhetoric (Warnick 2007), and Googling health issues (Siempos et al. 2008; Tang et al. 2006). We also read Susan Sontag's (1990) work on metaphor and illness and engaged disability perspectives by reading Shapiro (1993), Kleege (2007), Finger (2009), and Garland-Thomson (2009).

2. Starcevic and Aboujaoude (2015) note that issues of education, information processing, and technological ability may be at play in cyberchondria (97), though their suggestion that "mental health professionals" should serve as trainers is problematic.

3. Google has been shown to be more precise in providing health information than health-focused search engines (such as WebMD) (Lopes and Ribiero 2011). I chose Google because I figured it was where students would most likely start.

4. See Aiken and Kirwan (2012) for a reading of "cyberchondria by proxy."

5. Rosa included a photo of a Lyme-disease-like rash on her arm, so it may be that she was researching herself, though she was a creative student and did not formally disclose.

6. On productively repurposing disability simulation exercises, see Brueggemann (2001).

7. Similarly, studies overfocus on the relationship of health anxiety (HA) and cyberchondria (see Muse et al. 2012; Singh and Brown 2014; Norr et al. 2015; for a critique, Baumgartner and Hartmann 2011).

8. Judy Segal (2009) describes cyberchondriacs as those who go online, "sometimes late at night, often in a state of anxiety" (353), contrasted with "interested, inquiring, and rational" health seekers who likely have chronic conditions (362–63). See Fox and Purcell (2015) on online health research by those with chronic conditions.

9. Loos (2013) claims that searching online for health information does not constitute an "illness," (2013, 440). Still, I found few studies that claimed online health research was truly useful, one of which identified the internet as the number one source of information for patients (Tustin 2010; see also Paré et al. 2009; Reed 2002).

10. So might disability research disclose potentially enlightening and exciting possibilities and identities, though I feel most disability studies curriculum prepares students for such moments, and that such representations are less common in student research.

Chapter 16

1. These are pseudonyms selected by the students.

Chapter 17

1. To view the most up-to-date list of FSA approved comprehensive transition programs visit: http://studentaid.ed.gov/eligibility/intellectual-disabilities

Chapter 18

1. Some contents of this publication/presentation were developed under a grant from the U.S. Department of Education, National Institute on Disability and Rehabilitation Research (now the National Institute on Disability, Independent Living, and Rehabilitation Research) grant H133B100037 (Salzer, Principal Investigator). However, those contents do not necessarily represent the policy of the U.S. Department of Education, and endorsement by the federal government should not be assumed.

2. Following Price in *Mad at School* and "The Bodymind Problem," we use mentally disabled and with mental disability to indicate a variety of disabilities having to do mainly with the brain and/or mind. Such disabilities include cognitive impairments, intellectual disability, mental illness, autism, brain injury, and learning disability. In using this umbrella term, our intention is not to imply that all these diagnoses or identities are the same. Rather, we mean to indicate, and explore further, the commonalities among conditions that are, in Lewiecki-Wilson's phrase, "imagined to be located in the mind" (157). Being identified as a person whose mind is impaired implies all sorts of things about one's fitness as a liberal subject (Lewiecki-Wilson 2003). It should also be noted that we recognize that many so-called "physical" or "sensory" disabilities have mental aspects, and vice versa; we are not arguing for tightly controlled borders between these categories. However, at times, definitions must be operationalized for research to be practicable. On the survey described in this article, we operationalized "mental disability" as follows: "For the purposes of this survey, person with mental disability means someone who has received mental-health care and/or a mental-health diagnosis. You do not have to identify as 'disabled' to participate in this survey; you may alternatively identify as a mental-health services consumer, a psychiatric survivor, a person with mental illness, a psychocrip, or simply someone with your particular diagnosis."

3. We use "accommodation" and "modification" interchangeably in this essay.

4. For the purpose of this analysis, we focused on a U.S. sample because of dif-

ferences between U.S. higher education and postsecondary education in other parts of the world. However, we believe these differences are important to understand further, and other analyses that include our international sample are planned.

5. Although most of the examples in this article relate to physical or sensory disability, one could say "bodyminds" there, too (see Price 2015 for a detailed discussion of this point).

List of Contributors

Shahd Alshammari is Assistant Professor of English Literature at the Gulf University for Science and Technology (GUST, Kuwait). She has published in academic journals such as the *Journal of Literary and Cultural Disability Studies*, as well as various fiction. *On Love and Loss* is her poetry collection dealing with illness and love. Her first collection of short stories is *Notes on the Flesh* (2017), a biomythography that considers disability, love, and loss.

Eduardo Barragan was born in Mexico and immigrated to the United States at age twelve. Having been sheltered for most of his childhood and with no previous schooling, Eduardo began the challenging journey of ultimately obtaining his master's degree in rehabilitation counseling. His thesis on disability perception and understanding at a postsecondary institution portrays powerful revelations of the disability atmosphere from students identified as having a disability. Eduardo is currently living in the central valley of California and works for the Department of Social Services and individuals who receive various disability benefits.

Daisy L. Breneman holds a joint appointment with University Advising and Justice Studies at James Madison University, where she created and teaches a course on disability and justice. She also serves as the co-coordinator for the Disability Studies minor. Her scholarly and campus work focuses on disability studies, diversity, social justice, coalition building, academic advising, storytelling, ethical reasoning, digital media, and popular culture.

Rosalie Boone, Ed.D., has taught special education students and prepared special education personnel for almost four decades. She has authored and directed numerous grant-funded programs that supported the preparation of leadership personnel and the improvement of teaching. Her research and numerous publications reflect commitment to addressing the needs of exceptional students/families and educators from culturally and linguistically diverse backgrounds. In 2013, Dr. Boone retired as a full professor from the Howard University School of Education.

Elaine Bourne Heath, Ph.D., has an extensive background in educational management and administration with proven ability to successfully direct academic programs as chief academic Officer, department head, dean, and director. More than twenty years of instructional experience as a chaired professor, with special expertise in curricula design, course development, administration, research, strategic planning, management, and program evaluation. Her work as Dean of Student Services at Howard University focuses on delivery of services and advocacy for students with disabilities.

Moira A. Carroll-Miranda, Ph.D., has an earned doctorate from New Mexico State University in curriculum and instruction with a minor in special education. She is a part-time professor at the Graduate School of Education of the Universidad del Este Carolina, Puerto Rico. Moira has been an elementary teacher in inclusive settings at Nueva Escuela Montessori for fourteen years. Her research interest is related to disability studies and students living with disabilities participating in postsecondary education.

Angela M. Carter became a first generation college graduate in 2009 when she earned a BA in English from Truman State University. Now a Ph.D. candidate in feminist studies at the University of Minnesota, Angela's research explores dominant discourses of trauma through the intersecting analytics of queer theory and feminist disability studies.

R. Tina Catania is a Ph.D. student in geography at the Maxwell School of Citizenship and Public Affairs at Syracuse University, from where she has also obtained an MA in geography and a certificate of advanced studies in women's and gender studies. Her research interests lie at the intersections of immigration, identity, social justice, youth, and feminist theory and practice. She has conducted fieldwork in the United States and in Italy.

Joshua C. Collins, Ed.D., is assistant professor of human resource development and graduate and affiliate faculty in gender, women, and sexuality studies at the University of Minnesota-Twin Cities. He is the current chair of the Critical HRD and Social Justice Perspectives Special Interest Group of the Academy of HRD. His research focuses on linking individual and organizational learning to issues of equity and social justice in the workplace and in higher education.

Laura T. Eisenman is associate professor in the University of Delaware's School of Education and affiliated with the Center for Disabilities Studies. She coordinates an undergraduate disability studies minor. She teaches graduate and undergraduate courses about students' transitions to adult life and a senior seminar on disability studies. Her research interests include social and community experiences of young adults with disabilities and the integration of disability studies perspectives in interdisciplinary pre-service professional programs.

Brian Freedman is the associate director of the Center for Disabilities Studies at the University of Delaware (UD) and assistant professor in the School of Education. He directs the Career & Life Studies Certificate, UD's inclusive higher education program for students with intellectual disabilities. He has published as well as presented at national and international conferences on supports in postsecondary education for students with intellectual disabilities and autism. Learn more about his work at www.udel.edu/cds

Dr. Susan Ghiaciuc is an associate professor at James Madison University in the school of Writing, Rhetoric, and Technical Communication, and serves as co-director of the newly established (2017) undergraduate disability studies minor. She teaches graduate and undergraduate courses on topics, including: language, law, ethics, disability rhetoric, literacy studies, as well as first year writing. Her current research interests incorporate marginalized communities, justice, invisible disability, working class identity, and ethos.

Meg Grigal is a senior research fellow at the Institute for Community Inclusion at University Massachusetts Boston and the codirector of Think College, a national organization focused on research, policy, and practice in inclusive higher education and people with intellectual disability. At Think College, she serves as a principal investigator on a variety of research projects aimed at expanding college access for students with intellectual disability. To learn more about her work, visit www.thinkcollege.net

Wendy Harbour, Ed.D., is an associate executive director of the Association on Higher Education And Disability (AHEAD), where she directs the new federally funded National Center for College Students with Disabilities and the HBCU Disability Consortium. She has published in journals including *Innovative Higher Education, Review of Disability Studies*, and the *Journal of Postsecondary Education and Disability*. Her degrees are from the University of Minnesota and Harvard University, and she is currently teaching at the College of St. Catherine.

Debra Hart, M.S, is director of Education and Transition for the Institute for Community Inclusion at the University of Massachusetts, Boston. She has over thirty years of experience working with students with disabilities, their families, and professionals to support youth in becoming valued members of their community via participation in inclusive K-12 education, higher education, and competitive employment. She has published in the area of higher education for students with intellectual disability.

Kate Kaul is a doctoral candidate in social and political thought at York University, Toronto, writing on disability theory and interdisciplinarity, subjectivity, and experience. She is interested in a broad range of critical theory, as well as questions of form and content in pedagogy and accessible design. She teaches disability studies and writing in Toronto. This work was supported by York University through a CUPE 3903 Unit 2 Major Research Grant.

Stephanie L. Kerschbaum is associate professor of English at the University of Delaware and a faculty scholar with UD's Center for the Study of Diversity. Her book, *Toward a New Rhetoric of Difference* (NCTE 2014), won the 2015 Advancement of Knowledge Award from the Conference on College Composition and Communication, and her work on disability, narrative, interaction, and rhetorical agency has appeared in various journals and essay collections. Learn more about her work at http://sites.udel.edu/kersch

Amber Knight is assistant professor of political science at the University of North Carolina, Charlotte. Her research—which explores issues pertaining to feminist theory, disability studies, and contemporary political thought—has been featured in *The Journal of Politics* and *Hypatia: A Journal of Feminist Philosophy*. She is currently working on a book project, tentatively titled *Disability and the Politics of Parenthood*.

Sislena Grocer Ledbetter, Ph.D., is the associate vice president of student development and success at the University of the District of Columbia, in Washington, DC. Dr. Ledbetter has lectured, published, and presented in the fields of education, research, marketing, and psychology. Her research interests are in behavioral health with a focus on prevention and the reduction of stigma in African American college students with disabilities, HIV/AIDS, substance abuse, depression and suicide, and veteran's affairs. She also has research interests in women in leadership and workforce development in urban populations. She received her bachelor's degree from North Carolina Central University and her master's and doctorate from Howard University.

Bradley Lewis, MD, Ph.D., is associate professor at New York University's Gallatin School of Individualized Study and a practicing psychiatrist. He is affiliated with NYU's disability studies minor, Department of Social and Cultural Analysis, and Department of Psychiatry. Lewis writes and teaches at the interface of humanities, cultural studies, disability studies, medicine, psychiatry, and the arts. His recent books are *Narrative Psychiatry: How Stories Shape Clinical Practice* and *Depression: Integrating Science, Culture, and Humanities.*

Josh Lukin teaches first-year writing in the Department of English at Temple University. His articles, reviews, and interviews have appeared in *The Encyclopedia of American Disability History*, *The Disability Studies Reader*, *Journal of Modern Literature*, *Radical Teacher*, *Guernica*, and many other venues. He has served on the Modern Language Association's Committee on Disability Issues, Temple's Interdisciplinary Faculty Council on Disability, and the National Black Disability Coalition's Committee on Black Disability Studies. His website is http://joshlukinwork.wordpress.com

Ryan A. Miller, Ph.D., is assistant professor of educational leadership at the University of North Carolina at Charlotte. His research centers on creating inclusive campus cultures in higher education. Ryan's dissertation on intersections of disability and LGBTQ identities received the 2016 Melvene D. Hardee Dissertation of the Year Award from NASPA Student Affairs Administrators in Higher Education. He holds graduate degrees in education from the University of Texas at Austin and Harvard University.

Emily A. Nusbaum, Ph.D., is an assistant professor at University of San Francisco. Her current research focuses on the advancement of critical, qualitative methods as they relate to disability, the ideology of inclusive education, and experiences of postsecondary students who identify as disabled. She won the 2010 AERA Disability Studies in Education Special Interest Group Outstanding Dissertation award and the 2017 Ellen Brantlinger Emerging Scholar Award. Her work has been published in the *International Journal of Inclusive Education* and *Research and Practice for Persons with Severe Disabilities,* as well as edited volumes such as *Disability and the Politics of Education* and *Whatever Happened to Inclusion? The Place of Intellectual Disability in Education.*

Amber O'Shea received a Ph.D. in educational psychology in 2016. She is currently a research scientist in the Rehabilitation Sciences Department in the College of Public Health at Temple University. Her research focuses on understanding the psychological, social, and motivational processes related to learning, and promoting educational and occupational outcomes among individuals with disabilities in higher education. She can be reached by email at amber.oshea@temple.edu.

Dr. Therí A Pickens authored *New Body Politics* (Routledge, 2014). Her essays appear in *Disability Studies Quarterly, American Comparative Literature Journal,* and *Hypatia.* Currently, she is working on an edited collection on Arab American Aesthetics and the special issue of African American Review on Blackness and Disability. Her second monograph, *Mad Blackness/Black Madness* is forthcoming from Duke University Press. Learn more about her work at www.tpickens.org

Margaret Price is associate professor of rhetoric/composition and disability studies at the Ohio State University. Her book *Mad at School: Rhetorics of Mental Disability and Academic Life* (University of Michigan Press, 2011) won the Outstanding Book Award from the Conference on College Composition and Communication. She is a member of the Black Disability Studies Coalition and founding member of the Accessible Books Project (http://www.disstudies.org/Publishing%20Accessible%20Books). Margaret is at work on a book titled *Crip Spacetime.* http://margaretprice.wordpress.com

Tonette S. Rocco is professor and graduate program director of adult education and HRD, and director of the Office of Academic Writing and Publication Support, Florida International University. Dr. Rocco is a Cyril O. Houle scholar in adult and continuing education, a recipient of the Laura Bierema

Excellence in Critical HRD Award, and editor-in-chief of *New Horizons in Adult Education and Human Resource Development*. She examines the intersection of disability, work, privilege, and equity.

Mark Salzer, Ph.D., is professor and founding chair of the Department of Rehabilitation Sciences at Temple University. He is also the principal investigator and director of the Temple University Collaborative on Community Inclusion of Individuals with Psychiatric Disabilities, a rehabilitation research and training center (RRTC) funded by the National Institute on Disability, Independent Living, and Rehabilitation Research (tucollaborative.org). Dr. Salzer is an internationally recognized expert on community inclusion of individuals with psychiatric disabilities.

Rebecca Sanchez is an associate professor of English at Fordham University. Her book, *Deafening Modernism: Embodied Language and Visual Poetics in American Literature*, was published in 2015 with New York University Press. She was a recipient of a 2015–16 AAUW American fellowship, and her work on disability, modernism, and poetics has appeared in numerous journals including *American Literary Realism, Modern Language Studies*, and the *CEA Critic*.

Ellen Samuels is associate professor of gender and women's studies and English at the University of Wisconsin at Madison and the author of *Fantasies of Identification: Disability, Gender, Race* (NYU Press, 2014). Her critical work has appeared in numerous journals and anthologies, including *Signs: Journal of Women in Culture and Society, Feminist Disability Studies, GLQ, MELUS, Amerasia*, and *The Disability Studies Reader*. She is working on a new book, *Double Meanings: Representing Conjoined Twins*.

Sam R. Schmitt is a doctoral candidate in Multicultural Women and Gender Studies at Texas Woman's University. Sam's teaching and research interests include the prison industrial complex and trans prison activism; trans and intersex subjectivities in the field of women's studies; spiritual activism; disability/chronic illness; LGBTQIA politics; womanist self-recovery; epistemologies of whiteness; and feminist-womanist pedagogies.

Valerie L. Schoolcraft serves as director of the Office of Disability Services at James Madison University. In addition to supporting access and accommodations, her work on campus is highly collaborative with a focus on raising awareness of disability and diversity as well as supporting faculty and students, particularly in clinical field work and internships. She also serves on the Disability Studies minor steering committee.

Katherine D. Seelman, Ph.D., is Professor Emerita at the University of Pittsburgh. Until June 2016, she served as associate dean of disability programs and professor of rehabilitation science and technology. In 2015, she was a member of the inaugural group inducted into the Disability National Mentoring Hall of Fame, and in 2014, President Barack Obama appointed her to the National Council on Disability. In 2011, she was one of two from the U.S. serving with the World Health Organization to draft the first World Report on Disability.

Amanda Swenson is a Ph.D. student at Louisiana State University, where she studies twentieth and twenty-first century transatlantic and postcolonial literature. Her dissertation project interrogates the intersections of vulnerability and violence co-existing at the intersections of animality, disability, and otherness.

Keri Vandeberg is a disability advocate who graduated from James Madison University in May 2015 and is headed to law school to work in social justice. She won the Advocacy in Action Award from the JMU Department of Social Work for her disability advocacy work, including assisting with the planning and implementation of the 2012–2015 Disability Awareness Weeks, presenting at the Disability Disclosure in/and Higher Education Conference at the University of Delaware, and involvement in numerous other campus and community events.

Amy Vidali is associate professor of English at the University of Colorado Denver. Her research focuses on the rhetorical politics of disability in university texts, as well as metaphor, gastrointestinal rhetorics, stuttering, and infertility. Her work has appeared in *College English, Rhetoric Review, The Journal of Medical Humanities, Disability Studies Quarterly (DSQ)*, and elsewhere. She is currently working on an article entitled "Writing for Access: Disability and College Admissions," and a collection of essays on rhetorical disabilities.

Kristine Wiest Webb, Ph.D., is a professor at the University of North Florida in the Department of Exceptional, Deaf, and Interpreter Education.

Her interests are transition to postsecondary education for students with disabilities, inclusion on college campuses, and student empowerment. Kris was the UNF 2015 Distinguished Professor, and she was the co-editor of the *Handbook of Adolescent Transition Education for Youth with Disabilities* and co-author of *Transition to Postsecondary Education for Students with Disabilities.*

Tara Wood is assistant professor of English at Rockford University, where she teaches courses in rhetoric, body studies, and gender. Her work has appeared in several essay collections and journals, including *Composition Studies* and *Open Words: Access and English Studies.* She is currently working on a book project focused on access-centered writing pedagogies.

Dr. Richmond D. Wynn is associate professor and director of the clinical mental health counseling program at the University of North Florida. His research focuses on intersectionality of identity, traumatic stress, and health outcomes with an emphasis on historically marginalized social identity groups. He is specifically interested in the ways in which culturally diverse, lesbian, gay, bisexual, and transgender (LGBT) people negotiate their identities and manage their health.

Index